T0255344

Casebook of Dementia

A case-based approach to dementia care, especially one which is so thoroughly grounded in an up-to-date evidence base, is a perfect way for primary care professionals to enhance both their knowledge and skills in this complex area. Reviewing patient cases is a core learning technique for GPs and other primary care team members; the detailed approach presented in this book, in a wide variety of scenarios, offers both a learning from recent research and also practical tips from decades of experience in delivering early-interventions services in post-diagnostic dementia care. I hope this book will be of great use to primary care teams, wherever in the world they are working, in providing better-quality care to their patients living with dementia.

Professor Dame Louise Robinson
Regius Professor of Ageing
Newcastle University, UK

This is a book for all who care about people whose lives have been distorted by dementia. The book, based on 99 real case studies of people seeking help for suspected dementia, distinguished itself from others on similar topics in that the authors, being geriatric specialists, psychologists and occupational therapists themselves, show how to put together their efforts in providing those suspected of having dementia with early identification and subsequent management strategies, especially primary care. Though the 99 cases examined in the book all came from Hong Kong, it is, however, a work of reference value internationally. The book has my endorsement as it is one which adds to our knowledge about dementia, guides our strategies to provide help, and, most important of all, lightens up our hearts to care.

Nelson WS Chow
Emeritus Professor of Social Work and Social Administration
The University of Hong Kong

Casebook of Dementia

A Reference Guide for Primary Care

Gloria HY Wong
The University of Hong Kong

Bosco HM Ma
Hong Kong Alzheimer's Disease Association

Maggie NY Lee
Hong Kong Alzheimer's Disease Association

David LK Dai
Hong Kong Alzheimer's Disease Association

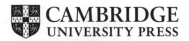

CAMBRIDGE
UNIVERSITY PRESS

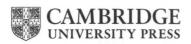

Shaftesbury Road, Cambridge CB2 8EA, United Kingdom

One Liberty Plaza, 20th Floor, New York, NY 10006, USA

477 Williamstown Road, Port Melbourne, VIC 3207, Australia

314–321, 3rd Floor, Plot 3, Splendor Forum, Jasola District Centre, New Delhi – 110025, India

103 Penang Road, #05-06/07, Visioncrest Commercial, Singapore 238467

Cambridge University Press is part of Cambridge University Press & Assessment,
a department of the University of Cambridge.

We share the University's mission to contribute to society through the pursuit of
education, learning and research at the highest international levels of excellence.

www.cambridge.org
Information on this title: www.cambridge.org/9781108984492

DOI: 10.1017/9781108989336

First published 2024

A catalogue record for this publication is available from the British Library

Library of Congress Cataloging-in-Publication Data
Names: Wong, Gloria Hoi-yan, author. | Ma, Bosco H. M., author. | Lee, Maggie N. Y., author. | Dai, David L. K., author.
Title: Casebook of dementia : a reference guide for primary care / Gloria H.Y. Wong, Bosco H.M. Ma, Maggie N.Y. Lee,
    David L.K. Dai.
Description: Cambridge ; New York, NY : Cambridge University Press, 2024. | Includes bibliographical references and index.
Identifiers: LCCN 2023041827 (print) | LCCN 2023041828 (ebook) | ISBN 9781108984492 (paperback) |
    ISBN 9781108989336 (epub)
Subjects: MESH: Dementia | Primary Care | Case Reports
Classification: LCC RC521 (print) | LCC RC521 (ebook) | NLM WT 155 | DDC 616.8/31–dc23/eng/20231213
LC record available at https://lccn.loc.gov/2023041827
LC ebook record available at https://lccn.loc.gov/2023041828

ISBN 978-1-108-98449-2 Paperback

Contents

Foreword

I am honoured to introduce this *Casebook of Dementia*, which serves as a valuable resource to promote the important role of primary healthcare for dementia. The case studies share practical experiences and insights gained from the unique healthcare setting of Hong Kong, and can benefit healthcare professionals and caregivers alike.

In recent years, the global community, including esteemed organisations like the World Health Organisation and Alzheimer's Disease International, has recognised dementia as a pressing public health concern. It is a chronic disease that requires long-term care and support. However, the problem of over-specialisation persists which hinders effective care delivery.

To address this problem, community-based primary healthcare models for dementia have been developed and tested, providing useful and valuable insights. By fostering knowledge exchange and reciprocal learning between the East and West, we can expedite progress in this field. This book serves as a guide that emphasises on community engagement and carer support, through early intervention enabled by primary healthcare.

Why advocate for primary healthcare in the management of dementia? I have openly expressed my concerns regarding the numerous challenges faced by individuals living with dementia and their caregivers. Limited resources and inadequate training of healthcare professionals often hinder access to appropriate care and support services. Family caregivers shoulder a significant burden, resulting in high levels of stress and burnout. By focusing on primary healthcare, we can address these challenges and alleviate the difficulties faced by those living with dementia and their families.

Primary healthcare plays a pivotal role in dementia care, serving as the gateway to comprehensive and coordinated approaches for early detection and effective management. Primary healthcare providers have crucial responsibilities, including identifying individuals at risk in a timely matter, facilitating interdisciplinary care, and making specialist referrals when necessary. To ensure that primary healthcare providers fulfil these roles effectively, both training and education are essential.

This book serves as a valuable training tool for primary healthcare providers, with real case examples to facilitate clinical learning. The book also offers practical assistance in using and interpreting cognitive and other screening assessments, highlighting collaborative care and the importance of interdisciplinary teams which comprise primary healthcare physicians, social workers, occupational therapists, and family caregivers. The provision of comprehensive care addressing the physical, emotional, and social needs of individuals and their caregivers is at the heart of this book.

The cases described and the primary healthcare model suggested in this book have been developed and tested within the unique context of Hong Kong by dedicated professionals from the Hong Kong Alzheimer's Disease Association. Hong Kong's specific features, such as strong filial piety values and the ongoing pursuit of 'Family doctor for all', contribute to the relevance of this model. Hong Kong benefits from a wealth of high-quality medical, allied health and social care professionals, as well as robust community support services. While each country and city has its own distinct primary healthcare context, the educational materials produced in Hong Kong have relevance to contexts both in the East and in the West, the rapidly ageing societies, and healthcare systems where the lack of human resources made innovation and collaboration an imperative for quality dementia care.

I am delighted to witness the fruition of this important work, made possible by the support of the Lee Hysan Foundation and the dedication of my long-term partners and friends from the Hong Kong Alzheimer's Disease Association. Developing a workable model of community dementia care in Hong Kong has been a journey spanning many years, and requires concerted efforts from patients, healthcare professionals, policy-makers, and the community at large to significantly improve the quality of life for people with dementia and their caregivers.

I wholeheartedly encourage readers from around the world to make the best use of this book to improve the provision of comprehensive care and support services to patients and their caregivers.

LI Kwok-tung, Donald, SBS, JP
Chairman, Elderly Commission, Hong Kong Special Administrative
Region of the People's Republic of China (HKSAR)
Past President, World Organisation of Family Doctors (WONCA)

Preface

This book is a collective effort over two decades in Hong Kong, of many dedicated primary care professionals and families of people living with dementia who trusted us with their care.

The early detection service described in this book – the contact point where we get connected with the 99 help-seeking families presented here – started as a small-scale service of the Hong Kong Alzheimer's Disease Association (HKADA) in 2006, which has since served thousands of people against a context of poor access to diagnostic services. The HKADA is a non-profit-making self-financed charitable organisation and the only member of Alzheimer's Disease International in Hong Kong, with a humble origin in the form of a self-help group established in 1995. With the generous support from the Lee Hysan Foundation, we piloted a shared primary care model in 2016 ('Project Sunrise'), which was built on the existing early detection service to form partnerships between allied health and social care professionals with primary care physicians.

This pilot model proved to be a rich source of inspiration and experiences. In Hong Kong, primary care physicians are mostly in private practice, who are not short of patient demand for their care with regular clinic services. This is why it is particularly encouraging to see many enthusiastic primary care physicians joining the pilot, spending many extra hours in training, consultations, case conferences, and communication with the allied care team. The social workers, occupational therapists, and primary care physicians who have participated in the pilot contributed to this book in multiple ways: they have showed us that the model is feasible, that the shared care helped to develop confidence in dementia care and treatment, and most importantly, why a reference guidebook like this is needed.

We learned from Project Sunrise that, in a busy primary care practice, clinic, or centres, staff training is at the same time an acute need and burden. While in-person, synchronised training sessions are valuable, reference materials for self-paced learning are just as important. We have also learned that clinical competences and confidence require time and experience to develop: over time, physicians and allied care professionals in the project managed to provide quality care for families impacted by Alzheimer's disease and needed minimal specialist support only with a few cases with atypical presentations. A pedagogy with brief induction training with continuous (low-level) post-training specialist support, supplemented with easy-to-read self-learning materials in the format of cases and practical tools, appears to fit the learning needs of our primary care team. Such was the motivation for our compilation of this book, with real cases and learning points from the piloted model and HKADA's 28 years of implementation experience.

Readers should be aware that all the cases presented here are from Hong Kong. While pseudonyms are used, we have decided to retain the use of Chinese surnames, although they may be less familiar to readers from other countries or regions. This serves as an attempt to remind ourselves of the importance of the cultural (and service) context in dementia care. Just as it is the case for learning materials developed in Western cultures, these backgrounds and contexts may or may not be directly applicable elsewhere (in our case, these may include family dynamics and public/private service configuration), although we trust that they are of reference value internationally when presented in context.

This is because the core of this book is people living with dementia and their families in real life. We have learned so much about dementia and care from the 99 families in Project Sunrise, who selflessly shared their help-seeking journey with us for education and research purposes. The brief descriptions of each case, so brief (with only essential information for clinical decision-making) that it feels brutal at times, did not do justice to all the complexities and nuances of the dementia experience in primary care. Even with such brutal treatment, each case presented here remains a great illustration of the clinical wisdom in dementia care and is worth a thousand (generalised, theoretical) words to many. We are truly thankful to all the people living with dementia and their families who made this book possible. We hope you enjoy learning from these families as much as we do.

Gloria Wong
Bosco Ma
Maggie Lee
David Dai

Background
Primary Care in Dementia

In the World Alzheimer's Report 2016: Improving Healthcare for People Living with Dementia, Alzheimer's Disease International (ADI) highlighted the role of primary care in dementia (1). With overly specialised healthcare systems and stretched specialist workforce, dementia is currently under-diagnosed and under-managed. There are 55 million people living with dementia globally, with an increase of nearly 10 million people each year (2). As a public health priority (3), dementia diagnosis and management need primary care involvement.

The idea of involving primary care in dementia is not something new or unconventional – similar developments have been witnessed in other chronic diseases such as diabetes. While various service models have been trialled in different parts of the world, several barriers remain; among them are (when it comes to dementia) a lack of a gatekeeping role for primary care in highly stretched healthcare systems and a perception that primary care is of a lower service quality (1). The two barriers can be interrelated: high-quality care (and the development of reputation and trust) requires sufficient clinical exposure supported with the right amount of training, while a reputation of high-quality care is needed for primary care to be entrusted with the gatekeeping role.

In the next two chapters, where readers will learn from 99 real cases of people with suspected dementia seeking help from a dementia early intervention service operated by a primary care team, the purpose is to share our experience and lessons learned from these clinical exposures – which can be used as part of a training programme to ensure high-quality dementia care in primary care. Before we move on to these cases, in this chapter we wish to briefly review and outline the possible roles of primary care, including gatekeepers, based on the concepts and practices of task-shifting or task-sharing in dementia care.

1.1 Concepts and Practices of Task-Shifting or Task-Sharing in Dementia Care

What Is Task-Shifting or Task-Sharing?

Task-shifting or task-sharing refers to the 'rational redistribution of tasks among the health workforce – specific tasks are moved, where appropriate, from highly qualified health workers to health workers with shorter training and fewer qualifications' (4). This redistribution of tasks can be to an existing group of healthcare professionals, with tailored training that is more narrowly focused (1, 5).

Task-shifting or -sharing in dementia care may involve reallocating tasks from specialists, who are more broadly trained in their respective specialities (e.g., geriatric medicine, psychiatry, and neurology), to primary care. As can be seen from the definition, the focus is one that concerns the allocation of human resources in healthcare, although there are other rationales for involving primary care in dementia care.

Why Shift/Share Tasks in Dementia?

In the Global Action Plan on the Public Health Response to Dementia 2017–2025 (6), a (justly) ambitious goal was set out to ensure people with dementia and their carers 'live well and receive the care and support they need to fulfil their potential with dignity, respect, autonomy, and equality'.

This goal is ambitious for at least two reasons. First, the current workforce is already struggling to meet the current needs for diagnosis and continuing care (1). Difficult-to-access services and long waiting times are common problems in dementia (7). With the projected increase in dementia prevalence, it is unrealistic to wish that the world will be able to meet the demand by continuing with the current way dementia care tasks are allocated (e.g., by training dementia care specialists only). Second, the societal impacts of dementia care are wide within and outside the healthcare system, and include carer support and labour force participation, housing and environmental design, and legal and financial planning, to name a few. The complexity of care needs in dementia means that without proper coordination, the care and service systems will be fragmented, if not impossible to navigate. Governments across the world are working to develop national dementia strategies (8).

Particularly for the second reason, primary care is in a good position to help – by minimising service fragmentation or transition and taking care of the person's other health and social care or support needs, with a person-centred approach and collaborative interdisciplinary care. In countries or areas where family physicians or primary care physicians have an existing rapport with the family, their involvement in dementia care may also reduce the barriers of fear and stigma surrounding the dementia diagnosis (see Section 5.3) to encourage timely help-seeking, as well as decrease the possibilities of the person dropping out from service (9–12).

Alongside these obvious reasons to promote primary care involvement in dementia care, some worries remain: is it feasible to shift/share the task with primary care? What tasks can be shifted/shared? Is such a model as effective and safe as services provided by specialists – a question about service quality (and equity, if both primary care and specialist care are available) – and in what ways?

Task-Shifting/-Sharing in Dementia Care: Real-World Implementation

The above are questions that many practitioners and researchers around the world have been trying to answer. Since the publication of the World Alzheimer's Report 2016 (1), experience is quickly accumulating in involving primary care in dementia care. As task-shifting/-sharing is essentially a complex intervention, its development and evaluation are still evolving with new methodological and theoretical approaches (13); nevertheless, some models have been implemented and evaluated, with evidence of improved service supply and maintained service quality in diagnosis and continuing care (7, 10, 11, 14–20).

In some countries such as New Zealand, a shift of the diagnosis and management of uncomplicated dementia cases to primary care has been recommended in their national framework, freeing up specialists who can then provide episodic support/advice to primary care (21). Elsewhere in other high-income countries such as the UK and Sweden, various services have been piloted and developed. Here is a snapshot:

- In the UK, the impacts of the National Dementia Strategy with a focus on increasing the dementia diagnostic rate with financial incentive schemes for primary care have been evaluated. The policy was introduced in 2009, and incentive schemes were introduced between 2013 and 2015 to increase the diagnosis of dementia by encouraging general practitioners to proactively identify undiagnosed cases and develop collaborative care packages. The incentives seem to have effectively boosted diagnostic rates (22) and the quality of drug treatment (23). More recently, applying the Quality and Outcomes Framework and patient experience measurements, the schemes have been shown to have a positive impact on quality outcomes, including spillover effects in other clinical areas, although there were also some unintended negative impacts on patient experience, such as continuity of care (possibly due to efforts being diverted away from other patients) (24).
- In Sweden, primary care was compared with specialist care for the diagnostic process and management of Alzheimer's disease, using data from the Swedish Dementia Registry (25). There were no differences in the use of cholinesterase inhibitors between the services, with primary care associated with a higher likelihood of home care or day care use. Primary care physicians were, however, less likely to have ordered neuroimaging or completed a Clock Drawing Test (see Section 1.3). Although these observations do not imply differences in service quality (as there were differences in patient characteristics between services), they provided some ideas about the existence of any important differences in practice.

With these accumulating experiences, we are witnessing burgeoning developments of primary care models in dementia. From a more forward-looking perspective, future generations of primary care physicians also appeared positive about having a role in early intervention for dementia with community-based care and post-diagnostic support services established (26).

In Section 1.2, we outline a few selected primary care models for reference. While it is not the goal of this book to provide a comprehensive review of these rapidly evolving service models and developing evidence, examples are included here to put the cases presented in this book in context for potential application in our readers' local setting. The cases involved participants from a primary care model with developing integrated health and social care in Hong Kong, which we will describe in Section 1.5.

1.2 Primary Care Models in Dementia: Some Examples

The below examples were selected to illustrate the diversity of possible models and where more detailed information can be found on their operations and outcomes. The examples are organised around the following models: (a) a primary care service with specialist outreach; (b) a specialist service with primary care support; and (c) an integrated multidisciplinary team. Readers who are interested in finding out more about these services are encouraged to visit the online resources provided.

Primary Care Service with Specialist Outreach: An Example

Gnosall Primary Care Memory Clinic in the UK (10, 12) (see www.england.nhs.uk/2015/09/leading-models-dementia/ for details in an NHS England report) is a primary care-based service, with specialist input to support the diagnosis, initial treatment, and ongoing patient review and to provide supervision. The service's ethos is to 'bring the best of secondary care into the primary care service'. A general practitioner would identify people with suspected dementia, who would then be referred to an eldercare facilitator for further assessments – including a Clock Drawing Test and the General Practitioner Assessment of Cognition (GPCOG; see Chapter 4) – and service coordination. When needed, a specialist (a consultant psychiatrist) who spends 3.5 hours per month on site would meet with the person with dementia, the carer, and the facilitator in a monthly memory clinic session to discuss the diagnosis and care. He/she would also provide support to the primary care through phone calls in between the monthly sessions. For the family of the person with dementia, the facilitator is their single point of contact, who works closely with the general practitioner and the specialist.

Benefits noted of the model include minimised delays in access to the service, a nearly 100 per cent attendance rate, identification and treatment of comorbidities, reduced secondary healthcare costs (mainly from reduced acute hospital service use), high levels of user satisfaction, and reduced stigma about seeing a psychiatrist. A key message for effective service is close collaboration with the local mental health partnership service.

Specialist Service with Primary Care Support: An Example

The Dementia Community Support Scheme in Hong Kong (27) (see www.communit ycarefund.hk/download/Evaluation_Report_Dementia_eng.pdf for details in an evaluation report of the pilot service) is a medical–social collaboration model to provide community care services for people with mild or moderate dementia and their carers. People living with dementia receive diagnostic and follow-up consultation services from a specialist outpatient clinic (psychiatry or geriatric medicine) in a public hospital, and are referred to a nearby District Elderly Community Centre, where he/she and the carers would receive a care planning service and corresponding activity support to enhance cognition, daily activity, physical and social functioning; to improve home safety; alleviate carer burden; and to maintain the quality of life of both the person with dementia and their carers. The service is provided by a multidisciplinary allied healthcare and social care team (mostly comprised of a nurse, a social worker, and an occupational therapist/physiotherapist) in the community centre, who work with the hospital specialist team through case conferences and other means of communication (e.g., phone calls). People with suspected dementia identified by the multidisciplinary team may also receive diagnostic consultation and follow-up by a trained primary care physician in private practice and be provided with the same community support.

Benefits of the model identified in the pilot phase include reduced carer burden, particularly among those experiencing a greater burden before reaching the service; a high level of user satisfaction; enhanced collaboration between specialist outpatient clinics and community centres; and maintained quality of life despite deterioration in functioning and symptom severity. Lessons learned from this model include the need for equal-status partnership, joint decision-making, and an information-sharing system when the service crosses the two sectors/settings (medical and social/hospital and community).

Integrated Multidisciplinary Team: An Example

Multispecialty Interprofessional Team (MINT) memory clinics (previously referred to as Primary Care Collaborative Clinics) in Canada (7, 17, 28–30) (see https://mintmemory.ca/ for details) are an integrated model with a team comprising the person's family doctor, nurses, social workers, pharmacists, and other related professionals (e.g., occupational therapists) who work with other specialists and representatives from local community groups such as the Alzheimer's Society. Upon referral to the memory clinics, the person's assessment results are reviewed by the team for an initial diagnosis and management plan, which are shared with the specialist, and complex cases are referred to the appropriate service. Professional team members have to go through standardised accredited training (28).

Benefits observed with this model include reduced costs in the healthcare system (including a reduction in inpatient and emergency department visit costs) and reduced waiting times of nearly 50 per cent. This model highlighted the need to equip the team with training and on-the-job education, to ensure care quality when the complex task of dementia care is shifted/shared with primary care; it also reflects the importance of service integration with a primary care and care management partnership, which was noted in a systematic review of the effectiveness of various post-diagnostic dementia care models delivered by primary care (31).

Learning Points from the Three Examples

The above examples illustrate the potential roles of primary care in dementia work-up, diagnosis, and management within various primary care models; family physicians, as part of a primary care team, should arguably be involved in all key aspects of dementia care (32), including prevention, providing a timely diagnosis, dementia staging, determining dementia subtypes, differentiating other conditions with similar presentations to dementia, communicating the diagnosis while protecting the person's dignity and balancing the family's needs, and providing person-centred, post-diagnosis management support.

1.3 Overview on Dementia: Work-up, Diagnosis, and Management

With the above-mentioned extensive role of primary care in dementia services, an in-depth review of each of the key aspects would be beyond the scope of this casebook (for more detailed reviews and clinical guides, see 33–36). As our purpose here is to share knowledge that would enable the primary care team to function as gatekeepers in the health and social care system to avoid secondary and tertiary care becoming overwhelmed, we will focus on work related to simple, uncomplicated Alzheimer's disease, while also touching on issues surrounding recognising complex cases when referral or collaboration beyond primary care is warranted.

Common Dementia Subtypes

There are various subtypes of dementia, reflecting different symptomatology and pathology. Alzheimer's disease is the most common subtype of dementia, accounting for 60 per cent to 80 per cent of cases (37). The condition is characterised by an insidious, slow onset and gradual progression over many years. The most common clinical presentation is episodic memory impairment, in which individuals have difficulty learning and recalling recently learned information. Cognitive dysfunction may also present in language ability, such as deficits in word finding, and executive dysfunction, including impaired reasoning, judgement, and problem-solving. Individuals may also present with visuospatial problems, such as object agnosia, impaired face recognition, simultanagnosia, and alexia (38, 39). The neuropathology of Alzheimer's disease is marked by the accumulation of plaques, which are extracellular deposits of β-amyloid peptides, and neurofibrillary tangles (40). The underlying cause of Alzheimer's disease is still unknown, but several possible pathological pathways have been suggested. According to the widely accepted 'amyloid cascade hypothesis' (41), the condition is initiated by the progressive accumulation and disposition of β-amyloid, leading to the formation of plaques and neurofibrillary tangles and ultimately neuronal death and dementia.

Vascular dementia is the most common comorbid condition with Alzheimer's disease (42, 43). The brain infarcts or white matter lesions associated with the condition can develop from cerebrovascular incidents, such as a stroke. The condition is diagnosed when there is a relationship between dementia and cerebrovascular disease, where the onset of dementia is within three months following a recognised stroke, an abrupt deterioration in cognitive functions, or a fluctuating, stepwise progression of cognitive deficits (44). Individuals with the condition show gait disturbances in the early stages, such as small-step gait or parkinsonian gait, a history of unsteadiness, and frequent, unprovoked falls. They may also experience early urinary frequency, urgency, and other urinary symptoms that are not explained by urologic disease. Other clinical features include pseudobulbar palsy, personality and mood changes, abulia, depression, emotional incontinence, and other subcortical deficits, including psychomotor retardation and abnormal executive function. Memory, language ability, motor skills, and insight are relatively intact in the early stages of the condition.

Other major subtypes of dementia include dementia with Lewy body (DLB) and frontotemporal dementia (FTD). The former has a slow onset and progresses gradually over months and years (45). Memory impairment may not necessarily occur in the early stages, but it usually increases as the disease progresses. Deficits in attention, executive function, and visuospatial ability may be especially prominent. The core features of DLB include fluctuating levels of attention and alertness, well-formed and detailed recurrent visual hallucinations, which are generally present in the early course of the disease, and spontaneous features of parkinsonism, such as bradykinesia and rigidity (45, 46). Individuals with DLB are likely to present with rapid eye movement (REM) sleep behaviour disorder, severe neuroleptic sensitivity, and low dopamine transporter uptake in the basal ganglia as demonstrated by SPECT or PET imaging. Other common features include repeated falls and syncope; transient, unexplained loss of consciousness; severe autonomic dysfunction (such as orthostatic hypotension and urinary incontinence); hallucinations in other modalities; systematised delusions; and depression. The pathology of the condition is marked by the presence of Lewy bodies and neurites, with the anatomical distribution of Lewy bodies rather than the severity of Lewy pathology more likely to determine the clinical presentation of the condition (47).

Frontotemporal dementia has an insidious onset and slow progression (48). Individuals with the condition exhibit early loss of personal awareness, such as neglect of personal hygiene and grooming; social awareness, including lack of social tact and misdemeanours such as shoplifting; and signs of disinhibition, which include unrestrained sexuality, violent behaviour, inappropriate jocularity, and restless pacing. They may have utilisation behaviour, exploring objects in the environment unrestrainedly.

Affected individuals may also show mental rigidity and inflexibility. Hyperorality, such as dietary changes, excessive smoking, and alcohol consumption, is common with the condition. Individuals may also demonstrate stereotyped and preservative behaviours, including wandering and mannerisms, such as clapping, singing, and dancing, and ritualistic preoccupations, such as hoarding, toileting, and dressing. They may be easily distracted, impulsive, and impersistent and lack insight into the altered condition due to a pathological change in their own mental state. Individuals with FTD may also have speech disorders. Examples might be progressive reduction of speech, including aspontaneity and economy of utterance; stereotypy of speech, such as repetition of a limited repertoire of words, phrases, or themes; echolalia and perseveration; and late mutism. The pathologic feature of the condition is focal brain atrophy in the frontal and/or anterior temporal lobes, while the other areas are relatively spared. The condition shows a slow onset and gradual progression over months or years (49).

Diagnosis and Differential Diagnosis

A number of established criteria are available to guide dementia diagnosis and subtyping (35), which are listed in Box 1.1 for readers who wish to read further. For the diagnosis of dementia, a few key points (49) are highlighted here:

- the diagnosis of dementia requires a *history* of

    . cognitive *decline* and
    . impairment in *daily activities*; and

- it necessitates

    . corroboration from a knowledgeable *informant* and
    . a cognitive *examination*.

Cognitive *decline* refers to a decline from the person's own previous level of function, which is why corroboration is needed. With many of the cognitive screening tests, if done only cross-sectionally (i.e., once), the scoring against locally validated cut-off scores essentially provides only a statistical reference for how likely or unlikely a person's performance is 'normal' compared with his/her peers, without giving information on the decline. It should also be noted that decline can be present in cognitive domains other than memory and learning, including executive function, attention, language, perceptual-motor, and social cognition.

The criteria for dementia differ from those for mild cognitive impairment: for mild cognitive impairment, the cognitive decline has yet to significantly impair the person's independence in daily living. For people with self-experienced cognitive decline with normal performance on standardised cognitive tests, the category 'subjective cognitive impairment' (50) can be considered. While there are debates over their clinical significance, subjective complaints in primary care settings may predict future dementia and should be taken seriously (51).

Work-up and further history are needed to determine the possible *aetiology* of dementia (49); some may be potentially treatable or reversible (such as depression, which has been referred to as 'pseudodementia'; see (52) for a review of the concept). These work-ups (see Chapter 4) include the following:

- neurological, general medical, and family history;
- physical examination of neurological signs and pertinent systemic signs;

- neuropsychological testing;
- laboratory testing, including thyroid function and vitamin B_{12};
- brain imaging if needed (e.g., to exclude other abnormalities such as a brain tumour).

Box 1.1   Criteria for Diagnosing and Subtyping Dementia: Further Reading

General Diagnostic Criteria
Diagnostic and Statistical Manual of Mental Disorders (DSM-5) (53)
International Statistical Classification of Diseases and Related Health Problems (ICD-11) (54).

Mild Cognitive Impairment
'The diagnosis of mild cognitive impairment due to Alzheimer's disease: recommendations from the National Institute on Aging – Alzheimer's Association workgroups on diagnostic guidelines for Alzheimer's disease' (55)

Alzheimer's Disease
NINCDS-ADRDA criteria: The diagnosis of dementia due to Alzheimer's disease: recommendations from the National Institute on Aging – Alzheimer's Association workgroups on diagnostic guidelines for Alzheimer's disease (56)

Vascular Dementia
Report of the National Institute of Neurological Disorders and Stroke and Association Internationale pour la Recherche et l'Enseignement en Neurosciences (NINDS-AIREN) International Workshop (57)
    https://doi.org/10.1212/WNL.43.2.250

Frontotemporal Dementia
Classification of primary progressive aphasia and its variants (58).
    Sensitivity of revised diagnostic criteria for the behavioural variant of frontotemporal dementia (59)
    https://doi.org/10.1093/brain/awr179.

Dementia with Lewy Bodies
Diagnosis and management of dementia with Lewy bodies: Fourth consensus report of the DLB Consortium (45)
    https://doi.org/10.1212/WNL.0000000000004058

Staging

The manifestation of Alzheimer's disease varies depending on the disease stage. Several clinical criteria have been developed to assess dementia severity, and some of the more widely used criteria are the Clinical Dementia Rating (CDR) (60), the Global Deterioration Scale (GDS) (61), and the Functional Assessment Staging (FAST) in Alzheimer's Disease (62, 63). In the early stages of Alzheimer's disease, individuals may present with memory impairments that interfere with daily activities, especially decreased knowledge of current and recent events. Orientation to time and place, as well as recognition of familiar people and faces, would be relatively intact; they may be able to travel to familiar places, but may have difficulty with time relationship. People with early Alzheimer's disease may have difficulty solving problems and engaging in abstract thinking about similarities and differences between things, although they are often intact in social judgements. In terms of community affairs, they may need some assistance in activities such as work, shopping, volunteering, or engaging in social groups. Even though impairments at this stage often remain mild, there can be obvious dysfunction at home, and the person may have given up more difficult or complicated chores, hobbies, and interests. They are, however, often still capable of personal care, although prompting may be needed.

In the moderate stage, individuals may show obvious memory impairments, with newly learned materials rapidly lost and only highly learned information retained. For example, people with moderate Alzheimer's disease may not recall an address or telephone number they have been using for many years, forgetting the names of their grandchildren or the high school they graduated from. Disorientation to date, time, and place is common at this stage, and people tend to have severe difficulty with time relationship. The ability to solve problems and judge similarities and differences between things, as well as social judgement, can be severely impaired. Although engaging in community affairs independently is unlikely at this stage, people with moderate Alzheimer's disease can be well enough to attend functions and events outside the home. At home, they may only be able to do simple chores and have very restricted interests. Regarding personal care, many require no assistance with toileting and eating, but may exhibit difficulty choosing proper clothing to wear.

In the severe stage, individuals would have severe memory impairment, with only fragments of memory remaining. They may be unaware of their surroundings and are oriented towards people only. While they may be able to distinguish familiar people from unfamiliar ones, they may occasionally forget the names of close family members such as their spouse. People at this stage are often unable to make a sound or safe judgement, solve problems, or engage in community affairs. They may also be too ill to be taken to events outside the home. People at this stage of Alzheimer's disease would be unable to function at home and require much assistance with personal care, including toileting and feeding. All verbal abilities are lost at this advanced stage, with only unintelligible utterances and rarely some pieces of words and phrases produced.

Communicating Diagnosis

It is not an uncommon practice to avoid direct and clear communication of the diagnosis, perhaps out of concerns for preserving hope; however, it would also compromise understanding and future planning (64), affecting the person's opportunities to getting proper support, such as early interventions that can maintain cognitive function and prolong community living (65).

Communication of the diagnosis should be handled with sensitivity, considering individual needs. An important point to note in the process is to explain in easy-to-understand language the symptoms, what to expect, and what can be done. It is good practice to allow time for processing the information and give written information with contact details of the service for reference.

Post-diagnostic Management

There is currently no cure or widely available disease-modifying treatment to slow or stop the progression of dementia; however, treatments that may change the experience of dementia by temporarily improving the symptoms are available (34). Drug treatments for cognitive symptoms of dementia have been approved for Alzheimer's disease, DLB, and Parkinson's disease dementia. They target biochemical abnormalities due to neuronal loss but do not alter the underlying neuropathology or its progression. Acetylcholinesterase inhibitors (AChEIs: donepezil, rivastigmine, and galantamine) have proven yet modest effects in maintaining or delaying cognitive decline (66–68). Donepezil and rivastigmine also have a positive effect on hallucinations in DLB. Memantine has a smaller effect in moderate to severe Alzheimer's disease (34). For people with mild to moderate Alzheimer's disease, the intervention goals include delaying cognitive decline, optimising functioning, and minimising secondary morbidity. It should be noted that depending on local regulations, primary care physicians may or may not be allowed to prescribe dementia drugs, which can have an effect on their engagement level in dementia work-up (69).

The effects of psychosocial interventions on improving cognitive symptoms of dementia have been reviewed (70). These include cognitive stimulation, cognitive training, cognitive rehabilitation, reality orientation, combined cognitive and exercise programmes, and computer-based cognitive interventions. Cognitive interventions can be categorised as follows (71):

- Cognitive stimulation is the engagement in activities and discussions with the aim of enhancing general cognitive and social functioning;
- Cognitive training is guided practice on a set of standard tasks designed to improve specific cognitive function, such as working memory;
- Cognitive rehabilitation is an individualised approach where personal goals are identified and the therapist works with the person and his or her family to create strategies to address the goals.

In people with mild to moderate dementia, more consistent evidence is available for cognitive stimulation, with group-based cognitive stimulation therapy (CST) (72) and a range of activities tailored to the person's preferences being recommended in clinical guidelines (35). Other strategies such as reminiscence therapy, cognitive rehabilitation, or occupational therapy are also recommended for consideration (35). Music for agitation (73), physical exercise for fitness (74), social interaction, a healthy diet, adequate sleep, safety, advance directives, and advance care planning (49) are potential strategies. As for carers, multicomponent carer support programmes such as Resources for Enhancing Alzheimer's Carer Health (REACH) (75) and STrAtegies for RelaTives (START) (76) are evidence-based, time-limited interventions that can improve carer outcomes such as burden and quality of life, as well as the distressed behaviours and neuropsychiatric symptoms of dementia.

The multitude of post-diagnostic interventions and care available and diverse individual situations require individual care plans and care coordination. The actual practice of care planning varies (see Section 1.5 for an example of a 'Certified Dementia Care Planner' in Hong Kong, with training content developed with support from Alzheimer's Disease International); in general, a named professional would be responsible for assessing the person's needs, strengths, and preferences; providing information about services; and developing (in collaboration with the family where appropriate), reviewing, and evaluating the individual care plan (35). As with a comprehensive geriatric assessment (77), in dementia an individual care plan is a tool used as a form of integrated care, where the care plan is formulated to address the issues of concern to the person and his/ her family members and carers, based on assessments that may cover physical/functional, psychosocial/behavioural, carer support needs, and environmental factors. The coordinated services may include the above pharmacological and non-pharmacological interventions, as well as legal and financial advice, education, and carer support groups.

1.4 Integrated Health and Social Care: Rationales and Evidence

Models of Dementia

In the primary care models and dementia management approaches described above, both biological and psychosocial aspects are emphasised. This reflects a shift over the past decades in the conceptualisation of dementia: from a focus on a medical perspective, moving to a dialectical view, and more recently to an integrated biopsychosocial model of dementia.

From a medical perspective, dementia is a condition caused by neurological problems, and management should therefore focus on biological factors (78). In the 1990s, Tom Kitwood introduced the concept that dementia is a manifestation of an interaction between neuropathology and psychological factors (including personality, biography, and social psychology), putting an emphasis on 'personhood' and person-centred care (the 'dialectic model') (79). This view has revolutionised the way people living with dementia are being cared for. Building on this theoretical foundation, the biopsychosocial model expanded the factors to include mental stimulation, sensory stimulation, environment, life events, and mood in the manifestation of dementia (80).

A range of interventions targeting each of the tractable factors can be effective dementia management strategies, based on the biopsychosocial model, to reduce excess disability and promote independence. Table 1.1 lists some suggested factors and interventions (modified from (80)). An integrated health and social care service allows for more efficient delivery of these psychosocial and biological interventions.

Service Integration: The Role of Primary Care

In countries where health and social care services are delivered by different organisations and monitored by different governmental departments/bureaus, provision and coordination of these psychosocial and biological interventions for people living with dementia can be challenging. Service fragmentation and overlap can result in gaps and inefficient resource use. Integrated care has been proposed in these situations for delivering services and implementing complex interventions (81), to enhance system efficiency while benefiting the person requiring care (82).

The integration of healthcare and social care can occur at various levels and care settings. In the healthcare system, it could range from general practice to a specialist clinic in the community, from subacute care to acute care; within social care, it could include community aged care services (e.g., social centres), home care, day care centres, and long-term care facilities. In people with mild dementia, community-based integrated health and social care may slow deterioration, maintain quality of life, and delay institutionalisation (83, 84). While existing models of integration vary in the involvement of primary and specialist care, an emphasis on early detection and integration into general health and social care has been recommended (85).

Table 1.1 Examples of tractable factors and interventions based on the biopsychosocial model

	Tractable factors	Possible interventions
Psychosocial	• Mental stimulation • Mood • Life events • Environment	• Cognitive intervention • Reminiscence • Carer support • Home modification
Biological	• Comorbidity • Sensory impairment	• Medication for comorbidity • Sensory aids

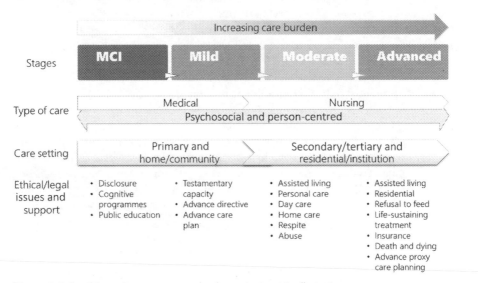

Figure 1.1 Possible service arrangements by dementia stage: An illustration

Depending on the dementia stage, integration of health and social care at the primary care level can represent an ideal option. Figure 1.1 illustrates a possible arrangement of services by dementia stage.

In this illustration, throughout the dementia trajectory, primary care (including primary health and social care) can serve as a base to provide early intervention services in the earlier stages of the illness, and signposting and transitioning to secondary and tertiary care as needs arise. Especially in simple, uncomplicated early Alzheimer's disease, with a relatively predictable disease trajectory, primary care could be the starting point for outreach detection, delivery of pharmacological and non-pharmacological intervention, and advance care planning to ensure a continuum of care. Here, the disease journey begins with early diagnosis and psychosocial support that is culturally appropriate. Families are supported by a care planner who can advise on the different needs of the person with dementia and the carer. At different dementia stages, the family is advised in advance on the next stage of management: as Alzheimer's disease has a predictable trajectory, according to the FAST staging, in the moderate stage the person would, for example, present with dressing apraxia and need more assistive care for getting dressed, proceeding to needing assistance in bathing and then in toileting. As s/he enters the advanced stage, more attention is needed for mobility and swallowing problems. Home care and the prospect of institutionalisation should therefore be discussed.

With an integrated care service, ethical and legal considerations are also taken care of. During the early stages, the will, powers of attorney, and advance directives are discussed, and consensus from the person and the family is gained. At the other extreme, end-of-life care and the related ethical issues need to be considered and discussed. Advance care planning is needed, considering the typical trajectory of Alzheimer's disease and the multidimensional needs at different stages. As regular interactions among the person living with dementia, the family, and the care provider are needed, a care planner in an integrated health and social care service can act as a moderator to coordinate all care issues. This arrangement has the potential to improve quality of life, while saving scarce secondary and tertiary care resources. An example of an integrated primary health and social care service is given in Section 1.5.

1.5 Lessons Learned from 15 Years of Early Intervention Service

Service Context and Design

In Hong Kong, an early detection scheme (EDS) was developed in 2005 by the Hong Kong Alzheimer's Disease Association as a community-based, territory-wide programme to provide early intervention for people with suspected dementia (86). The service was originally developed out of a need for earlier dementia diagnosis, especially Alzheimer's disease, to cut down the waiting time for establishing a diagnosis and to provide timely health and social care services.

As with many Asian areas, Hong Kong is one of the most rapidly ageing societies in the world. With a population of approximately 7 million, over 100,000 people were living with dementia in 2009, a number that is projected to reach over 330,000 by 2039 (87). The diagnostic rate in Hong Kong has been low, at 11 per cent, based on an earlier study (88). While the low diagnostic rate could be related to low awareness among people needing help, provider factors such as service accessibility (e.g., long waiting times for the first diagnostic consultation with a public memory clinic) are also barriers to help-seeking (89).

The EDS is accessible by open referral. People with suspected dementia and/or their carers can self-refer to arrange an assessment by trained social care professionals, such as occupational therapists and social workers, who would gather necessary information (such as history and complaints) and conduct a series of locally validated assessments that include clinical, neuropsychological, functioning, and mood measures (see Chapter 4 for details). The tools were selected balancing psychometric properties and appropriateness for use in service, including applicability in older people with no or very limited formal education (common in Hong Kong). By facilitating early help-seeking, which is linked with milder symptoms (86), the EDS serves as a useful component of a dementia triage system (86, 90) to promote early intervention.

Before 2015, people initially identified through EDS as probably having dementia would be referred to specialists for diagnosis. The barrier of long waiting times for diagnostic consultation remained: this contradicts the recommendation in the World

> **Box 1.2** Training curriculum for primary care physicians in dementia care: An example in Hong Kong
>
> Eighteen hours of in-depth training with lectures, case demonstrations, and case sharing:
>
> - Early clinical diagnosis of dementia – core clinical features and diagnostic criteria.
> - In-depth understanding of Alzheimer's dementia
> - Strategic pharmacological intervention for dementia
> - Neuropsychological assessments and multidisciplinary collaboration to facilitate the diagnostic process.
> - Neuropsychiatric behaviours and psychological symptoms of dementia.
> - Mental capacity assessments, financial planning, and legal and ethical issues.
> - Skills in disclosure of diagnostic results and care planning advice.
>
> With post-training support provided by a specialist, including advice on imaging/examination ordering and feedback on diagnosis.

> **Box 1.3** Training curriculum for a certified dementia care planner: An example in Hong Kong
>
> Four modules (80 hours) of training co-developed by Alzheimer's Disease International and the Hong Kong Alzheimer's Disease Association with support from The University of Hong Kong to equip healthcare and social service professionals with competence in assessment, care planning, management, family-caregiver support, and coordination of community resources:
>
> - Module 1 Essentials for understanding dementia.
> - Module 2 Getting prepared: pre-diagnostic social cognitive assessment and caregiver needs appraisal.
> - Module 3 Care planning and management: counselling and caregiver support.
> - Module 4 Advance care management.

Alzheimer's Report (1) that the majority of cases of early Alzheimer's disease can be diagnosed with treatment initiated by primary care, with only a small proportion requiring referral for secondary care. An enhanced, shared-care model was piloted ('Project Sunrise'), with the following additional features:

- training and support for primary care physicians in dementia diagnosis and management by an experienced specialist (geriatrician) (see Box 1.2 for the training curriculum);
- care planning, coordination, and family carer support by a certified dementia care planner (see Box 1.3 for training curriculum);
- information-sharing between EDS and the trained primary care physicians to facilitate diagnosis and management;
- rapid referral of atypical cases to other potentially appropriate services; and
- provision of post-diagnostic support with day centre services and primary care physicians.

This community-integrated health and social care model for dementia was designed with the aim of promoting task-shifting or task-sharing. By shifting some of the diagnosis workload to trained primary care physicians, with support from EDS, the waiting time for receiving a diagnosis among help-seekers could be cut down, with a smaller proportion of people requiring referral for secondary care. In this model, collaboration between primary and secondary care is also advocated, so that specialists provide mentorship and support for primary care physicians for complicated cases and if there is a change in the condition of the person requiring secondary care, while the primary care physician would also collaborate with the specialist for referral of appropriate cases, eventually achieving task-sharing across disciplines and between primary and secondary care.

Lessons Learned among Primary Care Physicians

Using action research, several key lessons learned were identified from this model of community-integrated health and social care involving task-shifting/-sharing with primary care, including the following:

1. Primary care physicians considered the support from social care essential: collaboration was needed for engaging the person with dementia in general practice. This seems to be true, particularly among families of lower socioeconomic status, some of whom would have otherwise opted out of receiving a diagnosis and intervention. Informational support (e.g., assessment reports) from social care has also allowed more focused consultation sessions, shortening the time requirement in a busy clinic.

2. There is a need to prepare society for the role of primary care in dementia care: a challenge noted is to engage potential patients or carers in general practice, as the public is generally unaware of/sceptical about the role of primary care physicians in dementia diagnosis and treatment.

3. Good-quality non-pharmacological interventions provided by social care (e.g., person-centred care and effective cognitive interventions) are an important consideration among primary care physicians for collaborative care. A regular feedback system with brief reports on service status (e.g., when a home visit was arranged) is desired.

4. With training and support from EDS, primary care physicians reported that diagnosing typical cases of Alzheimer's disease is straightforward in most cases. In cases with atypical presentations, where the diagnosis is less clear or when complications arise (e.g., mood symptoms) and an expert review would be needed, primary care physicians regarded themselves as having a clear understanding of when to refer. They also expressed confidence in providing medication treatment for early dementia, considering the stable and chronic nature of Alzheimer's disease, although a mechanism of transition to specialist care would be needed when the disease progresses or when there are complications requiring stabilisation. Comparing the expert review with the initial diagnosis made by the primary care physicians, agreement in diagnosis was observed in the majority (>80 per cent) of cases.

5. There is a need for practicum, pedagogy, and clinical guidelines for primary care physicians to help them make decisions (e.g., when an MRI is indicated) in their daily practice. Regular case conferences were considered crucial. Attachment to a few consultation sessions by specialists and continuous post-training specialist support at a low level, such as by monthly phone consultation, were considered useful in the training.

In summary, with appropriate training and an integrated health and social care service, task-shifting/-sharing of dementia care with primary care can be feasible; the key is to focus on 'simple, uncomplicated early Alzheimer's disease' in such a service model. In the next two chapters, we will review cases that fall into this category, and atypical cases in comparison, to facilitate an understanding of the target population of a primary care dementia service.

References

1. Prince M, Comas-Herrera A, Knapp M, Guerchet M, Karagiannidou M. World Alzheimer Report 2016: Improving Healthcare for People Living with Dementia: Coverage, Quality and Costs Now and in the Future. London: Alzheimer's Disease International. 2016.

2. World Health Organization. World Health Organization Fact Sheet: Dementia. 2023 (15 March). Available from: www.who.int/news-room/fact-sheets/detail/dementia.

3. World Health Organization. Dementia: A Public Health Priority. Geneva: World Health Organization. 2012.

4. World Health Organization. Task Shifting: Rational Redistribution of Tasks among Health Workforce Teams: Global Recommendations and Guidelines. Geneva: World Health Organization. 2007.

5. Kakuma R, Minas H, van Ginneken N, Dal Poz MR, Desiraju K, Morris JE, et al. Human resources for mental health care: Current situation and strategies for action. The Lancet. 2011;378 (9803):1654–63.

6. World Health Organization. Global Action Plan on the Public Health Response to Dementia 2017–2025. Geneva: World Health Organization. 2017.

7. Lee L, Hillier LM, Heckman G, Gagnon M, Borrie MJ, Stolee P, et al. Primary care-based memory clinics: Expanding capacity for dementia care. Canadian Journal on Aging/La Revue canadienne du vieillissement. 2014;33(3):307–19.

8. Alzheimer's Disease International. Policy Brief for Heads of Government: The Global Impact of Dementia 2013–2050. London: Alzheimer's Disease International. 2013.

9. Dodd E, Cheston R, Ivanecka A. The assessment of dementia in primary care. Journal of Psychiatric and Mental Health Nursing. 2015;22(9):731–7.

10. Greaves I, Greaves N, Walker E, Greening L, Benbow SM, Jolley D. Gnosall Primary Care Memory Clinic: Eldercare facilitator role description and development. Dementia. 2015;14(4):389–408.

11. Banerjee S, Willis R, Matthews D, Contell F, Chan J, Murray J. Improving the quality of care for mild to moderate dementia: An evaluation of the Croydon Memory Service Model. International Journal of Geriatric Psychiatry: A Journal of the Psychiatry of Late Life and Allied Sciences. 2007;22(8):782–8.

12. Hawkins J. Models of Dementia Assessment and Diagnosis: Indicative Cost Review. 2015. Available from: www.england.nhs.uk/wp-content/uploads/2015/09/mods-demntl-assessmnt-diag-cost.pdf.

13. Skivington K, Matthews L, Craig P, Simpson S, Moore L. Developing and evaluating complex interventions: Updating Medical Research Council guidance to take account of new methodological and theoretical approaches. The Lancet. 2018;392:S2.

14. Jolley D, Greaves I, Clark M, editors. Memory clinics and primary care: Not a question of either/or. BMJ; 2012: BMJ Group.

15. Banerjee S, Wittenberg R. Clinical and cost effectiveness of services for early diagnosis and intervention in dementia. International Journal of Geriatric Psychiatry. 2009;24(7):748–54.

16. Dodd E, Cheston R, Fear T, Brown E, Fox C, Morley C, et al. An evaluation of primary care led dementia diagnostic services in Bristol. BMC Health Services Research. 2014;14(1):592.

17. Lee L, Hillier LM, Stolee P, Heckman G, Gagnon M, McAiney CA, et al. Enhancing dementia care: A primary care-based memory clinic. Journal of the American Geriatrics Society. 2010;58 (11):2197–204.

18. Chibanda D, Mesu P, Kajawu L, Cowan F, Araya R, Abas MA. Problem-solving therapy for depression and common mental disorders in Zimbabwe: Piloting a task-shifting primary mental health care intervention in a population with a high prevalence of people living with HIV. BMC Public Health. 2011;11(1):828.

19. Joshi R, Alim M, Kengne AP, Jan S, Maulik PK, Peiris D, et al. Task shifting for non-communicable disease management in low and middle income countries: A systematic review. PLOS ONE. 2014;9(8):e103754.

20. Buttorff C, Hock RS, Weiss HA, Naik S, Araya R, Kirkwood BR, et al. Economic evaluation of a task-shifting intervention for common mental disorders in India. Bulletin of the World Health Organization. 2012;90(11):813–21.

21. New Zealand Ministry of Health. New Zealand framework for dementia care. 2013.

22. Mason A, Liu D, Kasteridis P, Goddard M, Jacobs R, Wittenberg R, et al. Investigating the impact of primary care payments on underdiagnosis in dementia: A difference-in-differences analysis. International Journal of Geriatric Psychiatry. 2018;33(8):1090–7.

23. Donegan K, Fox N, Black N, Livingston G, Banerjee S, Burns A. Trends in diagnosis and treatment for people with dementia in the UK from 2005 to 2015: A longitudinal retrospective cohort study. Lancet Public Health. 2017;2(3):e149–e56.

24. Liu D, Green E, Kasteridis P, Goddard M, Jacobs R, Wittenberg R, et al. Incentive schemes to increase dementia diagnoses in primary care in England: A retrospective cohort study of unintended consequences. British Journal of General Practice. 2019;69(680):e154–e63.

25. Garcia-Ptacek S, Modeer IN, Kareholt I, Fereshtehnejad SM, Farahmand B, Religa D, et al. Differences in diagnostic process, treatment and social Support for Alzheimer's dementia between primary and specialist care: Results from the Swedish Dementia Registry. Age Ageing. 2017;46(2):314–9.

26. Tang EYH, Birdi R, Robinson L. Attitudes to diagnosis and management in dementia care: Views of future general practitioners. International Psychogeriatrics. 2018;30(3):425–30.

27. Wong GHY, Lum TYS, Tang JYM, Kwan JSK, Chan WC, Cheung ACY, et al. Formative Evaluation Study on the Dementia Community Support Scheme (Pilot Scheme): Final Report. Hong Kong: Food and Health Bureau, The Government of the Hong Kong Special Administrative Region. 2019.

28. Lee L, Weston MW, Hillier ML. Developing memory clinics in primary care: An evidence-based interprofessional program of continuing professional development. Journal of Continuing Education in the Health Professions. 2013;33(1):24–32.

29. Lee L, Hillier LM, Weston WW. Ensuring the success of interprofessional teams: Key lessons learned in memory clinics. Canadian Journal on Aging. 2014;33(1):49–59.

30. Lee L, Kasperski MJ, Weston WW. Building capacity for dementia care Training program to develop primary care memory clinics. Canadian Family Physician. 2011;57(7):E249–E52.

31. Frost R, Walters K, Aw S, Brunskill G, Wilcock J, Robinson L, et al. Effectiveness of different post-diagnostic dementia care models delivered by primary care: A systematic review. British Journal of General Practice. 2020;70(695):e434–e41.

32. Moore A, Frank C, Chambers LW. Role of the family physician in dementia care.

Canadian Family Physician. 2018;64 (10):717–19.

33. Livingston G, Huntley J, Sommerlad A, Ames D, Ballard C, Banerjee S, et al. Dementia prevention, intervention, and care: 2020 report of the Lancet Commission. The Lancet. 2020;396 (10248):413–46.

34. Livingston G, Sommerlad A, Orgeta V, Costafreda SG, Huntley J, Ames D, et al. Dementia prevention, intervention, and care. The Lancet. 2017;390 (10113):2673–734.

35. National Institute for Health and Care Excellence. Dementia: Assessment, management and support for people living with dementia and their carers. 2018. Available from: www.nice.org.uk/ guidance/ng97/chapter/ Recommendations#diagnosis.

36. Barrett E, Burns A. Dementia Revealed: What Primary Care Needs to Know. UK: NHS England. 2014. Available from: www .england.nhs.uk/wp-content/uploads/ 2014/09/dementia-revealed-toolkit.pdf.

37. Alzheimer's Disease International. World Alzheimer Report 2015. London: Alzheimer's Disease International. 2015.

38. McKhann GM, Drachman D, Folstein M, Katzman R, Price D, Stadlan EM. Clinical diagnosis of Alzheimer's disease: Report of the NINCDS-ADRDA Work Group under the auspices of Department of Health and Human Services Task Force on Alzheimer's Disease. Neurology. 1984;34(7):939–44.

39. McKhann GM, Knopman DS, Chertkow H, Hyman BT, Jack CR, Jr Kawas, CH, et al. The diagnosis of dementia due to Alzheimer's disease: Recommendations from the National Institute on Aging-Alzheimer's Association workgroups on diagnostic guidelines for Alzheimer's disease. Alzheimer's & Dementia: The Journal of the Alzheimer's Association 2011;7(3):263–9.

40. Montine TJ, Phelps CH, Beach TG, Bigio EH, Cairns NJ, Dickson DW, et al. National Institute on Aging-Alzheimer's Association guidelines for the neuropathologic assessment of Alzheimer's disease: A practical approach. Acta Neuropathologica. 2012;123 (1):1–11.

41. Hardy JA, Higgins GA. Alzheimer's disease: The amyloid cascade hypothesis. Science. 1992;256 (5054):184–5.

42. Kapasi A, DeCarli C, Schneider JA. Impact of multiple pathologies on the threshold for clinically overt dementia. Acta Neuropathology. 2017;134 (2):171–86.

43. Brenowitz WD, Hubbard RA, Keene CD, Hawes SE, Longstreth Jr WT, Woltjer RL, et al. Mixed neuropathologies and estimated rates of clinical progression in a large autopsy sample. Alzheimer's & Dementia. 2017;13(6):654–62.

44. Roman GC, Tatemichi TK, Erkinjuntti T, Cummings JL, Masdeu JC, Garcia JH, et al. Vascular dementia: Diagnostic criteria for research studies. Report of the NINDS-AIREN International Workshop. Neurology. 1993;43(2):250–60.

45. McKeith IG, Boeve BF, Dickson DW, Halliday G, Taylor J-P, Weintraub D, et al. Diagnosis and management of dementia with Lewy bodies: Fourth consensus report of the DLB Consortium. Neurology. 2017;89(1):88–100.

46. Postuma RB, Berg D, Stern M, Poewe W, Olanow CW, Oertel W, et al. MDS clinical diagnostic criteria for Parkinson's disease. Movement Disorders: Official Journal of the Movement Disorder Society. 2015;30(12):1591–601.

47. Kon T, Tomiyama M, Wakabayashi K. Neuropathology of Lewy body disease: Clinicopathological crosstalk between typical and atypical cases. Neuropathology. 2020;40(1):30–9.

48. The Lund and Manchester Groups. Clinical and neuropathological criteria for frontotemporal dementia. Journal of Neurology, Neurosurgery and Psychiatry. 1994;57(4):416–18.

49. Arvanitakis Z, Shah RC, Bennett DA. Diagnosis and management of dementia: Review. JAMA. 2019;322(16):1589–99.

50. Jessen F, Amariglio RE, Buckley RF, van der Flier WM, Han Y, Molinuevo JL, et al. The characterisation of subjective cognitive decline. Lancet Neurology. 2020;19(3):271–8.

51. Numbers K, Crawford JD, Kochan NA, Draper B, Sachdev PS, Brodaty H. Participant and informant memory-specific cognitive complaints predict future decline and incident dementia: Findings from the Sydney Memory and Ageing Study. PLOS ONE. 2020;15(5): e0232961.

52. Brodaty H, Connors MH. Pseudodementia, pseudo-pseudodementia, and pseudodepression. Alzheimers Dementia (Amst). 2020;12(1): e12027.

53. American Psychiatric Association. (2022). Diagnostic and statistical manual of mental disorders (5th ed., text rev.). https://doi.org/10.1176/appi.books .9780890425787.

54 World Health Organization. (2022). ICD-11: International classification of diseases (11th revision). Available from: https://icd.who.int/.

55. Albert MS, DeKosky ST, Dickson D, Dubois B, Feldman HH, Fox NC, et al. The diagnosis of mild cognitive impairment due to Alzheimer's disease: Recommendations from the National Institute on Aging-Alzheimer's Association workgroups on diagnostic guidelines for Alzheimer's disease. Alzheimers Dementia. 2011;7(3):270–9.

56. McKhann GM, Knopman DS, Chertkow H, Hyman BT, Jack CR, Jr., Kawas CH, et al. The diagnosis of dementia due to Alzheimer's disease: Recommendations from the National Institute on Aging-Alzheimer's Association workgroups on diagnostic guidelines for Alzheimer's disease. Alzheimers Dementia. 2011;7 (3):263–9.

57. Roman GC, Tatemichi TK, Erkinjuntti T, Cummings JL, Masdeu JC, Garcia JH, et al. Vascular dementia: Diagnostic criteria for research studies. Report of the NINDS-AIREN International Workshop. Neurology. 1993;43(2):250–60.

58. Gorno-Tempini ML, Hillis AE, Weintraub S, Kertesz A, Mendez M, Cappa SF, et al. Classification of primary progressive aphasia and its variants. Neurology. 2011;76(11):1006–14.

59. Rascovsky K, Hodges JR, Knopman D, Mendez MF, Kramer JH, Neuhaus J, et al. Sensitivity of revised diagnostic criteria for the behavioural variant of frontotemporal dementia. Brain. 2011;134(Pt 9):2456–77.

60. Morris JC. The Clinical Dementia Rating (CDR): Current version and scoring rules. Neurology. 1993;43(11):2412–4.

61. Reisberg B, Ferris SH, de Leon MJ, Crook T. The Global Deterioration Scale for assessment of primary degenerative dementia. American Journal of Psychiatry. 1982;139(9):1136–9.

62. Reisberg B. Functional assessment staging (FAST). Psychopharmacology Bulletin. 1988;24(4):653–9.

63. Sclan SG, Reisberg B. Functional assessment staging (FAST) in Alzheimer's disease: Reliability, validity, and ordinality. International Psychogeriatry. 1992;4(Suppl 1):55–69.

64. Dooley J, Bass N, McCabe R. How do doctors deliver a diagnosis of dementia in memory clinics? British Journal of Psychiatry. 2018;212(4):239–45.

65. Alzheimer's Disease International. World Alzheimer Report 2011. London: Alzheimer's Disease International. 2011.

66. Birks J. Cholinesterase inhibitors for Alzheimer's disease. The Cochrane Database of Systematic Reviews. 2006(1): CD005593.

67. Mangialasche F, Solomon A, Winblad B, Mecocci P, Kivipelto M. Alzheimer's disease: Clinical trials and drug development. Lancet Neurology. 2010;9(7):702–16.

68. Prince M, Bryce R, Ferri C. World Alzheimer Report 2011: The Benefits of Early Diagnosis and Intervention. London: Alzheimer's Disease International. 2011.

69. Yaman H. Exploring dementia management attitudes in primary care:

A key informant survey to primary care physicians in 25 European countries – CORRIGENDUM. International Psychogeriatry. 2018;30(10):1577.

70. McDermott O, Charlesworth G, Hogervorst E, Stoner C, Moniz-Cook E, Spector A, et al. Psychosocial interventions for people with dementia: A synthesis of systematic reviews. Aging & Mental Health. 2018;23(4):393–403

71. Woods B, Aguirre E, Spector AE, Orrell M. Cognitive stimulation to improve cognitive functioning in people with dementia. Cochrane Database of Systematic Reviews. 2023(1):CD005562.

72. Woods B, Aguirre E, Spector AE, Orrell M. Cognitive stimulation to improve cognitive functioning in people with dementia. Cochrane Database of Systematic Review. 2012;2:CD005562.

73. Pedersen SKA, Andersen PN, Lugo RG, Andreassen M, Sutterlin S. Effects of music on agitation in dementia: A meta-analysis. Frontier in Psychology. 2017;8:742.

74. Lamb SE, Sheehan B, Atherton N, Nichols V, Collins H, Mistry D, et al. Dementia and physical activity (DAPA) trial of moderate to high intensity exercise training for people with dementia: Randomised controlled trial. BMJ. 2018;361:k1675.

75. Gitlin LN, Belle SH, Burgio LD, Czaja SJ, Mahoney D, Gallagher-Thompson D, et al. Effect of multicomponent interventions on caregiver burden and depression: The REACH multisite initiative at 6-month follow-up. Psychology and Aging. 2003;18 (3):361–74.

76. Livingston G, Barber J, Rapaport P, Knapp M, Griffin M, King D, et al. Clinical effectiveness of a manual based coping strategy programme (START, STrAtegies for RelaTives) in promoting the mental health of carers of family members with dementia: Pragmatic randomised controlled trial. BMJ. 2013;347:f6276.

77. Society BG. Comprehensive Geriatric Assessment Toolkit for Primary Care Practitioners 2019. Available from: www .bgs.org.uk/sites/default/files/content/ resources/files/2019-02-08/BGS% 20Toolkit%20-%20FINAL%20FOR% 20WEB_0.pdf.

78. Lyman KA. Bringing the social back in: A critique of the biomedicalization of dementia. Gerontologist. 1989;29 (5):597–605.

79. Kitwood T. Dementia Reconsidered: The Person Comes First. Philadelphia: Open University Press. 1997.

80. Spector A, Orrell M. Using a biopsychosocial model of dementia as a tool to guide clinical practice. International Psychogeriatry. 2010;22 (6):957–65.

81. Joint Commissioning Panel for Mental Health. Guidance for Commissioners of Older People's Mental Health Services. 2013.

82. World Health Organization. World report on ageing and health. World Health Organization. 2015. Report No.: 9241565047.

83. Maki Y, Yamaguchi H. Early detection of dementia in the community under a community-based integrated care system. Geriatrics & Gerontology International. 2014;14:2–10.

84. Michalowsky B, Xie F, Eichler T, Hertel J, Kaczynski A, Kilimann I, et al. Cost-effectiveness of a collaborative dementia care management-Results of a cluster-randomized controlled trial. Alzheimers Dementia. 2019;15(10):1296–1308.

85. Draper B, Low LF, Brodaty H. Integrated care for adults with dementia and other cognitive disorders. International Review of Psychiatry. 2018;30(6):272–91.

86. Tang JY, Wong GH, Ng CK, Kwok DT, Lee MN, Dai DL, et al. Neuropsychological profile and dementia symptom recognition in help-seekers in a community early-detection program in Hong Kong. Journal of American Geriatric Society. 2016;64(3):584–9.

87. Yu R, Chau PH, McGhee SM, Cheung WL, Chan KC, Cheung SH, et al. Trends in prevalence and mortality of dementia

in elderly Hong Kong population: Projections, disease burden, and implications for long-term care. International Journal of Alzheimers Diseases. 2012;2012:406852.

88. Dementia Care Seminar cum Kick-off Ceremony for Dementia Care Campaign [press release]. 2006.

89. Ng CKM, Leung DKY, Cai X, Wong GHY. Perceived help-seeking difficulty, barriers, delay, and burden in carers of people with suspected dementia. International Journal of Environmental Research and Public Health. 2021;18 (6):2956.

90. Xu JQ, Choy JCP, Tang JYM, Liu TY, Luo H, Lou VWQ, et al. Spontaneously reported symptoms by informants are associated with clinical severity in dementia help-seekers. Journal of American Geriatric Society. 2017;65 (9):1946–52.

Typical Alzheimer's Disease

2.1 Cases Illustrative of Pathognomonic Features

Case 001 Post-Brain Injury Memory Decline

Mrs Lee, an 82-year-old lady, presented with concerns raised by her daughter about her memory problems. Her daughter complained that Mrs Lee's memory had worsened (e.g., she would forget whether she had taken her medications, and she would misplace things) and that there is a general slowness in her behaviours observed after a fall earlier this year, when Mrs Lee sustained a subdural haematoma.

Findings from Screening Assessments by Allied Healthcare and Social Care Team

Cognitive functioning	Scored 24/30 on MMSE; after adjusting for education level (less than six months of formal education), results suggested no evidence of impairment. Findings from MoCA (15/30), however, indicated possible dementia, after adjusting for her education level. She was significantly impaired in naming (0/3), abstraction (0/2), and delayed recall (0/5) and had impaired visuospatial/executive performance (1/5). Language (2/3) and orientation (5/6) were slightly impaired. Findings from the Clock Drawing Test (Figure 2.1) suggested impairment in executive function, visuospatial ability, and conceptual thinking. Reversal of numbers was observed in the drawing but not in the copying condition. There was no indication of time in both conditions using the clock hands.
ADL/IADL	Some decline was observed in IADL performance (e.g., financial and medication management).
Staging and clinical rating	Results suggested a Global Deterioration Scale stage 4, indicating mild dementia. During the assessment, deficits in concentration were noted in the serial subtraction task. Her daughter reported a decreased ability to travel and handle finances, although orientation to time and place, as well as the ability to recognise familiar people and faces, were preserved.

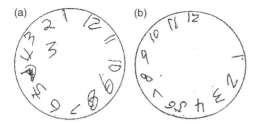

Figure 2.1 Findings from Mrs Lee's Clock Drawing Test. (a) Clock Drawing (3 o'clock). (b) Clock Copying (10 past 10)

History Taken with Carer by Primary Care Physician

Mrs Lee's daughter reported memory problems in her mother that had concerned her for seven months, although no delusional ideations were reported. Using the GPCOG Informant Interview, the following areas were noted to show more difficulties (✗) or were preserved (○) compared to about two years ago:

✗ Remembering recent events
✗ Recalling recent conversations
✗ Word finding
✗ Managing money and finances
✗ Managing medication independently
○ Using transport

There were no additional clinical features to consider for non-Alzheimer's dementia. Other medical history includes diabetes mellitus, hypertension, osteoarthritis of the knee, and gout. The subdural haematoma was drained earlier this year. No family history of dementia or psychiatric disorders was reported.

Diagnosis

Post-brain injury early Alzheimer's disease.

Management

A trial of low-dose cholinesterase inhibitors was recommended, alongside the prescription of an 18-month centre-based programme with cognitively stimulating activities to maintain cognitive functions and quality of life.

Suggestions for the Primary Care Team

This is an illustrative case of the interplay between ageing and cardiovascular risk factors for the development of Alzheimer's disease. Mrs Lee's age (82 years) falls into the age range when Alzheimer's disease is highly prevalent. In her case, the dementia may coincide with a subdural haematoma. Her difficulty in word finding, which is not a typical feature of early Alzheimer's disease, may be related to the subdural haemorrhage. Other features were compatible with early Alzheimer's disease: an IADL being affected was medication management, which is typical of early Alzheimer's disease. Although an MMSE score of 24 is not low, of note is the fact that her performance on the Clock Drawing Test was worse on the version requiring better executive functioning (drawing) than on the copying condition.

In early Alzheimer's disease, cholinesterase inhibitors are not necessarily indicated. Non-pharmacological interventions, such as cognitively stimulating activities and social engagement, can help. In this case, the management of the cardiovascular risk factors should also be optimised.

In terms of non-pharmacological intervention and care, Mrs Lee's strengths included satisfactory attention, the ability to handle immediate instructions, and orientation; areas of weakness needing more attention are limited short-term memory (compatible with forgetfulness in daily performance reported by the carer), executive functions (unable to follow or execute complicated instructions), and impaired abstract thinking (e.g., the concept of time). Based on this profile, it is likely that advance reminders may not work, and immediate verbal coaching with simplified reminders (e.g., step-by-step instructions) would be more helpful in maintaining Mrs Lee's existing ADL/IADL functions.

The primary care team is advised to pay attention to physical discomfort and mood, as Mrs Lee may not be able to express these feelings and sensations clearly, and close observation by carers would be needed. Mrs Lee could still benefit from cognitively stimulating, social, and physical activities to delay deterioration, and therefore these should be encouraged. Given her good orientation and ability to engage in community living activities, these should also be encouraged, although support with supervision and an anti-lost/location-tracking device would be needed to ensure safety.

Case 002   Repeated Buying of Groceries

Mrs Chak, an 81-year-old lady, presented with concerns raised by her daughter over her memory problems.

Findings from Screening Assessments by Allied Healthcare and Social Care Team

Cognitive functioning	Scored 14/30 on MMSE, results indicative of cognitive impairment after adjusting for education level. Mrs Chak's performance was impaired in orientation to time (1/5) and place (2/5), delayed recall (0/3), calculation (1/5), and visuospatial relationships (0/1); she showed slight problems in three-step commands (2/3). Her performance was, however, normal in registration (3/3) and language (5/5). The Clock Drawing Test showed minimal evidence that a clock face is drawn when given a blank circle (an Arabic numeral and a Chinese character '3' were written; Figure 2.2a); when a clock face was provided for copying, she was unable to draw two arms to indicate the time (Figure 2.2b). She was able to write numbers from 1 to 12 and able to read the time on a clock with minimal prompting.
ADL/IADL	Mrs Chak needed minimal help in stair climbing and dressing (she may select inappropriate clothing), although she was independent in other ADLs (Barthel Index 96/100). In terms of IADLs, she was independent in laundry (she could handwash and use the washing machine); she needed assistance in taking medications (her daughter and granddaughter prepared the medications for her); and she needed supervision in meal preparation (she was able to reheat meals), external communication (she was able to pick up calls only), housekeeping, community access (she could have lunch in a nearby restaurant), handling finances (she was given a small amount of money every day for meals and snacks), and grocery shopping (she would repeatedly purchase the same items) (Lawton IADL Scale 39/56).
Staging and clinical rating	Results suggested a Global Deterioration Scale stage 5, indicating moderate dementia. During the interview, Mrs Chak showed disorientation to time and place, was unable to recall the major relevant aspects of her current life (such as the address of her permanent residence) without prompting, and showed difficulty in counting backwards from 40 by 4s or from 20 by 2s.

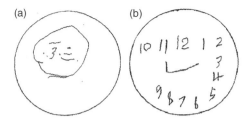

Figure 2.2 Findings from Mrs Chak's Clock Drawing Test. (a) Clock Drawing (3 o'clock). (b) Clock Copying (10 past 10) *A Chinese character 3 can be seen on the clock face, next to the Arabic number 3.

History Taken with Carer by Primary Care Physician

Mrs Chak's daughter reported noticing memory problems in her mother that had concerned her for two years, although no delusional ideations were reported. Using the GPCOG Informant Interview, the following areas were noted to show more difficulties (✗) or were preserved (○) compared to about two years ago:

✗ Remembering recent events
✗ Recalling recent conversations
○ Word finding
✗ Managing money and finances
✗ Managing medication independently
✗ Using transport

There were no additional clinical features to consider for non-Alzheimer's dementia. Mrs Chak had diabetes, bilateral cataract, and a left hip replacement three years ago. No family history of psychiatric disorders or dementia was reported. She was reported to have received more than six months but less than two years of education.

Diagnosis

Early Alzheimer's disease.

Management

Donepezil 5 mg every alternate night was prescribed. Mrs Chak was also recommended to join a centre-based programme with cognitively stimulating activities for 18 months for the maintenance of cognitive function.

Suggestions for the Primary Care Team

At 81 years old, Mrs Chak was at the usual age of symptom presentation for Alzheimer's disease. Although the MMSE score indicated a moderate severity of Alzheimer's disease, the Barthel Index score showed minimal help needed in her ADLs. She had problems managing her medications, which is an early sign of Alzheimer's disease. In the Clock Drawing Test, she could not perform on the executive part, but improved in copying. These suggest early-to-moderate Alzheimer's disease, in which a cholinesterase inhibitor is indicated. On top of pharmacological management, cognitively stimulating activities are always necessary. Fall prevention is also important in view of a history of left hip replacement and early-to-moderate dementia.

In terms of non-pharmacological intervention and care, Mrs Chak's strengths included her satisfactory ADL performance: she was still able to do simple household tasks (e.g., laundry, reheating food, and housekeeping) and had community access (e.g., going to a restaurant and grocery shopping), though her performance was affected by her short-term memory decline and needed supervision. She was also good at verbal expression and social communication, attention and following immediate instructions, and procedural memory in handling familiar daily living tasks. Her areas of weakness needing more attention included orientation and thus the risk of getting lost, poor short-term memory (she was able to encode but impaired in storage and retrieval), and an impaired concept of time.

The primary care team is advised to encourage Mrs Chak to continue engaging in daily living tasks to maintain functioning and quality of life, with simplified steps in the tasks to maintain her motivation by ensuring that the tasks are failure-free. It is likely that advanced reminders in appointments, taking medications, to-do tasks, etc., would not be applicable, and Mrs Chak would benefit more from immediate instructions or reminders: for example, immediate reminders can be inserted inside Mrs Chak's wallet to reduce repeated shopping of the same item; an audio reminder device can be placed at the entrance of the home to remind her about repeatedly going out for shopping. In view of her high risk of getting lost, an anti-lost device would be needed at home, and a location-tracking device would be needed when going out. As Mrs Chak's condition progresses, she may become more disoriented in time, day and night, so a well-structured daily routine and strategies for maintaining a regular circadian cycle would be important. Finally, public education and community engagement, such as educating nearby shopkeepers about dementia, would be helpful.

Case 003 Delayed Recall

Mr Lam, an 82-year-old man, presented with concerns raised by his homecare worker over his memory problems.

Findings from Screening Assessments by Allied Healthcare and Social Care Team

Cognitive functioning	Scored 20/30 on MMSE, suggestive of cognitive impairment after adjusting for education level. Mr Lam's performance was impaired in delayed recall (0/3), visuospatial relationships (0/1), and calculation (1/5). His performance was fair in orientation to time (3/5) and was normal in place orientation (5/5), registration (3/3), language (5/5), and three-step commands (3/3). The Clock Drawing Test showed a recognisable attempt to draw a clock face but with no clear denotation of time, impaired executive function, as well as conceptual and visual-spatial deficits (Figure 2.3).
ADL/IADL	Mr Lam needed moderate help in bathing due to physical impairment, but was independent in other ADLs (Barthel Index 97/100). In terms of IADLs, he was dependent in meal preparation; needed assistance in taking medications, doing laundry, housekeeping, community access, handling finances, and grocery shopping; and needed supervision on external communication (Lawton IADL Scale 24/56).
Staging and clinical rating	Results suggested a Global Deterioration Scale stage 4, indicating mild dementia. He showed decreased knowledge of current and recent events, decreased ability to travel and handle finances, and inability to perform complex tasks.

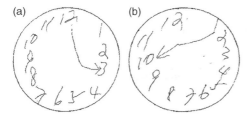

Figure 2.3 Findings from Mr Lam's Clock Drawing Test. (a) Clock Drawing (3 o'clock). (b) Clock Copying (10 past 10)

History Taken with Carer by Primary Care Physician

Mr Lam's homecare worker reported noticing memory problems in this client that had concerned her for two years, although no delusional ideations were reported. Using the GPCOG Informant Interview, the following areas were noted to show more difficulties (✗) or were preserved (○) compared to about two years ago:

✗ Remembering recent events

○ Recalling recent conversations

○ Word finding

✗ Managing money and finances

✗ Managing medication independently

○ Using transport

There were no additional clinical features to consider for non-Alzheimer's dementia. Mr Lam has hypertension. No family history of psychiatric disorders or dementia was reported. His level of education was unclear, except that he has probably received more than two years of education.

Diagnosis

Mild Alzheimer's disease.

Management

Donepezil 5 mg every alternate night was prescribed. Mr Lam was recommended to join a centre-based programme with cognitively stimulating activities for 18 months, to maintain cognitive and self-care functions; he was also encouraged to have regular exercise, a healthy diet and mental stimulation, and to stay socially active.

Suggestions for the Primary Care Team

We can note the usual age of presentation in this case: when Mr Lam was brought to seek medical attention, he was over 80 years old. Very often, the symptoms retrospectively reported by a knowledgeable informant upon direct questioning would date back one to two years before the person is brought to the clinic/service. Impaired short-term memory is the most common presentation of early Alzheimer's disease as it is easily noticed by carers. A typical pattern of this disease stage can be observed in Mr Lam's MMSE findings, with orientation to time more impaired than orientation to place, registration remaining intact, and serial subtractions often impaired (depending on education level); the more sensitive and telltale sign would be impaired delayed recall, which is observed in this case. Communication and speech are usually intact at this stage. The visuospatial ability as indicated by the interlocking pentagon result tends to be impaired, as in this case. While ADLs are largely independent at this stage, IADLs would be impaired. A cholinesterase inhibitor should be prescribed. Both pharmacological and non-pharmacological interventions are effective in early Alzheimer's disease.

Mr Lam's strengths included good ADLs despite his older age; continued engagement in these activities can therefore be used as a form of training or stimulation. Appropriate exercise to enhance physical strength, such as a morning walk in a park, should be encouraged, as better physical tolerance can be useful for keeping up his motivation in participating in daily activities. Another strength of Mr Lam is his generally satisfactory cognitive performance except for short-term memory. Engagement in regular daily cognitively stimulating activities based on his existing interests would help.

Family members may not always be available to provide history. In this case, a homecare helper can also be an important informant. Whenever possible, disclosing the diagnosis with a family member is helpful to ensure understanding and arrange future care through a collaborative process.

Case 004 How Many Children Do I Have?

Mr To, an 88-year-old man, presented with concerns raised by his grandson over his memory problems. He was noted to ask questions repeatedly, forgetting to turn the water off after use, and having problems with orientation and finding his way, and he was able to travel only to familiar places near his home.

Findings from Screening Assessments by Allied Healthcare and Social Care Team

Cognitive functioning	Scored 13/30 on MMSE, results indicative of cognitive impairment after adjusting for education level. He showed impaired performance in orientation to time (1/5) and place (0/5), delayed recall (0/3; unable to recall items even with cues), and calculation (1/5); he had slight problems in the three-step command task (2/3). His performance was, however, normal in registration (3/3), language (5/5), and visuospatial relationships (1/1). The Clock Drawing Test showed a slight impairment in the spacing of lines or numbers.
ADL/IADL	Mr To needed moderate help in dressing as he was unable to select appropriate clothing for the weather; he was independent in other ADLs (Barthel Index 95/100). In terms of IADL, he was dependent in taking medications (managed by his wife), meal preparation, and external communication; he also needed assistance in doing laundry and housekeeping (he was able to hold clothes and sweep the floor); and he needed supervision in community access, handling finances (he may repeatedly pay), and grocery shopping (for simple items) (Lawton IADL Scale 24/56).
Staging and clinical rating	Results showed a Global Deterioration Scale stage 5, suggestive of moderate dementia. He was unable to recall a major relevant aspect of his current life (e.g., address of long-term residence and names of close family members); he cannot recall how many children he has and was occasionally unable to recall the names of his grandson and the son with whom he lives; he showed frequent disorientation in time and place. Mr To also showed difficulties counting back from 40 by 4s or 20 by 2s. He can, however, recall his own name and his spouse's name; he required

no assistance with toileting or eating, but had difficulty choosing proper clothing to wear (and would forget that he had had meals).

History Taken with Carer by Primary Care Physician

Mr To's grandson reported noticing memory problems in his grandfather that had concerned him for three to four years. Delusional ideations and other distressed behaviours and neuropsychiatric symptoms of dementia were reported, including poor temper, the frequent scolding of family members, and waking up in the middle of the night to repeatedly look for items such as keys and money. Using the GPCOG Informant Interview, the following areas were noted to show more difficulties (×) or preserved (○) compared to about two years ago:

× Remembering recent events
× Recalling recent conversations
× Word finding
× Managing money and finances
× Managing medication independently
× Using transport

There were several additional clinical features to consider for non-Alzheimer's dementia, including an inability to control his mood and aggression, as well as overeating, especially sweet food. Mr To has hypertension, hypercholesterolaemia, and gout. No family history of psychiatric disorders or dementia was reported. Mr To's education level was unclear, except that he has probably received more than two years of education.

Investigations

CT brain (plain) was ordered.

Diagnosis

Moderate Alzheimer's disease.

Management

No medication was prescribed at the first consultation due to pending investigation results. Mr To was recommended to join a centre-based programme with cognitively stimulating activities for at least 18 months, for the maintenance of cognitive functions.

Suggestions for the Primary Care Team

Mr To presented at a slightly older age of 88 years. His MMSE findings showed a typical impairment pattern for Alzheimer's disease with impaired delayed recall, and his IADLs were more impaired than his ADL. The primary care team should note that Mr To's performance on the Clock Drawing Test was satisfactory even on the executive part, which is a strength. The reasons for seeking medical attention were also typical of Alzheimer's disease, including repeated questioning, forgetting to turn off the water, and getting lost easily. Taken together, this is a typical case of Alzheimer's disease occurrence in old age. A low-dose cholinesterase inhibitor is indicated in moderate Alzheimer's disease. Physicians may also consider using memantine to manage agitation and irritability. When the ageing process affects the temporal region and spreads to other areas of the brain, older people may develop symptoms mimicking other types of dementia, such as frontotemporal dementia. Nocturnal symptoms are hazardous to the person and their family members. In some cases, low-dose antipsychotics, such as quetiapine, may be used before sleep.

In terms of non-pharmacological intervention and support, considering his impairment in short-term memory and his inability to recall even with cues, reminders may not be a helpful option for Mr To. Adaptive strategies could be used to facilitate adapting to the dysfunctions, instead of relying on reminders or training. Aids such as sensor taps and location-tracking devices can be used; equipping carers with appropriate communication and caring skills would also be useful, to help them respond to Mr To's repeated questioning and other challenging behaviours. At an advanced age, Mr To's ADLs were satisfactory and well maintained (he was independent in most activities); his use of functions should be facilitated, and assistance should be provided only to compensate for the dysfunctions, to maintain his strengths for as long as possible. For example, as he was unable to choose appropriate clothes but able to dress himself, carers could help in preparing suitable clothes only, or in reducing the number of choices of clothes, and allow him to dress himself independently. In terms of safety, carers need to be reminded of the risk of getting lost; supervision in outdoor activities and the installation of an anti-lost sensor at home can be recommended. The fact that Mr To's grandson was involved in bringing him for consultation should lead to further exploration of family support and other potentially available resources that can be mobilised to support Mr To's care in the community.

Case 005 Deficits in Instrumental Activities of Daily Living

Mr Chow, a 94-year-old man, presented with concerns raised by his daughter over his memory problems.

Findings from Screening Assessments by Allied Healthcare and Social Care Team

Cognitive functioning	Scored 15/30 on MMSE, results indicative of cognitive impairment after adjusting for education level. He was impaired in orientation to time (0/5), delayed recall (0/3), calculation (1/5), and three-step commands (1/3); he had slight difficulties in orientation to place (4/5). Mr Chow's performance was, however, normal in registration (3/3), language (5/5), and visuospatial relationships (1/1). The Clock Drawing Test showed minimal evidence that a clock face is drawn, with impaired executive function and conceptual deficits (Figure 2.4).
ADL/IADL	He was independent in all ADLs (Barthel Index 100/100). In terms of IADL, he was dependent in laundry and housekeeping (relying on his carer); needed assistance in taking medications, handling finances, and grocery shopping; and needed supervision in meal preparation, external communication, and community access (Lawton IADL Scale 26/56).
Depressive symptoms	Scored 0/15 on GDS-15, no obvious depressive mood was noted.
Staging and clinical rating	Results showed a Global Deterioration Scale stage 5, suggestive of moderate dementia. He was unable to recall the names of his grandchildren and had difficulty counting backwards from 20 by 2s.

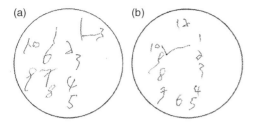

Figure 2.4 Findings from Mr Chow's Clock Drawing Test. (a) Clock Drawing (3 o'clock). (b) Clock Copying (10 past 10)

History Taken with Carer by Primary Care Physician

Mr Chow's daughter reported noticing memory problems in her father that had concerned her for one to two years. Delusional ideations were reported. Using the GPCOG Informant Interview, the following areas were noted to show more difficulties (×) or were preserved (○) compared to about two years ago:

× Remembering recent events
× Recalling recent conversations
× Word finding
× Managing money and finances
× Managing medication independently
× Using transport

There was an additional clinical feature to consider for non-Alzheimer's dementia: he has apraxia in self-care. Mr Chow has hypertension, gout, bronchiectasis, pancytopenia, and benign prostatic hyperplasia. No family history of psychiatric disorders or dementia was reported. He has received more than six months but less than two years of education.

Investigations

Calcium, VDRL, vitamin B_{12}, folate, and ECG were ordered.

Diagnosis

Alzheimer's disease.

Management

Rivastigmine transdermal system 4.6 mg daily was prescribed. Mr Chow was recommended to join a centre-based programme with cognitively stimulating activities for 18 months, for the maintenance of cognitive and self-care functioning; he was also encouraged to have regular exercise, a healthy diet, and mental stimulation, and to stay socially active.

Suggestions for the Primary Care Team

Mr Chow presented with cognitive symptoms at a very old age, at 94 years. He showed typical pattern deficits in cognitive functions and daily activities: his IADLs were much more affected than ADLs, and his performance in the Clock Drawing Test was worse in the executive part compared with the copying part. These patterns are compatible with Alzheimer's disease. It should be noted, however, that presentation in the 90s may indicate a different pathology other than amyloid: studies have shown that for symptoms occurring at an extremely old age, the underlying pathology may be hippocampal sclerosis rather than amyloid-driven disease (1, 2). His mild delusional ideas, mostly surrounding theft, may have arisen from poor memory and may relate to his personality. Taken together, Alzheimer's disease remains the most likely diagnosis, and a trial of a low-dose cholinesterase inhibitor (e.g., donepezil 2.5 mg) can be started, while the team observes for changes in cognition. Antipsychotics are not necessarily indicated if the delusional ideas can be handled by non-pharmacological means, such as distraction and the provision of cues.

In planning for non-pharmacological interventions and support/care, the following areas of strengths and weaknesses should be considered: Mr Chow's ADLs were well maintained in his old age; maintenance of ADLs can be used as a strength as part of his training, enhancing his physical strength through appropriate exercise (e.g., a morning walk in a park/garden), as better physical tolerance can help maintain his motivation in participating in daily activities. Deficits in IADLs are common in old age, and people living with dementia at this age might have been relying on carers (family members or helpers) over a long period of time and become deskilled. In such cases, it can be challenging for the person to return to an independent level of functioning; nevertheless, participation in outside activities with a carer should be encouraged as much as possible, to maintain community functioning. As the disease progresses and short-term memory becomes impaired further, it is foreseeable that Mr Chow's delusional ideation and other distressed behaviours and neuropsychiatric symptoms of dementia would worsen over time. The primary care team can advise his family to keep a regular schedule for Mr Chow, learn to cope psychologically and answer patiently when he asks questions repeatedly, help him to check his own belongings proactively in time or whenever he asks, and help Mr Chow develop a sense of security.

Case 006   Forgotten Home Address

Mrs Cheung, an 83-year-old lady, presented with concerns raised by her daughter over her memory problems. She was noted to have impaired short-term memory and disorientation to time and place.

Findings from Screening Assessments by Allied Healthcare and Social Care Team

Cognitive functioning	Scored 9/30 on MMSE, results suggesting cognitive impairment after adjusting for her education level. Her performance was impaired in orientation to time (0/5) and place (0/5), delayed recall (0/3; unable to recall even with categorical cueing given), visuospatial relationships (0/1), calculation (1/5), and three-step commands (1/3); she had a slight problem in language (4/5). Her performance was, however, normal in registration (3/3). The Clock Drawing Test showed significant impairment (Figure 2.5).
ADL/IADL	Mrs Cheung needed assistance in stair climbing and was dependent in bathing due to limb weakness and visual impairment (unrelated to

	her cognitive impairment); she was independent in other ADLs (Barthel Index 90/100). She needed assistance in external communication and required supervision in taking medication, which was related to her cognitive impairment. She was dependent in other IADLs (Lawton IADL Scale 16/56).
Depressive symptoms	Scored 2/15 on GDS-15, no indication of depression.
Staging and clinical rating	Results suggested a Global Deterioration Scale stage 5, indicating moderate dementia. She was unable to recall the major relevant aspects of her current life, such as her home address of long-term residence, and the names of her grandchildren. She had difficulty counting backwards from 40 by 4s and required assistance in choosing the proper clothing to wear.

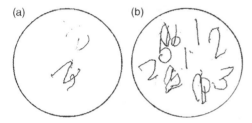

(a) (b)

Figure 2.5 Findings from Mrs Cheung's Clock Drawing Test. (a) Clock Drawing (3 o'clock). (b) Clock Copying (10 past 10)

History Taken with Carer by Primary Care Physician

Mrs Cheung's daughter reported noticing memory problems in her mother that had concerned her for three years. Delusional ideations were reported (she suspected her daughter of stealing her money). Using the GPCOG Informant Interview, the following areas were noted to show more difficulties (×) or were preserved (○) compared to about two years ago:

× Remembering recent events
× Recalling recent conversations
× Word finding
× Managing money and finances
× Managing medication independently
○ Using transport

There were no additional clinical features to consider for non-Alzheimer's dementia. Mrs Cheung has hypertension, diabetes, and a fractured left hip (total hip replacement was done three years ago). No family history of psychiatric disorders or dementia was reported. She has received less than six months of education.

Diagnosis

Moderate Alzheimer's disease.

Management

Donepezil 2.5 mg every alternate night and an 18-month centre-based programme with cognitively stimulating activities were prescribed to help Mrs Cheung maintain her cognitive and self-care functioning. Mrs Cheung was also encouraged to have regular exercise, a healthy diet, and mental stimulation, manage stress, and remain socially active. Non-pharmacological interventions were recommended to manage her distressed behaviours and neuropsychiatric symptoms of dementia.

Suggestions for the Primary Care Team

Mrs Cheung presented at a typical age of symptom presentation (in her 80s). Her performance was impaired in delayed recall and visuospatial relationships (copying an interlocking pentagon on MMSE), an impairment pattern that is compatible with Alzheimer's disease. Her ADLs were less impaired than IADLs, and in the Clock Drawing Test, she showed greater impairment in the executive part than in the copying part. Taken together, her presentation is typical of Alzheimer's disease. Considering that she was dependent in bathing, if not explained by other comorbid conditions (e.g., stroke), a moderate level of severity is suggested. Delusional ideas of theft against her carers (often against a paid informal carer such as a domestic helper, if there is one, or a family member), are common in moderately severe Alzheimer's disease. In this case, a cholinesterase inhibitor can be started (e.g., donepezil 2.5 mg, stepping up if needed), and the team should observe if Mrs Cheung's delusion (of her daughter stealing her money) improves with treatment. As the delusional idea or suspicion of a close family member can be disturbing to the family, if there is no improvement or if the delusional symptoms are severe, a low-dose antipsychotic may be considered.

Typical of cognitive deterioration in the moderate to severe stage of Alzheimer's disease, most of Mrs Cheung's higher-level cognitive functions and short-term memory were impaired, although she can still perform well in communication (language) and attention. The primary care team can therefore equip carers with appropriate caring and communication skills. For example, family members can be advised to avoid confrontation or correcting Mrs Cheung directly when she fails to recall a fact accurately; instead, carers can proactively provide her with the correct information whenever appropriate, such as her family members' names whenever they meet. Engaging her in more social activities, such as family gatherings and reminiscence groups, may also help.

Case 007 Forgotten Children's Names

Mrs Leung, an 88-year-old lady, presented with concerns raised by her daughter and son over her memory problems. She was reported to be unable to recall her children's names.

Findings from Screening Assessments by Allied Healthcare and Social Care Team

Cognitive functioning	Scored 10/30 on MMSE: cognitive impairment was suggested after adjusting for her education level. Her performance was impaired in delayed recall (0/3), calculation (0/5), visuospatial relationships (0/1), orientation to time (1/5) and place (1/5), and three-step commands (1/3); she had a slight problem in language (4/5). Her performance was, however, normal in registration (3/3). She showed significant impairment in the Clock Drawing Test; although her performance improved when a clock face was given for copying, she was unable to complete the test (see Figure 2.6).

Staging and clinical rating	Results suggested a Global Deterioration Scale stage 5, indicative of moderate dementia. Mrs Leung required assistance in most ADL and IADL tasks; she was unable to recall the address and telephone number of her long-term residence; she could not recall the names of her close family members, such as her son or her daughter; she showed disorientation to time and place during the interview; and she was reported to have difficulty choosing proper clothing to wear.

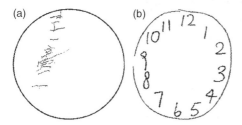

(a) (b)

Figure 2.6 Findings from Mrs Leung's Clock Drawing Test. (a) Clock Drawing (3 o'clock). (b) Clock Copying (10 past 10)

History Taken with Carer by Primary Care Physician

Mrs Leung's daughter and son reported noticing memory problems in their mother that had concerned them for two years, although no delusional ideations were reported. Using the GPCOG Informant Interview, the following areas were noted to show more difficulties (✗) or were preserved (○) compared to about two years ago:

✗ Remembering recent events
✗ Recalling recent conversations
✗ Word finding
✗ Managing money and finances
✗ Managing medication independently
✗ Using transport

Mrs Leung showed apraxia in self-care, which was an additional clinical feature to consider for possible non-Alzheimer's dementia. Mrs Leung has hypertension and diabetes. No family history of psychiatric disorders or dementia was reported. Her education level cannot be ascertained.

Diagnosis

Moderate Alzheimer's disease.

Management

Donepezil 2.5 mg every alternate night and an 18-month centre-based programme with cognitively stimulating activities were prescribed to maintain cognitive functions and quality of life; she was also encouraged to have regular exercise, a healthy diet, and mental stimulation, manage stress, and remain socially active.

Suggestions for the Primary Care Team

In this case of moderate Alzheimer's disease, the typical pattern of cognitive performance on the MMSE and Clock Drawing Test can be observed as discussed in earlier cases (e.g., poor performance on the executive part of the Clock Drawing Test, which improves on the copying part). What can also be noted in this case is the additional effect of age on cognitive performance: Mrs Leung presented in her late 80s; compared with individuals presenting at a younger age, cognitive screening test (e.g., MMSE and MoCA) scores among older individuals are often lower. The primary care team is advised to pay attention to the effects of ageing on cognition, which could play a collateral role in Alzheimer's pathology. In Mrs Leung's case, a moderate stage of Alzheimer's disease is likely, and the team can observe her response to donepezil 2.5 mg; if indicated, titrating up to 5 mg can be considered. Memantine may also be added on top of donepezil in moderate Alzheimer's disease.

Typical of cognitive deterioration in the moderate to severe stage of Alzheimer's disease, most of Mrs Leung's higher-level cognitive functions and short-term memory were impaired, although she can still perform well in communication (language) and attention. The primary care team can therefore equip carers with appropriate caring and communication skills, such as the avoidance of direct confrontation and correction if Mrs Leung fails to recall a fact, and providing information proactively. As Mrs Leung's inability to recall the names of her children can be emotionally distressing for her daughter and son, psychoeducation and counselling for the family (e.g., that feelings may be preserved even when episodic memory is impaired) may be helpful in facilitating psychological adjustment. Subtle reality orientation, such as providing Mrs Leung with the correct information in casual conversations whenever they meet (e.g., mentioning family members' names), could also help maintain her memories. Engaging Mrs Leung in family gatherings, reminiscence groups, or life review activities may also be useful.

Case 008 Repeated Questioning

Mr Chow, an 84-year-old man, presented with concerns raised by her daughter over his memory problems. He was reported to ask questions repeatedly and being forgetful of recent events. His daughter reported that Mr Chow has already received a diagnosis of Alzheimer's disease by a neurologist in his home town, although she cannot provide further details such as the name of the medication that Mr Chow was prescribed.

Findings from Screening Assessments by Allied Healthcare and Social Care Team

Cognitive functioning	Scored 22/30 on MMSE: adjusting for education level, results indicate cognitive impairment. Mr Chow's performance was impaired in delayed recall (0/3; unable to recall even with cues); his performance was affected in orientation to time (3/5) and place (3/5) and three-step commands (2/3). His performance was, however, normal in registration (3/3), calculation (5/5), language (5/5), and visuospatial relationships (1/1). Errors were observed in time denotation in the Clock Drawing Test: the clock arms were not provided in the executive (drawing) part of the test, although his performance was intact in the copying part (Figure 2.7).
ADL/IADL	He was independent in all ADLs (Barthel Index 100/100). He required assistance in community access and handling finances and needed supervision in taking medication and grocery shopping; he was, however, independent in other IADLs (Lawton IADL Scale 44/56).
Depressive symptoms	Scored 2/15 on GDS-15, no indication of depression.

Staging and clinical rating: Results suggested a Global Deterioration Scale stage 4, indicating mild dementia. He showed decreased knowledge of current and recent events; decreased ability to travel and handle finances; and an inability to perform complex tasks. He was, however, able to select the proper clothing to wear.

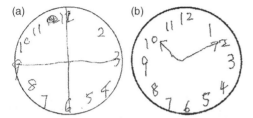

Figure 2.7 Findings from Mr Chow's Clock Drawing Test. (a) Clock Drawing (3 o'clock). (b) Clock Copying (10 past 10)

History Taken with Carer by Primary Care Physician

Mr Chow's daughter reported noticing memory problems in her father that had concerned her for over two years, although no delusional ideations were reported. Using the GPCOG Informant Interview, the following areas were noted to show more difficulties (×) or were preserved (○) compared to about two years ago:

× Remembering recent events
× Recalling recent conversations
× Word finding
× Managing money and finances
× Managing medication independently
○ Using transport

There were no additional clinical features to consider for non-Alzheimer's dementia. Mr Chow has hypercholesterolaemia. No family history of psychiatric disorders or dementia was reported. His exact education level cannot be ascertained, although according to his daughter Mr Chow has probably received more than two years of education.

Diagnosis

Early Alzheimer's disease.

Management

No medication was prescribed at this stage, as Mr Chow's carer claimed he was already on dementia medications and further information was pending. Mr Chow was recommended to join a centre-based programme with cognitively stimulating activities for 18 months to maintain his cognitive performance and self-care functions; he was also encouraged to have regular exercise, a healthy diet, and mental stimulation, and maintain an active social life.

Suggestions for the Primary Care Team

Repeated questioning is a common manifestation of impaired short-term memory. This case also illustrates a typical presentation of early Alzheimer's disease at a common age of symptom presentation in the early 80s: Mr Chow showed impairments in delayed recall, but was intact in registration, language, and calculation. It is typical for a person with early Alzheimer's disease to show more obvious impairments on the Lawton IADL scale, while results on the Barthel Index (ADL) would often appear more intact. What is noticeable in this case is that Mr Chow's visuospatial relationships (interlocking pentagon) performance was intact, while the Clock Drawing Test was positive. This illustrates the understanding that the Clock Drawing Test can be a more sensitive test for early Alzheimer's disease than the interlocking pentagon. As Mr Chow is likely taking anti-dementia medication already, physicians can observe and monitor his cognitive performance and step up the medications in the event of cognitive decline in the future.

In this case of the early stage of typical Alzheimer's disease, another illustrative point is that Mr Chow has more areas of strengths than weaknesses that the primary care team can leverage in his care plan. A key intervention target is to maintain his areas of strength, namely good daily functional performance in ADL and IADL, intact orientation, good attention, and other higher cognitive functions (e.g., calculation, as well as financial management, judgement, and problem-solving required for various IADL tasks). Mr Chow may still be able to develop new habits that can enhance his functioning and safety, such as keeping with him and using a mobile phone, a location-tracking device, and/or a smart watch. While he should still be able to function in terms of organising and executing daily living activities, carers should nevertheless be reminded about his emerging needs due to poor short-term memory: Mr Chow was able to encode, but unable to store and retrieve information. Timely reminders and other strategies to maintain his motivation to participate in daily activities would be the priority for intervention and support during this stage.

Case 009 Where Is My Wife?

Mr Tam, an 82-year-old man, presented with concerns raised by his son over his memory problems. He was noted to be misplacing items and asking about the whereabouts of his wife, with no recollection of the fact that she has been admitted to hospital.

Findings from Screening Assessments by Allied Healthcare and Social Care Team

Cognitive functioning	Scored 18/30 on MMSE: results were indicative of cognitive impairment, considering his education level. His performance was impaired in visuospatial relationships (0/1), orientation to time (1/5), and delayed recall (1/3; able to recall two items with categorical cues); his performance was slightly impaired in orientation to place (3/5), calculation (3/5), and three-step commands (2/3). His performance was, however, normal in registration (3/3) and language (5/5). The Clock Drawing Test showed abnormal clock face drawing, with reversal of numbers and inaccurate time denotation, which improved when a clock face was provided for copying (Figure 2.8).
ADL/IADL	He was independent in ADLs (Barthel Index 100/100). He required assistance in taking medication (his wife would prepare the medications for him, as he would sometimes forget to take medication), meal preparation (he was able to boil water only; he usually had meals in a community centre), handling finances, and grocery shopping; he also needed supervision in community access (he was able to go to the community centre and nearby area) (Lawton IADL Scale 31/56).

Staging and clinical rating	Results suggested a Global Deterioration Scale stage 4, indicating mild dementia. He showed clear deficits in cognition during the clinical interview, including difficulty in concentration elicited on the serial subtraction task. He was reported to have a decreased ability to travel and handle finances.

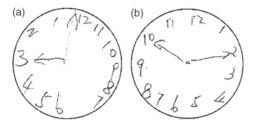

Figure 2.8 Findings from Mr Tam's Clock Drawing Test. (a) Clock Drawing (3 o'clock). (b) Clock Copying (10 past 10)

History Taken with Carer by Primary Care Physician

Mr Tam's son reported noticing memory problems in his father that had concerned him for four to five years, although no delusional ideations were reported. Using the GPCOG Informant Interview, the following areas were noted to show more difficulties (✗) or were preserved (○) compared to about two years ago:

✗ Remembering recent events
✗ Recalling recent conversations
○ Word finding
✗ Managing money and finances
✗ Managing medication independently
✗ Using transport

There were no additional clinical features to consider for non-Alzheimer's dementia. Comorbidity of hypertension was reported. No family history of psychiatric disorders or dementia was reported. His exact education level cannot be ascertained, although his son reported that he has probably received more than two years of education.

Investigations

VDRL, vitamin B_{12}, folate, CXR, TSH, and T4 tests were ordered.

Diagnosis

Early Alzheimer's disease.

Management

Rivastigmine transdermal system 5 mg daily and an 18-month programme of centre-based cognitively stimulating activities for maintaining cognitive ability and quality of life were prescribed.

Suggestions for the Primary Care Team

This is a typical case of early Alzheimer's disease. While Mr Tam presented at a typical age (early 80s) to the primary care team, in retrospect the age of onset could have been around his late 70s (informant noted four to five years of symptom history), with further deterioration in the past few years leading to medical attention. It is therefore likely that a mild cognitive impairment stage has preceded the onset of clinical Alzheimer's disease. In similar cases, if presented earlier during the mild cognitive impairment stage, non-pharmacological interventions such as mentally stimulating activities can be prescribed even if medication is usually not indicated. Non-pharmacological interventions could be helpful in delaying the onset of clinical Alzheimer's disease. In Mr Tam's case, the dose of transdermal rivastigmine can be escalated in the event of worsening cognitive function.

Repeatedly searching for loved ones who are not around is a common phenomenon in people with early to moderate dementia. The main cause of such behaviours is a deterioration in short-term memory, which makes remembering recent events and changes challenging. This phenomenon highlights the need to maintain consistency and regularity in the person's daily habits and living environment, which includes the social environment and the people around them. In Mr Tam's case, a strategy to help him overcome his repeated searching is to allow regular visits to his wife if possible. When Mr Tam asks, providing him with the fact that his wife is in hospital should be done with care to avoid triggering negative emotions such as depressive mood and anxiety: his search for his wife could reflect his anxiety at not having her around, and he could be missing his wife. Depending on the emotional needs, which should be understood on a case-by-case and person-centred basis, strategies to address the under-lying needs (e.g., engaging him in a discussion about his marriage or viewing a family photo) may be a validating response that helps more than factual correction. In the event that a negative mood is triggered and the person is in distress, sometimes carers and family members may find distraction and engaging the person in other enjoyable activities helpful. Regular, personally meaningful, and enjoyable daily activities can be used as a preventive strategy to reduce the repeated search of loved ones.

Case 010 Post-CVA Cognitive Decline

Mrs Pong, a 78-year-old lady, presented with concerns raised by her daughter over her memory problems. She was noted to have declining cognition after a cerebrovascular accident four years ago, with a more significant decline this year, including time orienta-tion, short-term memory (e.g., repeated questioning and looking for daily items), and wayfinding.

Findings from Screening Assessments by Allied Healthcare and Social Care Team

Cognitive functioning	Scored 20/30 on MMSE: results suggested cognitive impairment after adjusting for her education level. Her performance was impaired in recalling (0/3), visuospatial relationships (0/1), and calculation (1/5); Mrs Pong's performance was also slightly impaired in orientation to time (3/5). Her performance was, however, normal in orientation to place (5/5), registration (3/3), language (5/5), and three-step commands (3/3). The Clock Drawing Test showed abnormal clock face drawing with inaccurate denotation (Figure 2.9).
ADL/IADL	She was independent in ADLs (Barthel Index 100/100). She needed assistance in housekeeping, community access (she was anxious

	about going out by herself), handling finances, and grocery shopping; she also required supervision on taking medications (her medications were prepared by a helper) and meal preparation (she was able to reheat or make a very simple breakfast); she was modified independent in laundry (Lawton IADL Scale: 35/56).
Depressive symptoms	Scored 5/15 on GDS-15, no indication of depression.
Staging and clinical rating	Results suggested a Global Deterioration Scale stage 4, indicating mild dementia. She showed some deficits in remembering her personal history; a decreased ability to travel and handle finances; and a concentration deficit elicited on the serial subtraction task.

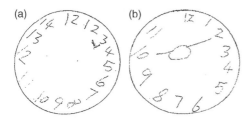

Figure 2.9 Findings from Mrs Pong's Clock Drawing Test. (a) Clock Drawing (3 o'clock). (b) Clock Copying (10 past 10)

History Taken with Carer by Primary Care Physician

Mrs Pong's daughter reported noticing memory problems in her mother that had concerned her for three years, although no delusional ideations were reported. Using the GPCOG Informant Interview, the following areas were noted to show more difficulties (×) or were preserved (○) compared to about two years ago:

× Remembering recent events
× Recalling recent conversations
○ Word finding
○ Managing money and finances
× Managing medication independently
× Using transport

There were no additional clinical features to consider for non-Alzheimer's dementia. Mrs Pong has hypertension, diabetes, hypercholesterolaemia, cerebrovascular accident (four years ago), arrhythmia, and bilateral cataract (operated on). No family history of psychiatric disorders or dementia was reported. Her exact education level cannot be ascertained, although her daughter reported that she has received more than six months but less than two years of education.

Investigations

CBP, ESR, R/LFT, calcium, vitamin B_{12}, folate, fasting sugar, fasting lipids, and TSH were ordered. Apart from ESR 26 (high), other investigations were normal. CT brain (plain) and MRI revealed a mixed picture of dementia: there were generalised cerebral age-related atrophy and microangiopathic changes over the subcortical white matter of bilateral frontal, parietal, and occipital regions.

Diagnosis

Early Alzheimer's disease.

Management

Rivastigmine transdermal system 5 mg and 10 mg alternate daily were prescribed. Mrs Pong was also recommended to join a centre-based programme with cognitively stimulating activities for 18 months for the maintenance of cognitive abilities.

Suggestions for the Primary Care Team

Compared with other cases in this cohort, Mrs Pong presented at a slightly younger age. Her history of a cerebrovascular accident four years before the current presentation may have advanced the onset of the clinical manifestation of dementia symptoms. The impairment pattern of cognition and ADL/IADL is compatible with typical Alzheimer's disease (e.g., impairment shown on the executive part of the Clock Drawing Test, which improved on the copying part). Of note in this case is the possible relationship between the cerebrovascular accident history and Alzheimer's disease: while the presence of stroke does not immediately lead to a diagnosis of vascular dementia, in some cases the possibility of vascular involvement may not be completely excluded. In the case of Mrs Pong, the duration between her cerebrovascular accident and the current significant decline suggests that Alzheimer's disease is more likely than vascular dementia. The CT brain scan showed bilateral microangiopathic changes: white matter disease is a risk factor for Alzheimer's disease (3). Treatment with a cholinesterase inhibitor is therefore indicated in Mrs Pong's case, while physicians may consider adding memantine on top of the rivastigmine transdermal patch.

As a person in her early stage of Alzheimer's disease, Mrs Pong was independent in her ADLs, although her IADLs showed a higher-than-expected level of dependency. While at this stage a person's short-term memory and complex cognitive processing would be affected, often procedural memory would remain intact. It should be noted that a person's IADL dependency level can be affected by mood states (e.g., anxiety and depression) and a low level of self-confidence or motivation. Carers and family members could try to encourage Mrs Pong to participate more in daily activities based on her interests and premorbid role. Social skills and communication appeared to be her current strengths, and social activities such as family gatherings and reminiscence may work by tapping into her strengths.

Case 011   Why Aren't My Grandchildren Visiting?

Mrs Ng, a 90-year-old lady, presented with concerns raised by her daughter over her memory problems. She was noted to have a decline in orientation, asking the same question repeatedly, misplacing valuable items, and forgetting recent events such as being visited by her grandchildren.

Findings from Screening Assessments by Allied Healthcare and Social Care Team

Cognitive functioning	Scored 11/30 on MMSE: results indicated cognitive impairment, adjusted for her education level. Her performance was impaired in delayed recall (0/3), calculation (0/5), visuospatial relationships (0/1), and orientation to time (1/5) and place (2/5), and she was also slightly impaired in registration (2/3), language (4/5), and three-step commands (2/3). In the

	Clock Drawing Test, she showed no reasonable or understandable attempt at drawing a clock face; she was able to write numbers from one to nine, but reported that she could not remember what a clock face looks like; results suggested executive function and conceptual deficits.
ADL/IADL	Mrs Ng needed minimal help in ambulation and stair climbing; she was independent in all other ADLs (Barthel Index 95/100). She required assistance in taking medications (needed to be reminded by calls); she also needed supervision in meal preparation (she was able to boil water and reheat meals and would usually use meal delivery), external communication, community access (she would go to nearby places only), handling finances, and grocery shopping (buying simple items only) and was modified independent in housekeeping (Lawton IADL Scale 41/56).
Staging and clinical rating	Results suggested a Global Deterioration Scale stage 4, indicating mild dementia. She showed some deficits in remembering her personal history; decreased knowledge of current and recent events; a concentration deficit elicited on the serial subtraction task; and a decreased ability to travel and handle finances.

History Taken with Carer by Primary Care Physician

Mrs Ng's daughter reported noticing memory problems in her mother that had concerned her for one to two years, although no delusional ideations were reported. Using the GPCOG Informant Interview, the following areas were noted to show more difficulties (✗) or were preserved (○) compared to about two years ago:

✗ Remembering recent events
✗ Recalling recent conversations
○ Word finding
✗ Managing money and finances
✗ Managing medication independently
✗ Using transport

There were no additional clinical features to consider for non-Alzheimer's dementia. Mrs Ng has hypertension and a benign gastrointestinal tumour. No family history of psychiatric disorders or dementia was reported. She has received less than six months of education. Mrs Ng currently lives alone, with her daughter staying with her on weekends.

Diagnosis

Mild dementia.

Management

Donepezil 5 mg every night and an 18-month centre-based programme of cognitively stimulating activities for maintaining cognitive ability were prescribed.

Suggestions for the Primary Care Team

Presenting at an old age, Mrs Ng's low MMSE score on presentation was within expectation. Mrs Ng showed the typical pattern of cognitive impairment and functional decline in Alzheimer's disease: greater impairment in orientation to time than to place; in

IADL than ADL; in the executive part than the copying part of the clock drawing; and impairments in delayed recall and visuospatial relationships (interlocking pentagon), with a history of one to two years in retrospect. Her clinical profile was compatible with early Alzheimer's disease. A trial of a cholinesterase inhibitor is indicated: a lower dose of donepezil (e.g., 2.5 mg) may be suitable for Mrs Ng considering the age factor, when physicians can monitor her clinical response to donepezil and escalate the dose in the event of further cognitive decline. A transdermal patch is preferred to oral formulation when patients develop side effects, such as reduced oral intake and gastrointestinal upset.

This is a good example to illustrate how ADL and even IADL functional levels may be maintained despite significant impairments in cognitive function. Particularly in people living with dementia who are active with a high level of premorbid independence in daily activities, a slower deterioration in functioning than in cognitive test performance can be seen. It highlights the importance of engaging people living with dementia in daily activities as much as possible to slow down functional deterioration. In Mrs Ng's case, most of her cognitive functions, especially short-term memory, were clearly impaired. With satisfactory attention and communication, however, most of the tasks requiring procedural memory in ADL and IADL remained intact. To encourage her continued participation in daily activities, the primary care team should equip her carers with the knowledge and psychological preparedness for deterioration, when Mrs Ng becomes 'clumsier' in self-care: instead of giving up the tasks, carers can start to facilitate by assisting or simplifying the tasks and by learning appropriate communication skills (e.g., giving Mrs Ng the information needed whenever she asks, avoiding direct confrontation for her 'mistakes').

Case 012 Which Room Is Which?

Ms Chan, a 74-year-old lady, presented with concerns raised by her daughter over her memory problem. She would sometimes forget about the conversations she had with others, mixing up events that happened in the past and needing to search for personal belongings frequently. She was aware of her own memory decline, which reportedly started about two years ago when she entered the wrong room at home and forgot what she was going to do in the room.

Findings from Screening Assessments by Allied Healthcare and Social Care Team

Cognitive functioning	Scored 23/30 on MMSE: results showed no indication of cognitive impairment, adjusted for education level. Ms Chan's performance was impaired in visuospatial relationships (0/1), and she had slight impairment in orientation to place (3/5), delayed recall (2/3), and calculation (2/5). Her performance was, however, good in orientation to time (5/5), registration (3/3), three-step commands (3/3), and language (5/5). The Clock Drawing Test showed obvious errors in time denotation, which improved in the clock copying part (Figure 2.10).
ADL/IADL	She was semi-independent in ADLs. Lower limb weakness affected her performance (Barthel Index 86/100). She was semi-independent in IADLs (Lawton IADL Scale 52/56). Ms Chan needed assistance in handling medications; she would sometimes forget to switch on the fire during cooking. She was

	able to shop, but would sometimes forget items or would buy the same items repeatedly.
Depressive symptoms	Scored 7/15 on GDS-15, suggestive of clinically significant depressive mood. She had limited social activities and made complaints about her health.
Staging and clinical rating	Scored 0.5/3 on Clinical Dementia Rating, indicating suspected dementia. She showed fair performance in memory, orientation, judgement and problem-solving, community affairs, and home and hobbies. She appeared normal in personal care.

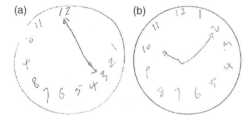

Figure 2.10 Findings from Ms Chan's Clock Drawing Test. (a) Clock Drawing (3 o'clock). (b) Clock Copying (10 past 10)

History Taken with Carer by Primary Care Physician

Ms Chan's daughter reported noticing memory problems in her mother that had concerned her for two years, although no delusional ideations were reported. Using the GPCOG Informant Interview, the following areas were noted to show more difficulties (✗) or were preserved (○) compared to about two years ago:

✗ Remembering recent events
✗ Recalling recent conversations
○ Word finding
○ Managing money and finances
○ Managing medication independently
○ Using transport

There were no additional clinical features to consider for non-Alzheimer's dementia. Ms Chan has hypertension, atrial fibrillation, dyslipidaemia, multinodular goitre, osteoporosis, and left hip fracture with a total hip replacement 12 years ago. She is currently on warfarin 2 mg daily, famotidine 20 mg daily, simvastatin 10 mg at night, alendronate sodium 70 mg once weekly, and cetirizine 10 mg daily. No family history of psychiatric disorders or dementia was reported. She has received primary education of P.2 (approximately two years of education).

Physical Examination Findings

General examination revealed no affect or hygiene problem. Atrial fibrillation was noted during CVS examination. There were no significant CNS findings.

Investigations

CBP, R/LFT, calcium, vitamin B_{12}, fasting sugar, fasting lipids, and TSH were ordered. CBP, vitamin B_{12}, and TSH were normal, whereas VDRL was negative. MRI revealed no evidence of disease.

Diagnosis

Mild cognitive impairment or early Alzheimer's disease.

Management

No medication was prescribed, as Ms Chan and her carer prefer not to start treatment at this stage. Ms Chan was recommended to join a specialised day care service for two days per week for two years, with a structured and tailored intervention programme and cognitively stimulating activities to delay deterioration.

Suggestions for the Primary Care Team

Ms Chan presented at a relatively younger age, and her higher MMSE score was within expectations. While her performance on the cognitive screening test showed a typical pattern of Alzheimer's disease, her ADL as shown in the Barthel Index was more impaired than expected, which was attributable to lower limb weakness. Her lower limb weakness needs to be medically assessed, as Alzheimer's disease in the early stages should not affect a person's mobility. It should also be noted that her GDS-15 assessment suggested depressive symptoms, which could have affected her cognitive and physical functioning. Ms Chan may have adjustment problems due to her cognitive impairment, which is common, especially in people with anxiety-prone personality traits, those who are younger, and individuals with insight into their cognitive problems. In this case, early Alzheimer's disease with adjustment disorder or depression should be suspected. Comorbid Alzheimer's disease and depression may also indicate a common neurologically based phenomenon. Considering Ms Chan's younger-than-usual age of presentation, lower limb weakness, and her strong vascular risk with atrial fibrillation, more advanced neuroimaging such as MRI is indicated to rule out significant vascular comorbidity. Close monitoring for further deterioration is needed.

Considering Ms Chan's preserved language and communication ability, a social worker in the primary care team can further assess any psychosocial factors contributing to her depressive mood. As anxiety and depressive moods in people with early stages of dementia with insight are quite common, if this is the case for Ms Chan, psychoeducation about dementia and strategies to facilitate support and adjustment may be helpful. In the event of more complicated or severe mood problems, counselling and psychotherapy can be considered, especially in view of her relatively intact cognitive functioning.

Her general functioning is satisfactory at this stage, with ADL and IADL largely independent, except for slight impairments that may be more related to physical than cognitive problems. The primary care team can equip Ms Chan with adaptive memory strategies, structured with cognitively stimulating activities to fit into her daily schedule as leisure activities, and a regular daily schedule to facilitate awareness of completed and unfinished tasks.

Case 013 Needing Help to Find Home

Mr Choy, a 79-year-old gentleman, presented with concerns raised by his son over his memory problems experienced for three years. His son complained about his repeated questioning, that Mr Choy would mix up day and night, and that he would be unable to find his way home sometimes, when he had to call his family members for assistance. He also noted that Mr Choy's hands would shake occasionally. Mr Choy had been aware of his own memory decline for about two years.

Findings from Screening Assessments by Allied Healthcare and Social Care Team

Cognitive functioning	Scored 21/30 on MMSE: results indicate cognitive impairment after adjusting for his education level. His performance was impaired in orientation to place (2/5) and delayed recall (0/3); he had slight problems in orientation to time (4/5), three-step commands (2/3), and calculation (4/5). His performance was, however, normal in registration (3/3), language (5/5), and visuospatial relationships (1/1). His Clock Drawing Test results were normal.
ADL/IADL	Mr Choy was independent in most ADLs. He needed to use an umbrella for going out due to lower limb weakness. He had occasional accidents with bladder control and needed to use an incontinence pad at night and when going out (Barthel Index 92/100). He has modified independence in IADLs. He was dependent in meal preparation. He would sometimes miss phone calls due to his hearing problem. He was not able to find his way home sometimes and needed to call family members for assistance. He would repeatedly buy the same style of clothing (Lawton IADL Scale 46/56).
Depressive symptoms	Scored 2/15 on GDS-15, no obvious depressive mood was noted.
Staging and clinical rating	Scored 1/3 on Clinical Dementia Rating, indicating possible mild dementia. He showed mild impairment in orientation to community affairs and personal care, but was fair in memory, judgement and problem-solving, and in home and hobbies.

History Taken with Carer by Primary Care Physician

Mr Choy's son reported noticing memory problems in his father that had concerned him for about three years, although no delusional ideations were reported. Using the GPCOG Informant Interview, the following areas were noted to show more difficulties (×) or were preserved (○) compared to about two years ago:

× Remembering recent events
× Recalling recent conversations
○ Word finding
× Managing money and finances
? Managing medication independently (carer was unaware of Mr Choy's ability)
× Using transport

There were no additional clinical features to consider for non-Alzheimer's dementia. No family history of psychiatric disorders or dementia was reported. He received secondary education up to Form 3 (approximately nine years of education). Mr Choy walks with an umbrella. He was living with his wife.

Physical Examination Findings

General examination revealed no affect or hygiene problem. Mr Choy had a blood pressure of 147/69 mm Hg. No other CVS or CNS findings were noted.

Investigations

TFT, vitamin B_{12}, CBP, R/LFT, and fasting lipids were ordered. MRI result showed small vessel disease.

Diagnosis

Early Alzheimer's disease.

Management

Rivastigmine transdermal system 4.6 mg daily was prescribed. Mr Choy was also recommended to join a specialised day care service for two days per week for two years, with structured and tailored intervention programme and cognitively stimulating activities to delay deterioration.

Suggestions for the Primary Care Team

Mr Choy presented at the age of 79 years, which was slightly younger than others in the cohort, although his MMSE results showed a typical pattern for Alzheimer's disease. Considering the normal results from the Clock Drawing Test and his intact ability in the visuospatial relationships (interlocking pentagon in MMSE), this is likely a case of early Alzheimer's disease. His impairment in orientation to place in the test needs to be interpreted with caution, as his performance may be affected if the test took place in an unfamiliar location for Mr Choy. On the other hand, the earlier presentation of symptoms may also suggest a more aggressive amyloid load. As Mr Choy is self-aware with insight into his own cognitive or memory problem, it may indicate good premorbid cognitive functioning, with the disease in an early phase. Physicians should watch out for mood problems, as adjustment disorder is common in these patients.

Although Mr Choy showed intact orientation in time on MMSE, the primary care team should also pay attention to the carer's complaint of his mixing up of day and night. The team should observe if there is any tendency for dysregulation in the circadian cycle. Mr Choy has a history of (and thus high risk for) getting lost, which should be carefully attended to. A strength that the primary care team can leverage is his ability to use the phone. As it is foreseeable that his risk of getting lost will increase as the disease progresses, he may no longer be able to describe his location to family members if he gets lost again in the future. Installing a location-tracking app on his mobile phone or using a smart watch or device with a GPS function should be encouraged.

Case 014 Reminders for Shower

Mr Chan, an 82-year-old gentleman, presented with concerns raised by his wife over his memory problems and involuntary muscle movements. Mr Chan would sometimes have hand tremors, and he would be seen opening and closing his mouth for no reason. His wife had noticed his memory decline for a year, when he became unable to use transportation by himself and would forget about his convervstions with others and appointments, and frequently forget to take personal belongings with him when going out.

Findings from Screening Assessments by Allied Healthcare and Social Care Team

| Cognitive functioning | Scored 19/30 on MMSE: results suggested cognitive impairment, adjusting for education level. His performance was impaired in orientation to time (0/5), delayed recall (0/3), and visuospatial relationships (0/1); he showed slight impairment in orientation to place (4/5) and three-step commands (2/3). His performance was, however, normal in calculation (5/5), registration (3/3), and language |

	(5/5). The Clock Drawing Test showed impaired executive function. He drew 10 lines with arrows of different directions. In the copying part of the test, his improved performance showed that he was able to read the clock (Figure 2.11).
ADL/IADL	He was modified independent in ADLs (Barthel Index 84/100). He needed help in selecting clothing; reminders for taking showers; and a companion when going out and using the stairs due to lower limb weakness. He was dependent in meal preparation, laundry, and housekeeping. Mr Chan was unable to use a phone; he needed supervision in taking medications; and he needed assistance for community access, handling finances, and grocery shopping (Lawton IADL Scale 22/56, assisted in IADLs).
Depressive symptoms	Scored 2/15 on GDS-15, no obvious depressive mood was noted.
Staging and clinical rating	Scored 1/3 on Clinical Dementia Rating, indicating possible mild dementia. He showed mild impairment in memory, orientation, judgement and problem-solving, community affairs, and home and hobbies.

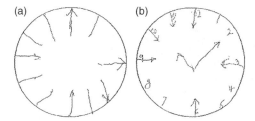

Figure 2.11 Findings from Mr Chan's Clock Drawing Test. (a) Clock Drawing (3 o'clock). (b) Clock Copying (10 past 10)

History Taken with Carer by Primary Care Physician

Mr Chan's wife reported noticing memory problems in her husband that had concerned her for about two years, although no delusional ideations were reported. Using the GPCOG Informant Interview, the following areas were noted to show more difficulties (×) or were preserved (○) compared to about two years ago:

× Remembering recent events
× Recalling recent conversations
○ Word finding
× Managing money and finances
× Managing medication independently
× Using transport

There were no additional clinical features to consider for non-Alzheimer's dementia. Mr Chan was on pantoprazole 40 mg daily, folic acid 5 mg once per week, methotrexate 7.5 mg once a week, and Calcichew 1000 mg daily. No family history of psychiatric disorders or dementia was reported. He received primary education to P.5 (approximately five years of education).

Physical Examination Findings

General examination revealed no affect or hygiene problem. Mr Chan had a normal blood pressure of 123/64 mm Hg. No other significant CVS or CNS findings.

Investigations

A CT brain scan was ordered.

Diagnosis

Early dementia, possible Alzheimer's disease.

Management

Rivastigmine transdermal system 4.6 mg daily was prescribed. He was also recommended to join a specialised day care service for two days per week, with a structured and tailored intervention programme and cognitively stimulating activities to delay deterioration.

Suggestions for the Primary Care Team

Mr Chan's symptomatology is suggestive of early Alzheimer's disease. Physicians should also look for features of parkinsonism, such as resting tremors, cogwheel rigidity, bradykinesia, and gaze palsy. During history-taking, physicians should try to delineate the timing of the onset of cognitive impairment and shaking mouth; the presence of any visual hallucinations should be elicited. Both Alzheimer's disease and Parkinson's disease are neurodegenerative conditions. The differential diagnoses in this case are Alzheimer's disease with parkinsonism and atypical parkinsonism (e.g., dementia with Lewy's body). Presenting at the age of 82 years, Mr Chan was at a typical age of dementia onset. Although his cognitive impairment was greater than expected, his impairment pattern on MMSE, Barthel Index and Lawton IADL, and the Clock Drawing Test was typical of early Alzheimer's disease.

Mr Chan's engagement in community living activities and IADL tasks may diminish over time due to his parkinsonism. At the current stage, his ADLs remained satisfactory, and that should be the focus of intervention: support should be provided to keep up his motivation and initiation in these tasks. Despite his disorientation in time, he was able to orient in place: this is a strength that the primary care team can focus on maintaining. Care should be taken to minimise the risk of Mr Chan giving up on activities outside the home due to his physical condition. Meanwhile, it would be appropriate to start preparing the family carers in advance psychologically for deterioration, and in terms of caring skills needed for a moderate stage of dementia.

Case 015   How to Use the Door Lock?

Mr Chan, an 85-year-old gentleman, presented with concerns raised by his son about his memory problems. His son complained of Mr Chan's memory decline, which he had noticed for about three years. Mr Chan was reported to be frequently forgetful about the conversations he had with others, always needing to look for his personal belongings, and forgetting about how to use the door lock of his home.

Findings from Screening Assessments by Allied Healthcare and Social Care Team

Cognitive functioning	Scored 16/30 on MMSE: results suggested cognitive impairment, adjusted for education level. His performance was impaired in

	orientation to time (0/5) and place (1/5), delayed recall (0/3), and visuospatial relationships (0/1); he had slight impairment in calculation (4/5); his performance was, however, normal in three-step commands (3/3), registration (3/3), and language (5/5). The Clock Drawing Test results showed impaired placement of numbers, with numbers missing. Poor executive function was observed, with little improvement in the copying part (Figure 2.12).
ADL/IADL	Mr Chan was modified independent in ADLs (Barthel Index 93/100). He would wear the same clothing for a few days and needed reminders to change his clothes. He would sometimes take a shower repeatedly because of forgetfulness. He was dependent in laundry, housekeeping, and handling finances and needed supervision in taking his medications. He was able to receive calls but was unable to make phone calls. He was able to shop but would sometimes forget items (Lawton IADL Scale 28/56, assisted in IADLs).
Depressive symptoms	Scored 5/15 on GDS-15, no indication of clinically significant depressive mood, although he was noticed to have low volition.
Staging and clinical rating	Staging and clinical rating assessment was not done as no family carer was available during the assessment with Mr Chan.

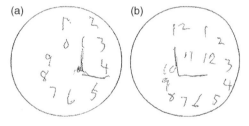

Figure 2.12 Findings from Mr Chan's Clock Drawing Test. (a) Clock Drawing (3 o'clock). (b) Clock Copying (10 past 10)

History Taken with Carer by Primary Care Physician

Mr Chan's son reported noticing memory problems in his father that had concerned him for about three years, although no delusional ideations were reported. Using the GPCOG Informant Interview, the following areas were noted to show more difficulties (×) or were preserved (○) compared to about two years ago:

× Remembering recent events
× Recalling recent conversations
○ Word finding
× Managing money and finances
× Managing medication independently
× Using transport

There were no additional clinical features to consider for non-Alzheimer's dementia. Mr Chan has hypertension. He is currently on nifedipine retard 20 mg twice daily, prazosin 0.5 mg twice daily, and allopurinol 100 mg daily. No family history of psychiatric disorders or dementia was reported. He received primary education to P.6 (approximately six years of education). Mr Chan was noted to have few social activities.

Physical Examination Findings

General examination revealed hygiene problems but no affective problem. No significant CVS or CNS findings.

Investigations

R/LFT, vitamin B_{12}, folate test, TSH/FT4, and H'stix were ordered. Apart from H'stix 6.6, all other investigations were normal. A CT brain (plain) scan revealed cerebral atrophy.

Diagnosis

Alzheimer's disease.

Management

Rivastigmine transdermal system 5 mg daily was prescribed. Mr Chan was also recommended to join a specialised day care service for two days per week for two years, with a structured and tailored intervention programme and cognitively stimulating activities to delay deterioration.

Suggestions for the Primary Care Team

The scenario in this case typifies early Alzheimer's disease, with a typical pattern of cognitive impairment shown on MMSE, and differential impairment on the Barthel Index versus the Lawton IADL Scale. The dose of rivastigmine can be escalated in the event of worsening cognitive function.

Low volition and hygiene problems were noted, and Mr Chan has mild impairment in initiating changes of clothes and taking showers. The primary care team should pay attention to the potential development of common distressed behaviours and neuropsychiatric symptoms of dementia, namely resistance to care. At this stage, intervention and support should focus on improving Mr Chan's volition in participating in daily living activities. Building up a daily routine based on his premorbid interests or lifestyle and scheduling regular cognitively stimulating activities at home or in the day care centre would be helpful. Family carers can be equipped with the caring skills that can promote functioning and facilitate self-care, such as by placing Mr Chan's belongings in a fixed place, using signs and cues to remind him about locations, changing the doors of cabinets into transparent ones to make searching easier, providing Mr Chan with lockable drawers with keys to increase his sense of security, and keeping spare keys in case they are misplaced or lost. Although Mr Chan's depressive symptoms did not reach a clinically significant level on assessment, because of the possible association between depressive mood and low motivation and self-neglect, the primary care team should explore if there may be any unmet psychosocial needs that can be addressed. Mr Chan attended the screening assessment unaccompanied by a family carer who could serve as an informant; whether Mr Chan has sufficient social support and the extent to which his son and other family members would be available to support his future care needs to be explored as part of his care plan.

2.2 Understanding Cognitive, Functioning, and Clinical Assessment Findings

Case 016 Whose Kids Are These?

Mrs Wong, a 75-year-old lady, presented with concerns raised by her daughter over her memory problems.

Findings from Screening Assessments by Allied Healthcare and Social Care Team

Cognitive functioning	Scored 14/30 on MMSE: results suggested cognitive impairment after adjusting for education level. Mrs Wong's performance was impaired in orientation to time (0/5), place (2/5), delayed recall (0/3), calculation (2/5), and three-step commands (1/3). Her performance was, however, normal in registration (3/3), language (5/5), and visuospatial relationships (1/1).
ADL/IADL	She needed assistance in bathing but was independent in other ADLs (Barthel Index 99/100). She needed assistance in taking medications, meal preparation, laundry, and housekeeping; needed supervision in external communication; and she was dependent in community access, handling finances, and shopping (Lawton IADL Score of 20/56).
Depressive symptoms	Scored 1/15 on GDS-15, no indication of depression.
Staging and clinical rating	Results suggested a Global Deterioration Scale stage 5, indicating moderate dementia. Mrs Wong was unable to recall major relevant aspects of her current life such as the address and telephone number of her long-term residence. She was also unable to recall the names of her grandchildren, and she needed assistance in choosing proper clothing to wear.

History Taken with Carer by Primary Care Physician

Mrs Wong's daughter reported noticing memory problems in her mother that had concerned her for two years, although no delusional ideations were reported. Using the GPCOG Informant Interview, the following areas were noted to show more difficulties (✗) or were preserved (○) compared to about two years ago:

✗ Remembering recent events
✗ Recalling recent conversations
○ Word finding
✗ Managing money and finances
✗ Managing medication independently
✗ Using transport

There were no additional clinical features to consider for non-Alzheimer's dementia. No comorbidity was reported. Her exact education level cannot be ascertained, although she has probably received more than two years of education according to her daughter.

Diagnosis

Alzheimer's disease.

Management

Mrs Wong was recommended to join a centre-based programme with cognitively stimulating activities for 18 months to maintain cognitive and self-care functioning; she was encouraged to have regular exercise, a healthy diet, and mental stimulation, manage stress, and maintain an active social life.

Suggestions for the Primary Care Team

At age 75, Mrs Wong was presenting at a relatively young age for the onset of dementia. While her impairment pattern was typical of Alzheimer's disease and her performance in the visuospatial relationships task (interlocking pentagon in MMSE) appeared intact, her MMSE score of 14/30 was lower than expected at this age, which may reflect a lower cognitive reserve against amyloid pathology. A cholinesterase inhibitor is indicated.

Mrs Wong has little comorbidity or physical health issues that may complicate her care and intervention, and her general good health is a strength. Mrs Wong's major area of weakness is her impaired short-term memory. Given her high level of independence in ADL, it is likely that her procedural memory remains intact. Her performance on IADL tasks can therefore be enhanced by simplifying tasks. Mrs Wong would also benefit from scheduled social activities or daily routines based on her premorbid interests or lifestyle. While her task initiation would be affected by her poor short-term memory, family carers can leverage her good attention, communication, and language ability and provide her with opportunities to handle hands-on tasks with immediate and step-by-step instructions.

Case 017 Time and Place Orientation

Mrs Yip, an 82-year-old lady, presented with concerns raised by her son over her memory problems: she was said to have poor short-term memory, difficulty in finding words, and problems remembering names.

Findings from Screening Assessments by Allied Healthcare and Social Care Team

Cognitive functioning	Scored 14/20 on MMSE: results indicative of cognitive impairment, adjusted for education level. Her performance was impaired in orientation to time (0/5) and place (2/5), delayed recall (0/3; she was unable to recall items even with prompting), and calculation (1/5); she had slight problems in three-step commands (2/3). Her performance was, however, normal in registration (3/3), language (5/5), and visuospatial relationships (1/1). The Clock Drawing Test showed a slight impairment in the spacing of lines and numbers only.
ADL/IADL	Mrs Yip showed a notable decline from a previous level of function in IADLs such as handling finances. No ADL impairments were noted.
Staging and clinical rating	Results suggested a Global Deterioration Scale stage 4, indicating mild dementia. She showed decreased knowledge of current and recent events, a decreased ability to travel and handle finances, and a concentration deficit elicited on the serial subtraction task. She was irritable and defensive during the assessment and interview.

History Taken with Carer by Primary Care Physician

Mrs Yip's son reported noticing memory problems in his mother that had concerned him for about one year, although no delusional ideations were reported. Using the GPCOG Informant Interview, the following areas were noted to show more difficulties (✗) or were preserved (○) compared to about two years ago:

✗ Remembering recent events
✗ Recalling recent conversations
✗ Word finding

× Managing money and finances
○ Managing medication independently
× Using transport

There were no additional clinical features to consider for non-Alzheimer's dementia. A pacemaker has been implanted. Mrs Yip's exact education level cannot be ascertained, although his son reported that she has probably more than two years of education.

Investigations

CBP, ESR, R/LFT, calcium, vitamin B_{12}, folate, fasting sugar, fasting lipids, MSU × R/M and culture test, CXR, and ECG were ordered.

Diagnosis

Mild Alzheimer's disease.

Management

Mrs Yip was recommended to join a centre-based programme with cognitively stimulating activities for 18 months to maintain her cognitive ability and quality of life.

Suggestions for the Primary Care Team

Mrs Yip presented at a typical age of presentation, in her early 80s. Although her MMSE score was lower than expected, the pattern of her impairment was typical of Alzheimer's disease: orientation to place was better than orientation to time, with impaired delayed recall and intact registration, language, and visuospatial relationships. This pattern indicates early Alzheimer's disease. With no other information explaining her low MMSE score, the presentation may be related to a lower cognitive reserve against amyloid pathology. It is worth noting here that Alzheimer's disease is not a homogeneous disease, and there may be interactions between cognitive reserve and pathological processes, with amyloid pathology being only one of the many pathologies. Physicians may consider cholinesterase inhibitors and/or memantine if Mrs Yip has worsening cognition on follow-up. Given that Mrs Yip was easily irritated when being confronted, as noted in the screening assessment, the need for memantine is indicated.

The fact that Mrs Yip was irritable and defensive during the assessment could also suggest possible self-awareness and denial of her cognitive deterioration and functional impairment. Alternatively, it could also indicate a complete lack of insight, when the assessment and interview may be viewed as something ungrounded, causing her annoyance. It is worth investigating further if any reasons can be identified for her irritation and defensiveness to inform further intervention and care strategies. This is also a good example to illustrate how some people living with dementia would react when meeting strangers (the assessor in this case), when he/she may not feel comfortable sharing personal information and feelings. Understanding whether the irritability and defensiveness were limited to the assessment setting or were more pervasive, for example, by using carer-reported questionnaires such as the Neuropsychiatric Interview Questionnaire (NPI-Q) and the Cornell Scale for Depression in Dementia, may provide useful clues to inform care planning.

Case 018 Inability to Draw a Clock

Mrs Mak, an 86-year-old lady, presented with concerns raised by her daughter-in-law about her memory problems. She was reported to have incidents of not being able to find her way home and not knowing where her money had gone.

Findings from Screening Assessments by Allied Healthcare and Social Care Team

Cognitive functioning	Scored 14/30 on MMSE: results indicate cognitive impairment, after adjusting for education level. Her performance was impaired in delayed recall (0/3), calculation (1/5), three-step commands (1/3), and visuospatial relationships (0/1); problems in orientation to time (2/5); and slight problems in orientation to place (3/5). Her performance was, however, normal in registration (3/3). The Clock Drawing Test showed no reasonable or understandable attempt at drawing a clock face, suggesting executive function, conceptual, and visual-spatial deficits; similar impairments can be observed in the copying part of the test (Figure 2.13).
ADL/IADL	IADL performance showed a notable decline; however, no formal assessment results were available.
Staging and clinical rating	Results suggested a Global Deterioration Scale stage 4, indicating mild dementia. She showed decreased knowledge of current and recent events, a decreased ability to travel and handle finances, deficits in memory of personal history, and an inability to perform complex tasks. A depressive mood was observed during the interview, although no formal assessment was conducted.

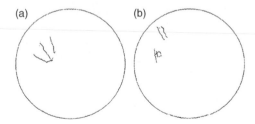

Figure 2.13 Findings from Mrs Mak's Clock Drawing Test. (a) Clock Drawing (3 o'clock). (b) Clock Copying (10 past 10)

History Taken with Carer by Primary Care Physician

Mrs Mak's daughter-in-law reported noticing memory problems in her mother-in-law that had concerned her for about six months, although no delusional ideations were reported. Using the GPCOG Informant Interview, the following areas were noted to show more difficulties (✗) or were preserved (○) compared to about two years ago:

- ✗ Remembering recent events
- ✗ Recalling recent conversations
- ○ Word finding
- ○ Managing money and finances
- ○ Managing medication independently
- ✗ Using transport

There were no additional clinical features to consider for non-Alzheimer's dementia. Mrs Mak has hypertension, hyperlipidaemia, atrial fibrillation, and gout. She is currently on allopurinol, colchicine, digoxin, amlodipine, rivaroxaban, simvastatin, and donepezil 10 mg daily. She has never received any education.

Investigations

ESR, R/LFT, calcium, and vitamin B_{12} were ordered. All investigations were normal. MRI revealed GCA scale 2, selective prominence in posterior parietal, inferior frontal, and medial temporal lobe atrophy, MTL R = 0.66, L = 0.45, Scheltens R = L = 2–3, ARWMC 3/3, and possible microhaemorrhages.

Diagnosis

Early Alzheimer's disease.

Management

Donepezil 10 mg daily and an 18-month programme of centre-based cognitively stimulating activities were prescribed. Mrs Mak was also encouraged to have regular exercise, a healthy diet, and mental stimulation, and maintain an active social life.

Suggestions for the Primary Care Team

Mrs Mak's onset of symptoms presented at a slightly older age, and a lower MMSE score is within expectations. Her pattern of impairment was typical of early Alzheimer's disease. Her prominent impairment in the Clock Drawing Test and visuospatial relationships (interlocking pentagon on MMSE) was remarkable at this stage, which may be related to her lack of formal education. Mrs Mak's inability to handle complicated tasks and draw may reflect impaired executive functions, which are common in Alzheimer's disease, and in this case more prominent in the absence of formal education. It would also be helpful to check her ability in clock reading to understand the nature of the impairment. There is also a significant vascular risk in her comorbidities, and the vascular element may have contributed to further cognitive impairment on top of her Alzheimer's disease.

Given the significant impairments as shown on MMSE, Mrs Mak's cognitive decline should have been noticeable much earlier than the six-month period reported by her daughter-in-law. Mrs Mak's family support would therefore be something worth exploring, for example, whether she is living with a carer and how often family members visit. Identifying existing resources and potential support networks is needed for care planning. While her short-term memory impairment is evident, which is common at this stage of Alzheimer's disease, her inability to recall her personal history (tapping on her long-term memory) is less compatible. With a depressive mood noted during the clinical interview, there is a possibility that Mrs Mak was unwilling to share her personal history, instead of being unable to recall it. The primary care team is recommended to conduct a more systematic assessment of her depressive mood. Good rapport and sensitivity towards potential mood symptoms would help ascertain or exclude the role of depression in Mrs Mak's impairments, with implications for the focus of her care and treatment plan.

Case 019 Perseveration Error in Clock Drawing

Mrs Chan, an 85-year-old lady, presented with concerns raised by her daughter about her memory problems, such as asking the same question repeatedly, for about a year.

Findings from Screening Assessments by Allied Healthcare and Social Care Team

Cognitive functioning	Scored 8/30 on MMSE: results indicative of cognitive impairment, adjusted for education level. Mrs Chan was incapable in orientation to time (0/5), delayed recall (0/3), calculation (0/5), and visuospatial relationships (0/1); she had impaired performance in orientation to place (1/5) and three-step commands (1/3) and slight problems in registration (2/3) and language (4/5). The Clock Drawing Test showed some evidence that a clock face is drawn, with noticeable impairments in executive function (planning and organisation), conceptual deficits, and perseveration error (Figure 2.14).
ADL/IADL:	She required assistance in choosing proper clothing to wear; she was, however, independent in other ADLs (Barthel Index 98/100). She was dependent in taking medication, meal preparation, and housekeeping; she required assistance in external communication, laundry, handling finances, and grocery shopping and needed supervision in community access (Lawton IADL Scale 20/56).
Depressive symptoms	Scored 0/15 on GDS-15, no depressive mood was noted.
Staging and clinical rating	Results suggested a Global Deterioration Scale stage 5, indicating moderate dementia. She was unable to recall major relevant events of her life, such as the names of her grandchildren; she had difficulty counting backwards from 20 by 2s; she was impaired in IADLs and needed assistance in choosing proper clothing due to cognitive impairments.

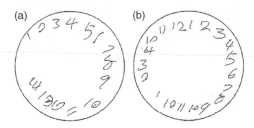

Figure 2.14 Findings from Mrs Chan's Clock Drawing Test. (a) Clock Drawing (3 o'clock). (b) Clock Copying (10 past 10)

History Taken with Carer by Primary Care Physician

Mrs Chan's daughter reported noticing memory problems in her mother that had concerned her for about a year, although no delusional ideations were reported. Using the GPCOG Informant Interview, the following areas were noted to show more difficulties (✗) or were preserved (○) compared to about two years ago:

✗ Remembering recent events
✗ Recalling recent conversations
✗ Word finding
○ Managing money and finances
✗ Managing medication independently
✗ Using transport

There were no additional clinical features to consider for non-Alzheimer's dementia. Mrs Chan has hypertension, diabetes, and a fracture of the right hip (operated on

10 years ago). No family history of psychiatric disorders or dementia was reported. There was no exact information on her education level, except that she probably received less than six months of education.

Investigations

CT scan was ordered.

Diagnosis

Moderate Alzheimer's disease.

Management

Mrs Chan was recommended to join a centre-based programme with cognitively stimulating activities for 18 months to maintain cognitive and self-care functions; she was also encouraged to have regular exercise, a healthy diet, and mental stimulation, remain socially active, and was recommended to have a community access evaluation. She was provided with an anti-lost device.

Suggestions for the Primary Care Team

Mrs Chan presented at the usual age of symptom presentation for Alzheimer's disease. Although at age 85, her presentation was leaning towards late presentation, with only one year's history of significant symptoms, her MMSE score was markedly low and her impairment pattern was compatible with Alzheimer's disease. It should be noted, however, that her ADLs were largely preserved, and the Clock Drawing Test did not show the usual pattern (of better performance on the copying part than the executive part). This case should be treated clinically as Alzheimer's disease; physicians can prescribe a cholinesterase inhibitor and memantine for moderate Alzheimer's disease.

This is a good example illustrating the possible dissociation between cognitive impairment and ADL functional level. In some people living with dementia, especially those who were active and independent in their premorbid daily activities, a good functional level of ADL could be well maintained despite significant cognitive impairment or later-stage dementia, with ADL functions declining much slower than other functions.

The relatively late help-seeking in Mrs Chan's case should alert the primary care team to explore her social support network. In countries or areas where good public awareness and early assessment services are in place, late help-seeking at a moderate stage may be unusual and suggest insufficient social support. If this is the case, enhancing Mrs Chan's support network and mobilising community resources to compensate for insufficient support would be an important component of her care planning.

Case 020 Forgetting to Get Dressed after Bathing

Mr Lai, a 91-year-old man, presented with concerns raised by his daughter over his memory problems, for example, forgetting about his appointments, particularly in the past two years.

Findings from Screening Assessments by Allied Healthcare and Social Care Team

Cognitive functioning	Scored 14/30 on MMSE: results suggested cognitive impairment, adjusted for education level. Mr Lai was incapable of performing in delayed recall (0/3) and visuospatial relationships (0/1); he was impaired in orientation to time (1/5) and place (2/5), calculation (2/5), and three-step commands (1/3); his performance was, however, normal in registration (3/3) and visuospatial relationships (Figure 2.15).

ADL/IADL	Mr Lai was independent in ADLs (Barthel Index 100/100). He was dependent in meal preparation (relied on carers); needed assistance in taking medications, community access, and handling finances; and needed supervision in external communication, housekeeping, and grocery shopping; he was, however, independent in laundry (Lawton IADL Scale 32/56).
Staging and clinical rating	Results suggested a Global Deterioration Scale stage that was approaching stage 5, indicating moderate dementia. He was unable to recall major relevant aspects of his life, such as the names of his grandchildren; he had difficulty counting backwards from 40 by 4s; his cognitive impairment affected his IADLs significantly and ADLs slightly; for example, he would sometimes forget to get dressed after taking a shower. Mild irritability was reported.

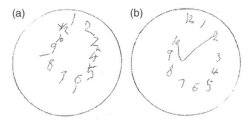

Figure 2.15 Findings from Mr Lai's Clock Drawing Test. (a) Clock Drawing (3 o'clock). (b) Clock Copying (10 past 10)

History Taken with Carer by Primary Care Physician

Mr Lai's daughter reported noticing memory problems in her father that had concerned her for seven to eight years, which appeared to be getting worse in the last two years. Delusional ideations were reported. Using the GPCOG Informant Interview, the following areas were noted to show more difficulties (✗) or were preserved (○) compared to about two years ago:

✗ Remembering recent events
✗ Recalling recent conversations
○ Word finding
○ Managing money and finances
○ Managing medication independently
✗ Using transport

There were no additional clinical features to consider for non-Alzheimer's dementia. Mr Lai has hypercholesterolaemia and ischaemic heart disease with percutaneous coronary intervention. He was followed up at a geriatric medicine outpatient clinic for ischaemic heart disease. No family history of psychiatric disorders or dementia was reported. His exact education level cannot be ascertained, although he probably has less than six months of education according to his daughter.

Investigations

Calcium, ESR, VDRL, vitamin B_{12}, folate, fasting sugar, ECG, and TSH were ordered. Results showed Ca 2.01, TSH 1.19, vitamin B_{12} 184, Hb 11.7 NcNc, and ESR 25. A CT brain (plain) scan revealed MTL atrophy R = 0.92, L = 0.81, Scheltens score R = 2 L = 2, ARWMC 3/3, and right frontal infarct.

Diagnosis

Mixed dementia.

Management

Mr Lai was recommended to join a centre-based programme with cognitively stimulating activities for 18 months to maintain cognitive functions; he was also encouraged to have regular exercise, a healthy diet, and mental stimulation, manage stress, and maintain an active social life.

Suggestions for the Primary Care Team

Mr Lai presented at a relatively old age, with symptom onset dating back seven or eight years; a lower MMSE score is therefore expected. His impairment pattern is compatible with Alzheimer's disease: with intact performance in the interlocking pentagon (visuospatial relationships on MMSE) and better performance in clock copying than the executive part of the Clock Drawing Test, which was in keeping with Alzheimer's disease. The physiological influence of age should be taken into consideration. A low dose of donepezil 2.5 mg can be started, and his progress should be monitored. The presence of irritability should raise attention to possible comorbid depressive symptoms, with a more detailed assessment indicated. Physicians may prescribe memantine for both irritability and mixed dementia. Concomitant use of cholinesterase inhibitors and memantine is suggested for mixed dementia (and moderate to severe Alzheimer's disease) by some experts (1, 2). Antipsychotics could also be considered when delusional ideas cannot be managed by non-pharmacological means.

While Mr Lai's cognitive decline was largely observed in his short-term memory, there is evidence that the impairment affects his orientation in time, his awareness of current events, and his long-term memory of his family members. It is therefore worth exploring whether his irritable mood and behaviours may be related to or preceded by the disorientation, which could cause a sense of insecurity. The fact that Mr Lai's ADL was well maintained suggested intact procedural memory; his impairment in getting dressed probably reflected poor short-term memory and deterioration in attention only, when he might be easily distracted and forget about the current tasks. With strategies to support concentration and short-term memory, Mr Lai's problem of forgetting to get dressed after a shower could be improved.

Case 021 Choosing Proper Clothes

Mr Tam, an 83-year-old man, presented with concerns raised by his wife about his memory problems. His wife complained about his disorientation to place, forgetfulness of recent events, and repeated questioning.

Findings from Screening Assessments by Allied Healthcare and Social Care Team

Cognitive functioning	Scored 12/30 on MMSE, suggestive of cognitive impairment after adjusting for education level. Mr Tam was incapable in orientation to time (0/5) and delayed recall (0/3); he had impaired performance in calculation (1/5); three-step commands (1/3); and slight problems in orientation to place (3/5), registration (2/3), and language (4/5). His performance was, however, normal in visuospatial relationships (1/1). The Clock Drawing Test showed minimal evidence that a clock face

	was drawn, with impaired executive function, conceptual deficits, and visual-spatial deficits suggested (Figure 2.16).
ADL/IADL	Mr Tam needed supervision in bathing due to cognitive impairment; he needed assistance in outdoor mobility and stair climbing due to lower limb weakness, but was independent in other ADLs (Barthel Index 91/100). He needed assistance in external communication and handling finances and was dependent in other IADLs due to cognitive impairments (Lawton IADL Scale 12/56).
Depressive symptoms	Scored 3/15 on GDS-15, no indication of depression.
Staging and clinical rating	Results suggested a Global Deterioration Scale stage 5, indicating moderate dementia. He was unable to recall major relevant aspects of his current life, such as the names of his grandchildren. He also showed difficulty choosing proper clothing to wear.

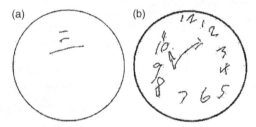

Figure 2.16 Findings from Mr Tam's Clock Drawing Test. (a) Clock Drawing (3 o'clock). (b) Clock Copying (10 past 10) *A Chinese character '3' was written on the clock face

History Taken with Carer by Primary Care Physician

Mr Tam's wife reported noticing memory problems in her husband that had concerned her for over a year. Delusional ideations were reported: Mr Tam was suspicious about strangers stealing his money. Using the GPCOG Informant Interview, the following areas were noted to show more difficulties (×) or were preserved (○) compared to about two years ago:

× Remembering recent events
× Recalling recent conversations
× Word finding
× Managing money and finances
× Managing medication independently
× Using transport

There were no additional clinical features to consider for non-Alzheimer's dementia. Mr Tam has hypertension and diabetes. No family history of psychiatric disorders or dementia was reported. His education level cannot be ascertained, although he has probably received more than two years of education.

Investigations

CBP, R/LFT, VDRL, vitamin B_{12}, folate, fasting sugar, fasting lipids, TFT, and a CT scan were ordered.

Diagnosis

Moderate Alzheimer's disease.

Management

No medication was prescribed as further investigation was pending. Meanwhile, Mr Tam was recommended to join a centre-based programme with cognitively stimulating activities for 18 months to maintain cognitive and self-care functions. Non-pharmacological interventions to manage his distressed behaviours and neuropsychiatric symptoms of dementia were also recommended.

Suggestions for the Primary Care Team

Mr Tam presented at a typical age of symptom onset for Alzheimer's disease, with a typical pattern of impairment noted in the Clock Drawing Test (worse performance in the clock drawing compared with the clock copying task). It is likely that amyloid load is a major factor in Mr Tam's pathology. It should be noted, however, that his MMSE score was lower than expected, and impairment in registration is unusual in early Alzheimer's disease. Also considering the fact that he was already showing difficulties choosing appropriate clothing, the presentations taken together would put Mr Tam in a moderate stage of Alzheimer's disease, when he would be expected to require assistance in putting on clothes in the next stage. This is a typical case of Alzheimer's disease going into a moderate stage; a cholinesterase inhibitor should be started. On top of a cholinesterase inhibitor, physicians may consider the use of a low-dose antipsychotic, such as quetiapine, if Mr Tam's delusional idea does not subside with a cholinesterase inhibitor and non-pharmacological interventions.

Mr Tam's functional impairment can be understood in the context of moderate Alzheimer's disease, with the typical presentation of cognitive impairment mostly related to short-term memory, such as orientation to time, following instructions, and continuous calculation. His impairment in the Clock Drawing Test reflected impaired executive functions and related higher cognitive functions, such as abstraction, conceptual thinking, and judgement. These impairments would help explain his inability to choose proper clothes, which involves executive function. With foreseeable further deterioration in ADLs and IADLs, support for his wife should be arranged, and the primary care team should support the identification and engagement of other family members if available. Assessment of the strengths and needs of Mr Tam's wife would be an important first step in working with them to develop a future care plan.

Case 022 Reversed Clock Numbers

Mrs Ko, an 80-year-old lady, presented with concerns raised by her daughter about her memory problems. She was noted to ask the same questions repeatedly and appeared forgetful of recent events.

Findings from Screening Assessments by Allied Healthcare and Social Care Team

| Cognitive functioning | Scored 18/30 on MMSE: results indicative of cognitive impairment, adjusted for education level. Mrs Ko's performance was impaired in delayed recall (0/3) and orientation to time (1/5) and place (1/5); she had slight problems in three-step commands (2/3). Her performance |

	was, however, normal in registration (3/3), calculation (5/5), language (5/5), and visuospatial relationships (1/1). The Clock Drawing Test showed abnormal clock face drawing, with reversal of numbers and no indication of time; results suggested impairments in executive function and conceptual deficits (Figure 2.17).
ADL/IADL	Mrs Ko was independent in ADLs (Barthel Index 100/100). She needed assistance in community access and handling finances; she also required supervision in taking medication, meal preparation, external communication, and grocery shopping (Lawton IADL Scale 40/56).
Depressive symptoms	Scored 2/15 on GDS-15, no indication of depression.
Staging and clinical rating	Results showed a Global Deterioration Scale stage 4, indicating mild dementia. Mrs Ko showed decreased knowledge of current and recent events; a decreased ability to travel and handle finances; and an inability to perform complex tasks; she was, however, able to select proper clothing to wear.

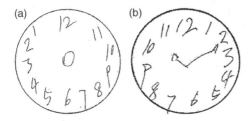

Figure 2.17 Findings from Mrs Ko's Clock Drawing Test. (a) Clock Drawing (3 o'clock). (b) Clock Copying (10 past 10)

History Taken with Carer by Primary Care Physician

Mrs Ko's daughter reported noticing memory problems in her mother that had concerned her for about three years. Delusional ideations were reported: she was suspicious about strangers stealing her money. Using the GPCOG Informant Interview, the following areas were noted to show more difficulties (×) or were preserved (○) compared to about two years ago:

× Remembering recent events
× Recalling recent conversations
× Word finding
× Managing money and finances
× Managing medication independently
○ Using transport

There were no additional clinical features to consider for non-Alzheimer's dementia. Mrs Ko had no comorbid chronic illness. No family history of psychiatric disorders or dementia was reported. Her education level cannot be ascertained, except that she has probably received more than two years of education according to her daughter.

Investigations

CBP, ESR, VDRL, calcium, vitamin B_{12}, folate, and CXR were ordered.

Diagnosis

Early Alzheimer's disease.

Management

Oral rivastigmine 1.5 mg four times a day was prescribed. Mrs Ko was also recommended to join a centre-based programme with cognitively stimulating activities for 18 months to maintain cognitive and self-care functions; she was also encouraged to have regular exercise, a healthy diet, and mental stimulation, and maintain an active social life; non-pharmacological interventions to manage her distressed behaviours and neuropsychiatric symptoms of dementia were also suggested to her carers.

Suggestions for the Primary Care Team

At a typical age of presentation, Mrs Ko's cognitive impairment pattern was compatible with Alzheimer's disease: she had an intact performance on the visuospatial relationships (as shown in the interlocking pentagon on MMSE), although findings from the Clock Drawing Test were positive, with greater impairment shown on the clock drawing part compared with the clock copying part. The primary care physician is recommended to start with a low-dose cholinesterase inhibitor and observe her progress. The daily dose of rivastigmine can also be titrated up if Mrs Ko does not experience any side effects.

The primary care team is also advised to investigate further the nature (content) of Mrs Ko's delusional ideations. If the ideations were likely caused by poor memory (e.g., forgetting where belongings were placed and confusion in money management), caring strategies such as increased environmental cues, reminders, and better organisation of personal belongings may help. On the other hand, although her daughter reported that Mrs Ko had no problem using transportation in the GPCOG, there is nevertheless a high risk of her getting lost, in view of her obvious deficits in orientation as shown on MMSE, impaired community access, and decreased ability to travel as shown in the IADL and staging assessment, suggesting a potential underestimation of risk by the carer. Mrs Ko's daughter should be advised to use a location tracker on a smartphone or other device to ensure safety.

Case 023 Wearing Shirts Unbuttoned

Mrs Chung, an 89-year-old lady, presented with concerns raised by her daughter about her memory problems. She was noted to have poor memory (e.g., repeated questioning), deteriorated hygiene at home (e.g., did not clean dishes thoroughly), and issues with personal attire (e.g., leaving her shirt unbuttoned).

Findings from Screening Assessments by Allied Healthcare and Social Care Team

Cognitive functioning	Scored 10/30 on MMSE: results indicative of cognitive impairment, adjusted for education level. Mrs Chung was incapable of performing in orientation to time (0/5) and place (0/5), delayed recall (0/3), calculation (0/5), and visuospatial relationships (0/1); she also had slight problems in language (4/5). Her performance was, however, normal in registration (3/3) and three-step commands (3/3). The Clock Drawing Test was not completed: she did not know how to write or read numbers, and when a clock was presented to her, she was unable to read the time correctly.

ADL/IADL	Mrs Chung was unsafe in stair climbing by herself; she also needed moderate help in ambulation (outdoors) and minimal help in feeding, bed/chair transfers, and dressing (she could select her own clothes with limited choices) (Barthel Index 78/100). In terms of IADLs, she was dependent in handling finances and grocery shopping; she required assistance in taking medications, housekeeping, and community access; she also needed supervision in meal preparation, external communication, and laundry (but she was able to handwash her clothes by herself) (Lawton IADL Scale 26/56).
Staging and clinical rating	Results showed a Global Deterioration Scale stage 4 approaching 5, indicating mild to moderate dementia. She had decreased knowledge of current and recent events; a decreased ability to travel and handle finances; an inability to perform complex tasks; and an inability to recall major relevant aspects of her current life, such as the address and telephone number of her home, without prompting.

History Taken with Carer by Primary Care Physician

Mrs Chung's daughter reported noticing memory problems in her mother that had concerned her for about two years. Delusional ideations were reported. Using the GPCOG Informant Interview, the following areas were noted to show more difficulties (×) or were preserved (○) compared to about two years ago:

× Remembering recent events
× Recalling recent conversations
× Word finding
× Managing money and finances
× Managing medication independently
× Using transport

There were some additional clinical features to consider for non-Alzheimer's dementia, which included complex visual hallucinations (seeing mild movement), apraxia in self-care (she cannot dress properly), an inability to control mood (she would use foul language, which was a change in behaviour), overeating (especially sweet food), and early swallowing problems (unable to swallow bigger tablets). Deterioration in the hygiene of her home (e.g., did not clean dishes thoroughly) and personal attire (e.g., wearing shirt unbuttoned) was reported by her daughter. Mrs Chung has a bilateral cataract and she is currently being followed up at a geriatric medicine outpatient clinic for hypertension. No family history of psychiatric disorders or dementia was reported. Her exact education level cannot be ascertained, except that she has probably received less than six months of education according to her daughter.

Investigations

CBP, R/LFT, calcium, VDRL, vitamin B_{12}, folate, fasting sugar, fasting lipids, and ECG were ordered.

Diagnosis

Moderate Alzheimer's disease.

Management

Donepezil 5 mg daily was prescribed. Mrs Chung was also recommended to join a centre-based programme with cognitively stimulating activities for 18 months for the maintenance of cognitive abilities and quality of life.

Suggestions for the Primary Care Team

Mrs Chung presented at a slightly older age, with a low MMSE score and typical cognitive impairment pattern in keeping with Alzheimer's disease. It should be noted, however, that her ADLs were already quite impaired on presentation, and her physical functioning was more impaired. She showed some frontal lobe features on top of the typical features of Alzheimer's disease. These presentations could suggest a frontal variant of Alzheimer's disease: the primary care team should be aware that presence of frontal symptoms can also occur in Alzheimer's disease. The treatment remains the same as in Alzheimer's disease without frontal lobe features. A trial of cholinesterase inhibitors is indicated, although the primary care physician should watch out for worsening in the behavioural symptoms, and adjust the medication when needed. Selective serotonin reuptake inhibitors can be considered when frontal lobe features are florid.

In this case, the physical deterioration in old age further affected Mrs Chung's ADL/IADL performance. It should also be noted that, although most of her cognitive functions were affected, she was still good at communication (language) and attention. These represent her strengths, which are worth leveraging to promote continued participation in social activities to maintain a stable mood and cognition. Although the quality of her household and self-care tasks was reported to have deteriorated, Mrs Chung still has motivation, which should be maintained: carers can be advised to focus on the process of her participation and use of functions, instead of focusing on the quality and outcomes of her performance (e.g., whether the washed dishes are cleaned thoroughly).

Case 024 Lines for Numbers

Mrs Ho, an 83-year-old lady, presented with concerns raised by her daughter about her memory problems. Her daughter complained of her repetitive conversational content and misplacement of valuable items; she was noted to have had a decline in cognitive functions for a year.

Findings from Screening Assessments by Allied Healthcare and Social Care Team

Cognitive functioning	Score 13/30 on MMSE: results indicative of cognitive impairment, adjusted for education level. Mrs Ho was incapable of performing in delayed recall (0/3), calculation (0/5), and visuospatial relationships (0/1). Her performance was impaired in orientation to time (1/5), and she had slight problems in orientation to place (3/5), language (4/5), and three-step commands (2/3). Her performance was, however, normal in registration (3/3). The Clock Drawing Test showed minimal evidence that a clock face was drawn; she has never received any formal education and was unable to write numbers, although she made attempts to draw spokes to represent the 12 numbers (Figure 2.18).

ADL/IADL	Mrs Ho needed minimal help in ambulation and stair climbing; she was independent in other ADLs (Barthel Index 95/100); she needed assistance in housekeeping (showed a decline in environmental hygiene); and she required supervision in taking medications (she needed to be reminded), meal preparation (she was able to make simple meals only), community access, handling finances (she would go to the bank with her daughter), and grocery shopping (she was able to buy simple items) (Lawton IADL Scale 42/56).
Depressive symptoms	Scored 1/15 on GDS-15, results showing no indication of depression.
Staging and clinical rating	Results suggested a Global Deterioration Scale stage 4, indicating mild dementia. She showed decreased knowledge of current and recent events; a concentration deficit was elicited on the serial subtraction task; and a decreased ability to travel and handle finances was noted.

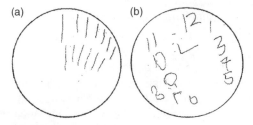

Figure 2.18 Findings from Mrs Ho's Clock Drawing Test. (a) Clock Drawing (3 o'clock). (b) Clock Copying (10 past 10)

History Taken with Carer by Primary Care Physician

Mrs Ho's daughter reported noticing memory problems in her mother that had concerned her for about a year. Delusional ideations were reported. Using the GPCOG Informant Interview, the following areas were noted to show more difficulties (×) or were preserved (○) compared to about two years ago:

× Remembering recent events
× Recalling recent conversations
○ Word finding
× Managing money and finances
× Managing medication independently
× Using transport

There were no additional clinical features to consider for non-Alzheimer's dementia. Mrs Ho has hypertension, hypercholesterolaemia, and bilateral cataract (operated on). No family history of psychiatric disorders or dementia was reported. Her exact education level was unknown, although her daughter reported that she had probably received no formal education. Mrs Ho lived alone.

Investigations

CBP, ESR, R/LFT, calcium, vitamin B_{12}, folate, fasting sugar, fasting lipids, MSU × R/M & culture test, ECG, and T4 were ordered. A CT brain (plain) scan was ordered.

Diagnosis

Mild Alzheimer's disease.

Management

No medication was prescribed as further investigation was pending. Mrs Ho was recommended to join centre-based cognitively stimulating activities for 18 months for the maintenance of cognitive abilities and quality of life.

Suggestions for the Primary Care Team

This is a typical case of early Alzheimer's disease. Despite her low MMSE score, Mrs Ho presented at a typical age of symptom onset, with an impairment pattern in keeping with Alzheimer's disease, as suggested in the differential Barthel Index and Lawton IADL scores and Clock Drawing Test results, taking into consideration her lack of formal education. The low MMSE score therefore possibly suggested a low brain reverse against the amyloid load. A low-dose cholinesterase inhibitor can be tried.

In Mrs Ho's case, although her deterioration appeared obvious according to cognitive screening test results, her general functions in daily living activities were good. Apart from a lack of formal education, which may explain part of the cognitive performance, this pattern may also be related to her premorbid lifestyle with a high level of independence in self-care. With relatively good physical health and a low cognitive requirement for daily activities, Mrs Ho's ADL and IADL functioning is largely satisfactory despite her cognitive impairment. At this stage, only minimal or supervisory support is needed, which her daughter has been handling.

However, as her disease progresses, there will be increasing risks in ADL and IADL tasks with Mrs Ho living alone; her deficits in orientation also pose a risk of her getting lost. The primary care team should work with Mrs Ho's daughter to explore options that can ensure safety, which would also enable Mrs Ho's continued participation in self-care, as this is her strength that should be enhanced and supported. The primary care team should also discuss with Mrs Ho and her daughter key intervention goals, including the main concerns that have prompted the help-seeking, such as advice for the misplacement of valuable items.

Case 025 Which Stage?

Ms Wong, an 88-year-old lady, presented with concerns raised by her daughter about her memory problems noted for about 12 months: she was reported to be forgetful of appointment dates, misplacing personal items, and showing difficulties in money and medication management. There was an incident when Ms Wong suspected her neighbour of stealing her safety box keys. Ms Wong expressed awareness of her own memory decline.

Findings from Screening Assessments by Allied Healthcare and Social Care Team

Cognitive functioning	Scored 14/30 on MMSE: results indicated cognitive impairment, adjusted for education level. Her performance was impaired in calculation (1/5), orientation in time (1/5) and place (1/5), delayed recall (1/3), and visuospatial relationships (0/1). Her performance was slightly impaired in three-step commands (2/3) and language (4/5). She was, however, intact in registration (3/3). The Clock Drawing Test

	showed that she was able to write sets of numbers in the correct sequence, although impairments were noted in arranging the numbers properly on the clock face and indicating the time; her performance improved on the clock copying task, which showed that she was able to copy the clock (Figure 2.19).
ADL/IADL	She was independent in most ADLs (Barthel Index 92/100), except that her lower limb weakness has affected her walking ability. She was semi-independent in IADLs. She required assistance in meal preparation, external communication, handling finances, and grocery shopping (Lawton IADL Scale 46/56).
Depressive symptoms	Scored 1/15 on GDS-15, no obvious depressive mood was found.
Staging and clinical rating	Scored 0.5/3 on Clinical Dementia Rating, indicating questionable dementia. She had mild impairment in memory and orientation.

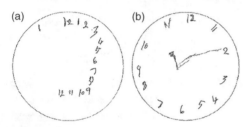

Figure 2.19 Findings from Ms Wong's Clock Drawing Test. (a) Clock Drawing (3 o'clock). (b) Clock Copying (10 past 10)

History Taken with Carer by Primary Care Physician

Ms Wong's daughter reported noticing memory problems in Ms Wong that had concerned her for about a year. Delusional ideations were reported. Using the GPCOG Informant Interview, the following areas were noted to show more difficulties (×) or were preserved (○) compared to about two years ago:

× Remembering recent events
× Recalling recent conversations
○ Word finding
× Managing money and finances
× Managing medication independently
× Using transport

There were no additional clinical features to consider for non-Alzheimer's dementia. Ms Wong has hypertension and dyslipidaemia. No family history of psychiatric disorders or dementia was reported. She did not receive any education.

Physical Examination Findings

General examination revealed no affect or hygiene problem. Ms Wong had a blood pressure reading of 134/70 mm Hg. No CVS or CNS findings.

Diagnosis

Mild to moderate Alzheimer's disease. No mood symptoms.

Management

Rivastigmine transdermal system 4.6 mg daily was prescribed. She was also recommended to join a specialised day care service for two days per week, with a structured and tailored intervention programme and cognitively stimulating activities to delay deterioration.

Suggestions for the Primary Care Team

Ms Wong presented at a slightly older age, with 12 months of symptom presentation. Her impairment pattern was typical (e.g., worse performance on the drawing part of the Clock Drawing Test, but improving on the copying part). The short time from symptom presentation to the current impairment level may suggest an aggressive amyloid load. In the case of deteriorating cognition, physicians may consider escalating the dose of cholinesterase inhibitors or adding memantine. Depending on the staging criteria used and whether assistance in getting dressed is needed (i.e., dressing apraxia), this can be a case of mild or mild to moderate Alzheimer's disease.

A point to note in this case is that very often clinical rating scales rely heavily on carers' impressions: with the Clinical Dementia Rating, for example, half of the assessment ratings were based on the carers' subjective report. In this case, the primary care team should pay attention to the possibility of a discrepancy between carers' subjective reports and objective assessment findings: the cognitive and functional assessments for Ms Wong appeared consistent with a moderate stage of dementia. This did not match well with merely 12 months of significant deterioration according to the carer's report, and the Clinical Dementia Rating of 0.5 was heavily based on her daughter's impression. It is possible that Ms Wong's symptoms have occurred for more than 12 months, although a low awareness of the early signs and symptoms or infrequent interaction might have caused a delay in symptom identification. The primary care team is therefore advised to explore the carer's awareness and understanding of dementia, provide education as needed, and assess the level of support available within Ms Wong's family.

Case 026 Clinical Dementia Rating Score of 1

Ms Ng, a 76-year-old lady, presented with concerns raised by her husband about her memory problems for about two years. Her husband complained about her forgetfulness of conversation with others, appointments, and past events. Ms Ng was aware of her own memory decline.

Findings from Screening Assessments by Allied Healthcare and Social Care Team

Cognitive functioning	Scored 17/30 on MMSE: results indicative of cognitive impairment, adjusted for education level. Ms Ng's performance was impaired in orientation to time (0/5), visuospatial relationships (0/1), and calculation (1/5); she was slightly impaired in delayed recall (2/3) and language (3/5); her performance was, however, normal in registration (3/3), orientation to place (5/5), and three-step commands (3/3). The Clock Drawing Test showed impaired executive function (abstract thinking), while she was able to read the clock during the clock copying task (Figure 2.20).
ADL/IADL	Ms Ng was modified independent in ADLs (Barthel Index 98/100): she needed reminders to take meals. She has modified independence in IADLs: she needed assistance in medications; she can shop but would sometimes forget items (Lawton IADL Scale 49/56).

| Depressive symptoms | Scored 1/15 on GDS-15, no obvious depressive mood was found. |
| Staging and clinical rating | Scored 1/3 on Clinical Dementia Rating, indicating mild dementia. She showed mild impairments in memory, orientation, judgement and problem-solving, and personal care. She also showed questionable impairments in communication affairs and in home and hobbies. |

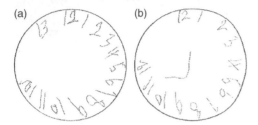

Figure 2.20 Findings from Ms Ng's Clock Drawing Test. (a) Clock Drawing (3 o'clock). (b) Clock Copying (10 past 10)

History Taken with Carer by Primary Care Physician

Ms Ng's husband reported noticing memory problems of his wife that had concerned him for about two years, although no delusional ideations were reported. Using the GPCOG Informant Interview, the following areas were noted to show more difficulties (✗) or were preserved (○) compared to about two years ago:

✗ Remembering recent events
✗ Recalling recent conversations
○ Word finding
✗ Managing money and finances
✗ Managing medication independently
○ Using transport

There were no additional clinical features to consider for non-Alzheimer's dementia. Ms Ng has diabetes and hypertension. No family history of psychiatric disorders or dementia was reported. She has received primary education. She plays card games with neighbours every day.

Physical Examination Findings

General examination revealed no affect or hygiene problem. Ms Ng had a normal blood pressure of 117/69 mm Hg. No other CVS or CNS findings.

Diagnosis

Alzheimer's disease.

Management

Rivastigmine transdermal system 4.6 mg daily was prescribed. Ms Ng was also recommended to join a specialised day care service for two days per week, with a structured and tailored intervention programme and cognitively stimulating activities to delay deterioration.

Suggestions for the Primary Care Team

Ms Ng presented at a slightly younger age of symptom onset for Alzheimer's disease, and her MMSE score was lower than expected for her age. Nevertheless, the impairment pattern (e.g., worse performance in clock drawing than clock copying in the Clock Drawing Test) was typical of Alzheimer's disease. The lower MMSE score and slightly younger age of presentation may reflect a more aggressive amyloid load. Physicians may consider escalating the dose of rivastigmine in the event of worsening cognitive function.

Considering the typical pattern of cognitive deterioration in Alzheimer's disease, with higher cognitive functions (e.g., executive functions) and short-term memory often being impacted early, Ms Ng's overall functional levels were satisfactory. Her strengths include insight into her cognitive decline, which can be used as a motivating factor to encourage participation in various cognitively stimulating activities and to ensure compliance with treatment and interventions. The fact that she plays card games with neighbours every day is also a strength, suggesting an active social life and a potential support network, which should be maintained and enhanced. With the new routine of going to a day care centre two days per week, care should be taken to ensure the existing social connection with her neighbours is not disrupted. The primary care team should also be sensitive to the possible negative psychological impacts associated with self-awareness of deterioration, which may include anxiety, depression, and adjustment problems. Managing Ms Ng's and her family's realistic expectations about intervention outcomes, while fostering a sense of hope and control, would be important elements in her care.

Case 027 Refusing to Draw

Ms Kong, an 84-year-old lady, presented with concerns raised by her granddaughter about her memory problems. Her memory decline was noted for about two years, when she started to show forgetfulness about the conversations she had with others and needed to look frequently for personal belongings.

Findings from Screening Assessments by Allied Healthcare and Social Care Team

Cognitive functioning	Scored 13/30 on MMSE: results suggested cognitive impairment, after adjusting for education level. Ms Kong was significantly impaired in orientation to time (0/5), calculation (1/5), visuospatial relationships (0/1), and delayed recall (0/3); she showed some impairments in orientation to place (3/5) and had slight difficulties in three-step commands (2/3) and language (4/5). Her performance was, however, normal in registration (3/3). The Clock Drawing Test was not completed: she refused to draw or copy the clock after starting (Figure 2.21).
ADL/IADL	She was assisted in ADLs (Barthel Index 83/100). She had difficulties in getting dressed and would mix up clean and dirty clothes. She also had slight difficulties using the stairs because of foot pain. She was generally dry in both daytime and night-time, but would have occasional accidents for bladder and bowel control. She needed supervision in taking medications and assistance in laundry, housekeeping, grocery shopping, and using phones. She was also unable to cook (Lawton IADL Scale 28/56, assisted in IADLs).

Depressive symptoms	Scored 2/15 on GDS-15, no depressive mood was found.
Staging and clinical rating	Scored 2/3 on Clinical Dementia Rating, indicating moderate dementia. She showed moderate impairment in orientation, home and hobbies, and personal care and mild impairment in memory, judgement and problem-solving, and community affairs.

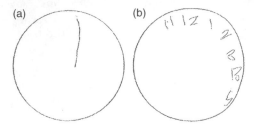

Figure 2.21 Findings from Ms Kong's Clock Drawing Test. (a) Clock Drawing (3 o'clock). (b) Clock Copying (10 past 10)

History Taken with Carer by Primary Care Physician

Ms Kong's granddaughter reported noticing memory problems in her grandmother that had concerned her for about two years, although no delusional ideations were reported. Using the GPCOG Informant Interview, the following areas were noted to show more difficulties (×) or were preserved (○) compared to about two years ago:

× Remembering recent events
× Recalling recent conversations
× Word finding
× Managing money and finances
× Managing medication independently
× Using transport

There were no additional clinical features to consider for non-Alzheimer's dementia. Ms Kong has hypertension. She has gout and would have foot pain occasionally, although she can walk unaided. No family history of psychiatric disorders or dementia was reported. She did not receive any education.

Physical Examination Findings

General examination revealed no affect or hygiene problem. Ms Kong had a blood pressure reading of 130/76 mm Hg. No other CVS or CNS findings.

Diagnosis

Alzheimer's disease.

Management

Rivastigmine transdermal system 4.6 mg daily was prescribed. Ms Kong was also recommended to join a specialised day care service for two days per week, with a structured and tailored intervention programme and cognitively stimulating activities to delay deterioration.

Suggestions for the Primary Care Team

This is a typical case of early Alzheimer's disease, in which a cholinesterase inhibitor is indicated. Ms Kong presented at a typical age of symptom onset for Alzheimer's disease, with a usual duration of retrospective onset of symptoms dating back to around two years ago. Her MMSE score was lower than expected, although the impairment pattern was in keeping with Alzheimer's disease, with the Clock Drawing Test also showing a pattern of worse performance in the drawing part than the copying part. Her Barthel Index score was lower than expected for her stage of Alzheimer's disease and may reflect physical frailty. The primary care team should pay attention to the interaction between physical and cognitive frailty in the presentation of Alzheimer's disease.

While Ms Kong's functional level in general reflected the common functional profile of people with Alzheimer's disease, her self-care impairment appeared to be worse than expected for her stage. The primary care team should investigate further the underlying cause(s) of the specific impairments, paying attention to possible motivational factors, physical frailty, premorbid daily habits, and roles. The Clinical Dementia Rating results suggested a moderate stage, which was based heavily on the carer's subjective report, and the primary care team may also explore the possibility that Ms Kong has become accustomed to being cared for by others, which could result in a lower level of functional performance than her actual functioning potential. A scheduled daily routine may be considered, which would also help prevent or reduce confusion in the later stages of the disease.

Case 028   Never Went to School

Ms Cheung, an 85-year-old lady, presented with concerns raised by her daughter-in-law about her memory over the last two years: she was noted to be unable to find her way home and got lost once, and she was unable to recognise her daughter and grandchildren. Ms Cheung was aware of her own memory decline.

Findings from Screening Assessments by Allied Healthcare and Social Care Team

Cognitive functioning	Scored 14/30 on MMSE: results indicative of cognitive impairment, after adjusting for education level. Ms Cheung's performance was impaired in orientation to time (2/5) and place (3/5), three-step commands (1/3), calculation (0/5), delayed recall (0/3), and visuospatial relationships (0/1). Her performance was, however, normal in registration (3/3) and language (5/5). The Clock Drawing Test was not completed: she refused to draw due to illiteracy. She had slight difficulties in reading the clock: she read a clock that showed 10:10 as 11:15 on the first attempt and changed her answer to 2 o'clock on the second attempt.
ADL/IADL	Ms Cheung was semi-independent in ADLs (Barthel Index 87/100). She has weakness in both her upper and lower limbs. She was also unable to select appropriate clothing according to the weather. Ms Cheung was assisted in IADLs (Lawton IADL Scale 30/56): she was dependent in meal preparation, laundry, housekeeping, and handling finances; she needed company for community access (she got lost once in the community) and grocery shopping.

| Depressive symptoms | Scored 7/15 on GDS-15, obvious depressive mood was noted. |
| Staging and clinical rating | Scored 1/3 on Clinical Dementia Rating, indicating mild dementia. She showed mild impairment in memory, orientation, judgement and problem-solving, community affairs, home and hobbies, and personal care. |

History Taken with Carer by Primary Care Physician

Ms Cheung's daughter-in-law reported noticing memory problems in her mother that had concerned her for about two years, although no delusional ideations were reported. Using the GPCOG Informant Interview, the following areas were noted to show more difficulties (×) or were preserved (○) compared to about two years ago:

× Remembering recent events
× Recalling recent conversations
× Word finding
× Managing money and finances
× Managing medication independently
× Using transport

There were no additional clinical features to consider for non-Alzheimer's dementia. Ms Cheung was reported to have depressive symptoms by her family member. She is currently on a calcium supplement. No family history of psychiatry disorders or dementia was reported. She did not receive any education. She was living alone, even though she was unable to take care of herself.

Physical Examination Findings

General examination revealed no affect or hygiene problem. Ms Cheung's blood pressure was 142/78 mm Hg. No other CVS or CNS findings.

Investigations

CBP, ESR, R/LFT, calcium, VDRL, vitamin B_{12}, fasting sugar, MSU × R/M, and culture test were ordered.

Diagnosis

Moderate Alzheimer's disease with a depressive mood.

Management

Ms Cheung was recommended to join a specialised day care service for two days per week, with a structured and tailored intervention programme and cognitively stimulating activities to delay deterioration.

Suggestions for the Primary Care Team

Ms Cheung's presentation was compatible with moderate Alzheimer's disease. She presented at a typical age of symptom onset for Alzheimer's disease, with two years of symptom presentation in retrospect. Her MMSE results showed a usual pattern of impairment. However, her physical functioning was quite impaired, and she was unable to take care of herself. In view of the presence of an obvious depressive mood, depression should be treated at this stage. Ms Cheung has probable dementia and depression, a combination that is not uncommon in older people. In this case the potential interaction between depression and Alzheimer's disease, and the timing of their respective onsets, should be noted. In Ms Cheung's case, if the symptoms of depression and those of Alzheimer's disease occurred within two years of each other, the two conditions may have shared neural substrates and could be part of the same disease process. Physicians can prescribe both cholinesterase inhibitors and antidepressants in one go. Alternatively, physicians can consider treating her depression first, while paying attention to any changes in her cognitive symptoms, and use a concomitant cholinesterase inhibitor if there is no improvement in cognition. The primary care team should also monitor Ms Cheung's weakness of the limbs and check for abnormalities in blood tests.

Ms Cheung's ADL was worse than expected, which may be attributable to her depressive mood and low motivation. It may also be a result of other physical discomforts or weakness instead of her cognitive impairment. While Ms Cheung may be unfit to be living alone and social support is obviously needed to maintain her living in the community, it is possible that she may not be receptive to the arrangement of having a carer or domestic helper at home. In that case, other suitable long-term care services and facilities in the community should be explored. The primary care team should discuss the options with the family, providing advice that balances the needs of Ms Cheung and the family carer(s), after a detailed assessment considering the interplay between cognition, mood, and physical factors.

Case 029 Cognitive vs Clinical Assessment Findings

Ms Yau, an 89-year-old lady, presented with concerns raised by her son about her memory problems for the past six months. She was noted to be forgetful, with poor short-term memory and was unable to recognise her grandchildren. Ms Yau was aware of her own memory decline.

Findings from Screening Assessments by Allied Healthcare and Social Care Team

Cognitive functioning	Scored 11/30 on MMSE: results indicate cognitive impairment, after adjusting for education level. Ms Yau's performance was impaired in orientation to time (0/5), delayed recall (0/3), visuospatial relationships (0/1), and calculation (1/5); she showed difficulties in recalling the residual sum; she showed some problems in orientation to place (2/5) and had slight difficulties in language (4/5). The Clock Drawing Test was not completed: she refused to draw, claiming that she was illiterate. She was, however, able to read the clock, although she was slow in response.
ADL/IADL	She was independent in most ADLs (Barthel Index 92/100), although because of knee pain she needed longer to finish the tasks. She occasionally needed reminding to take medications; she cannot remember phone numbers, but was still able to travel within the community, such as going to the aged care centre (Lawton IADL Scale 48/56).
Depressive symptoms	Scored 1/15 on GDS-15, no obvious depressive mood was noted.

Staging and clinical rating	Scored 1/3 on Clinical Dementia Rating, indicating mild dementia. She showed moderate impairment in memory and orientation, and mild impairment in judgement and problem-solving, and in home and hobbies.

History Taken with Carer by Primary Care Physician

Ms Yau's son reported noticing memory problems in his mother that had concerned him for about half a year, although no delusional ideations were reported. Using the GPCOG Informant Interview, the following areas were noted to show more difficulties (×) or were preserved (○) compared to about two years ago:

× Remembering recent events
× Recalling recent conversations
○ Word finding
× Managing money and finances
× Managing medication independently
○ Using transport

There were no additional clinical features to consider for non-Alzheimer's dementia. Ms Yau has diabetes, hypertension, and gout. No family history of psychiatric disorders or dementia was reported. She did not receive any education. She was living alone and able to walk independently with a stick.

Physical Examination Findings

General examination revealed no affect or hygiene problem. Ms Yau's blood pressure was 160/70 mm Hg. No other CVS or CNS findings.

Diagnosis

Mild to moderate Alzheimer's disease.

Management

Ms Yau was recommended to join a specialised day care service for two days per week for two years, with a structured and tailored intervention programme and cognitively stimulating activities to delay deterioration.

Suggestions for the Primary Care Team

What is notable in this case is the relatively short time (approximately six months) of symptom presentation before help-seeking by a carer, which is unusual in Alzheimer's disease given the often insidious nature of cognitive and functional decline. While treating Ms Yau as having mild to moderate Alzheimer's disease, with the use of a cholinesterase inhibitor, neuroimaging such as MRI is indicated to look for other comorbid conditions and investigate if this is a case of pure Alzheimer's disease. It is not uncommon for cognitive deterioration to go unnoticed by family carers, especially when the cognitive deterioration or signs and symptoms of dementia may be masked by a high level of independence in ADL or IADL: in Ms Yau's case, her high functional status appeared to be relatively unaffected by her cognitive impairment. Her low education level may also have lowered the expectations for her cognitive performance by her carers. Therefore, it is also possible that Ms Yau's cognitive symptoms had an onset much earlier than six months, although the help-seeking was delayed due to symptom masking and low expectations combined with a low level of awareness.

Good self-care ability despite cognitive impairment is commonly seen, especially among those who have a long-standing independent living style and reside in a familiar environment and community, with well-established habits and routines. If these factors remain unchanged, Ms Yau will be able to continue to take good care of herself for a long period of time, which is a strength and a good prognostic factor. The primary care team should nevertheless pay attention to potential safety concerns: although Ms Yau currently has no problem using transportation and is able to go out in familiar places, there is a risk of her getting lost in the future. She should therefore be accompanied when going out and/or have a location-tracking device in place to minimise such a risk.

Case 030 Reasons for Reduced Independence

Mr Hung, an 80-year-old gentleman, was recently noted to have memory deterioration by a social worker in his housing estate. He was reported to have poor short-term memory, appeared forgetful, and was becoming more and more confused recently. Mr Hung was aware of his own memory problems.

Findings from Screening Assessments by Allied Healthcare and Social Care Team

Cognitive functioning	Scored 19/30 on MMSE: results indicative of cognitive impairment, adjusted for education level. Mr Hung's performance was impaired in three-step commands (1/3), calculation (1/5), delayed recall (1/3), and visuospatial relationships (0/1); he had some problems in orientation to time (3/5); his performance was, however, normal in orientation to place (5/5), registration (3/3), and language (5/5). The Clock Drawing Test was not completed: he could not draw because of hand tremor and gave up in the middle of an attempt. He was able to read the clock; he was also aware of his mistake when told (Figure 2.22).
ADL/IADL	He was independent in most ADLs (Barthel Index 92/100), although completion of the tasks may take longer due to asthma and lower limb weakness. He needed assistance from his wife in bathing, because he was slow in the process, and his wife was worried about him getting cold. He was independent in most IADLs, except that he needed occasional reminders to take medications (Lawton IADL Scale 55/56).
Depressive symptoms	Scored 0/15 on GDS-15, no depressive mood was noted.
Staging and clinical rating	Staging and clinical rating was not completed as Mr Hung attended the assessment session unaccompanied by a carer/informant.

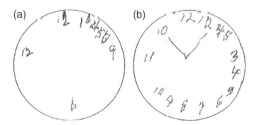

Figure 2.22 Findings from Mr Hung's Clock Drawing Test. (a) Clock Drawing (3 o'clock). (b) Clock Copying (10 past 10)

History Taken with Carer by Primary Care Physician

Mr Hung's wife reported that she did not notice any memory problems in her husband. No delusional ideations were reported. Using the GPCOG Informant Interview, the following areas were noted to show more difficulties (✘) or were preserved (○) compared to about two years ago:

○ Remembering recent events
○ Recalling recent conversations
○ Word finding
○ Managing money and finances
○ Managing medication independently
○ Using transport

There were no additional clinical features to consider for non-Alzheimer's dementia. Mr Hung has asthma and benign prostatic hyperplasia. He is currently on prazosin 1 mg daily, salbutamol two puffs three times a day, beclometasone dipropionate two puffs twice a day, and ipratropium bromide two puffs three times a day. No family history of psychiatric disorders or dementia was reported. He received education to P.6 (approximately six years of education). He was able to walk independently with a cane. He has limited social activity except for sitting outside a nearby supermarket to chat with friends.

Physical Examination Findings

General examination revealed no affect or hygiene problem. No CVS or CNS findings.

Investigations

No investigation was ordered as Mr Hung refused blood taking or a CT brain scan.

Diagnosis

Early Alzheimer's disease.

Management

Rivastigmine transdermal system 4.6 mg daily was prescribed. Mr Hung was also recommended to join a specialised day care service for two days per week for two years, with a structured and tailored intervention programme and cognitively stimulating activities to delay deterioration.

Suggestions for the Primary Care Team

This is a typical case of mild Alzheimer's disease. Mr Hung presented at a common age of symptom onset for Alzheimer's disease, and his impairment pattern was also typical. Although he could not complete the Clock Drawing Test due to hand tremor, there was evidence of impaired executive function and abstract thinking, and his assessment results were largely in keeping with the usual profile of early Alzheimer's disease. What can be noted in this case is that Mr Hung has chronic obstructive pulmonary disease, and this case illustrates how the chronic illness may aggravate and complicate his cognitive impairment. In the same vein, the intervention and care plan should therefore focus also on maintaining a stable physical condition for Mr Hung, which can be equally important as intervening for his cognitive functions.

This case also illustrated the potentially important role of social workers or other personnel in detecting cognitive impairment in the community. In Mr Hung's case, his wife might not have been able to recognise the signs and symptoms of early dementia due to low awareness: relying on the Clinical Dementia Rating or GPCOG alone, the primary care team may not have been able to detect the cognitive impairment until a later stage. While public education would help to promote early detection, education targeting potential 'gatekeepers' other than family carers (e.g., a social worker in this case) is also an important strategy and can be part of a triage system for cases needing diagnosis and further intervention in a dementia-friendly community. Such needs may be particularly profound for people living alone or with an older spouse only (who may also need care and support).

2.3 Indications for Investigations

Case 031 Apraxia in Self-Care

Mrs Ko, an 82-year-old lady, presented with concerns raised by her daughter-in-law about her memory problems. She was noted to have poor short-term memory, such as forgetting about what she had eaten a while ago, and repeatedly looking for items.

Findings from Screening Assessments by Allied Healthcare and Social Care Team

Cognitive functioning	Scored 11/30 on MMSE: results indicating cognitive impairment, adjusted for education level. Mrs Ko's performance was impaired in orientation to time (1/5) and place (1/5), delayed recall (0/3), calculation (0/5), and visuospatial relationships (0/1); she had slight problems in language (4/5) and three-step commands (2/3). Her performance was, however, normal in registration (3/3). The Clock Drawing Test showed significant impairment: she was only able to write the numbers 1–3 independently; her performance improved slightly in the copying part (Figure 2.23).
ADL/IADL	Mrs Ko required minor assistance for bathing and getting dressed (e.g., she may forget how to turn on the water heater for bathing or to choose appropriate clothing, although she was able to choose when given a limited number of choices); she also required a little help for ambulation and stair climbing due to her physical condition. She was independent in other ADL tasks (Barthel Index 90/100). She was dependent in taking medication, handling finances, and shopping; she needed assistance in meal preparation, laundry, housekeeping (simple chores), and community access; and she needed supervision in external communication (able to pick up calls only) (Lawton IADL Score 20/56).
Depressive symptoms	Scored 0/15 on GDS-15, no obvious depressive mood was found.
Staging and clinical rating	Results suggested a Global Deterioration Scale stage 5, indicating moderate dementia. During the interview, she was unable to recall a major relevant aspect of her current life (e.g., home address or with whom she lived) and showed frequent disorientation to time or to place.

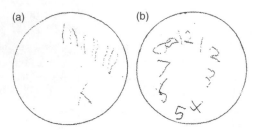

Figure 2.23 Findings from Mrs Ko's Clock Drawing Test. (a) Clock Drawing (3 o'clock). (b) Clock Copying (10 past 10)

History Taken with Carer by Primary Care Physician

Mrs Ko's daughter-in-law reported noticing memory problems in Mrs Ko that had concerned her for about three years, although no delusional ideations were reported. Using the GPCOG Informant Interview, the following areas were noted to show more difficulties (✗) or were preserved (○) compared to about two years ago:

- ✗ Remembering recent events
- ✗ Recalling recent conversations
- ○ Word finding
- ✗ Managing money and finances
- ✗ Managing medication independently
- ✗ Using transport

Mrs Ko may have apraxia in self-care, which might be a clinical feature to consider for non-Alzheimer's dementia. Mrs Ko has hypertension. No family history of psychiatric disorders or dementia was reported. Her exact education level cannot be ascertained, although she probably had less than six months of education.

Investigations

CT brain and MRI scans revealed cerebral atrophy with atrophic changes in medial temporal lobe.

Diagnosis

Alzheimer's disease.

Management

Donepezil 5 mg daily was prescribed. Mrs Ko was recommended to join an 18-month, centre-based programme with cognitively stimulating activities for the maintenance of cognitive function and quality of life; carer education was also provided with advice for adjusting activities to support Mrs Ko's continued participation and engagement in daily activities.

Suggestions for the Primary Care Team

Mrs Ko presented at a common age of symptom onset for Alzheimer's disease, with a typical impairment pattern: her performance was impaired in higher cognitive functions (such as executive function) and short-term memory, intact in attention and language, and she was able to follow instructions. Her ADL performance was much better than her IADLs. These presentations are compatible with the usual profile of Alzheimer's disease, while her low Barthel Index score would put her in the moderate stage. Mrs Ko's MMSE score was on the low side, with a slightly longer-than-usual delay in help-seeking (three years, compared to a median of one year in the same early intervention service). The reasons for the delay should be explored, including low awareness of the carer or infrequent interaction, which should be addressed in the care plan (e.g., carer education and family/social support).

Mrs Ko was able to maintain her ADL functioning with only minimal assistance needed, which should be considered her strength. Equipping her carers with the suitable skills to engage Mrs Ko in daily living activities should be a priority at this stage, which would help to reduce the risk of confusion and the development of distressed behaviours and neuropsychiatric symptoms of dementia: the latter may involve the rejection of care and refusal of ADL tasks, for example, refusal of bathing.

Apraxia in self-care is common in moderate Alzheimer's disease. In Mrs Ko's case, the apraxia may be linked with temporal lobe degeneration, although this is less likely considering that her ADLs were not grossly impaired. It may nevertheless be worth further investigation and clarification to inform her care plan.

Case 032 Comorbid Anaemia

Mrs Lau, an 88-year-old lady, presented with concerns raised by her daughter related to her memory problems over the last three years. Her daughter complained about Mrs Lau's repeated questioning.

Findings from Screening Assessments by Allied Healthcare and Social Care Team

Cognitive functioning	Scored 18/30 on MMSE, suggestive of cognitive impairment after adjusting for education level. Mrs Lau's performance was impaired in calculation (0/5) and delayed recall (1/3); she had slight problems in orientation to time (3/5) and place (4/5), language (4/5), and three-step commands (2/3). Her performance was, however, normal in registration (3/3) and visuospatial relationships (1/1). Impairment was observed in the Clock Drawing Test, with improvement in the copying part (Figure 2.24).
ADL/IADL	Mrs Lau was independent in ADLs (Barthel Index 100/100). She needed supervision on community access, handling finances, and grocery shopping; she has modified independence in taking medication; she was independent in other IADLs (Lawton IADL Scale: 49/56).
Staging and clinical rating	Results suggested a Global Deterioration Scale stage 4, indicating mild dementia. She showed decreased knowledge of current and recent events, a concentration deficit elicited on the serial subtraction task, a decreased ability to travel and handle finances, and an inability to perform complex tasks.

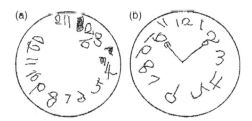

Figure 2.24 Findings from Mrs Lau's Clock Drawing Test. (a) Clock Drawing (3 o'clock). (b) Clock Copying (10 past 10)

History Taken with Carer by Primary Care Physician

Mrs Lau's daughter reported noticing memory problems in her mother that had concerned her for three to four years, although no delusional ideations were reported. No distressed behaviours and neuropsychiatric symptoms of dementia were noted. Using the GPCOG Informant Interview, the following areas were noted to show more difficulties (×) or were preserved (○) compared to about two years ago:

× Remembering recent events
× Recalling recent conversations
○ Word finding
× Managing money and finances
× Managing medication independently
× Using transport

There were no additional clinical features to consider for non-Alzheimer's dementia. Mrs Lau has macrocytic anaemia and left carotid bruit and was having follow-up consultations at a geriatric medicine outpatient clinic in hospital for her anaemia. No family history of psychiatric disorders or dementia was reported. She has never received any education and was noted to have poor social support.

Investigations

CBP, ESR, R/LFT, calcium, vitamin B_{12}, and folate were ordered. All investigations were normal except for globulin 40, B_{12} 178, and TSH 0.58. MRI revealed MTLA R = 7.8, L = 8.7, Scheltens score R = L = 2, ARWMC 3/3, and GCA scale 2.

Diagnosis

Early Alzheimer's disease with small vessel disease.

Management

A daily dosage of donepezil 5 mg and mecobalamin 500 μg was prescribed. She was also recommended to join a centre-based programme with cognitively stimulating activities for 18 months to maintain cognitive functions and quality of life and was encouraged to have regular exercise, a healthy diet, and mental stimulation, manage stress, and develop an active social life.

Suggestions for the Primary Care Team

This is a case with the typical impairment pattern of early Alzheimer's disease. Mrs Lau showed intact visuospatial ability on MMSE (interlocking pentagon), but her Clock Drawing Test was positive, suggesting an early stage of dementia with impaired executive functions and other higher cognitive functions. Her short-term memory was beginning to show impairment, although her functioning was still satisfactory in general. Physicians should note that white matter disease is a known risk factor for Alzheimer's disease (3). In Mrs Lau's case, there is a significant comorbidity of anaemia; although her CBC was normal, considering that she is being followed up at a geriatric clinic for anaemia, there are uncertainties regarding the contribution of white matter pathology to her cognitive impairment, which needs to be clarified.

Considering that her symptoms were first noticed three to four years ago, help-seeking in Mrs Lau's case was a little later than usual (compared to a median of one year in the same early intervention service). The best time to equip Mrs Lau with skills to self-manage the insidious deterioration, which is during the symptom onset phase, would have been missed; nevertheless, she was still quite independent in her ADLs and IADLs. The primary care team can make use of her remaining memory and cognitive functioning ability and try to use reminders, cues, and adaptive aids in maintaining her independence, such as using an alarm clock with an audio reminder function for daily scheduling and organising her belongings in a way that items can be easily found. This is also a good time to discuss with Mrs Lau and her family a future care plan, although the team should pay attention to her mood and any post-diagnostic depressive and/or anxiety symptoms that may occur.

Case 033 History of Small Vessel Disease

Mrs Hung, a 70-year-old lady, presented with concerns raised by her husband over her memory problems. She was noted to be forgetful about grocery items, the content of conversations, and having problems in handling her medications.

Findings from Screening Assessments by Allied Healthcare and Social Care Team

Cognitive functioning	Scored 21/30 on MMSE, indicating cognitive impairment after adjusting for her education level. Mrs Hung's performance was impaired in delayed recall (0/3) and visuospatial relationships (0/1); she had slight problems in orientation to time (3/5) and place (4/5), calculation (4/5), and three-step commands (2/3). Her performance was, however, normal in registration (3/3) and language (5/5). The Clock Drawing Test showed incorrect denotation of time with correct number placement.
ADL/IADL	Mrs Hung was independent in ADLs (Barthel Index 100/100). She needed assistance in taking medication (prepared by her husband) and housekeeping (done by her husband); she needed supervision in community access and had modified independence in handling finances (bills managed by her husband and pocket money given by her son); she was independent in other IADLs (Lawton IADL Scale 45/56).
Depressive symptoms	Scored 0/15 on GDS-15, no obvious depressive mood was found.
Staging and clinical rating	Results suggested a Global Deterioration Scale stage 4, indicating mild dementia. A concentration deficit was elicited on serial subtractions.

History Taken with Carer by Primary Care Physician

Mrs Hung's husband reported noticing memory problems in his wife that had concerned him for about three years. No delusional ideations were reported. Using the GPCOG Informant Interview, the following areas were noted to show more difficulties (✗) or were preserved (○) compared to about two years ago:

✗ Remembering recent events
✗ Recalling recent conversations
○ Word finding
○ Managing money and finances

✗ Managing medication independently
○ Using transport

There were no additional clinical features to consider for non-Alzheimer's dementia. Mrs Hung has gout and hypercholesterolaemia. An MRI scan performed the previous year revealed small vessel disease and mild cortical atrophy, with an MTA score of 2. No family history of psychiatric disorders or dementia was reported. Her education level was unclear, although it is known that she had received more than two years of education. .

Investigations

CBP, R/LFT, calcium, VDRL, vitamin B_{12}, folate, ECG, and TSH were ordered.

Diagnosis

Early Alzheimer's disease.

Management

Mrs Hung was recommended to join a centre-based programme with cognitively stimulating activities for 18 months to maintain her cognitive function and quality of life. She was also encouraged to have regular exercise, a healthy diet, and mental stimulation, manage stress, and maintain an active social life.

Suggestions for the Primary Care Team

Mrs Hung is relatively young for the presentation of symptoms of Alzheimer's disease. While her impairment pattern was typical of Alzheimer's disease, the primary care team can also watch out for symptoms that may suggest other types of dementia in subsequent follow-ups. For Alzheimer's disease to present at this younger age around the 70s, it is possible that a heavy amyloid load is present, which can no longer be masked by the person's cognitive reserve. Meanwhile, Mrs Hung's medication treatment can start off with a low dose of cholinesterase inhibitor, such as donepezil 2.5 mg daily, while the primary care team monitors her progress.

Mrs Hung has quite satisfactory performance in various cognitive functions, except for an obvious impairment in short-term memory. Her ADL was also good and should be maintained as far as possible: the primary care team could equip her carers with appropriate caring skills for ADL maintenance, for example, by providing verbal reminders or guidance when Mrs Hung became 'clumsier' in her daily living activities, instead of discouraging her attempts and providing direct help with all ADL tasks too early. Mrs Hung's IADL performance was worse than expected for her age and disease stage; one possible reason is that she might have been well cared for by her husband over a long time, which could have built up a habit of relying on others; in such a case, the care could become a barrier to active participation, leading to a lower level of perform- ance than her actual ability or potential, or 'excess disability'. The primary care team should guide her husband on how to empower and increase Mrs Hung's interest and engagement in IADL tasks. The team should also assess carer stress and the mood of Mrs Hung's husband and prepare him for the foreseeable increase in his caring role and task demands in the future. The possibility that it may eventually become overwhelming for him to be handling all care by himself should be mentioned. This is an important stage to start a family review and planning for supportive services and future care.

Case 034 CT Evidence of Small Vessel Ischaemia

Mrs Lai, an 84-year-old lady, presented with concerns raised by her son over her memory problems. She was noted to be forgetful about grocery items when shopping, misplacing items and accusing her son of taking them, showing a decline in finding her way, and having low motivation in meal preparation. A cognitive assessment done the previous year showed an MMSE score of 14/30 with results suggesting possible early dementia.

Findings from Screening Assessments by Allied Healthcare and Social Care Team

Cognitive functioning	Scored 13/30 on MMSE: results indicated cognitive impairment, adjusted for education level. Mrs Lai's performance was impaired in recall (0/3; cannot recall even with cues), calculation (0/5), visuospatial relationships (0/1), orientation to place (1/5), and three-step commands (1/3); she was slightly impaired in orientation to time (3/5). Her performance was, however, normal in registration (3/3) and language (5/5). The Clock Drawing Test showed abnormal clock face drawing with inaccurate time denotation, suggestive of executive function deficits, which showed improvement in the clock copying task (Figure 2.25).
ADL/IADL	Mrs Lai was independent in ADLs (Barthel Index 100/100). For IADLs, she required supervision in taking medication, community access, and handling finances; she was modified independent in meal preparation (she was able to cook a simple dinner and would usually eat out for lunch), housekeeping, and grocery shopping (she would sometimes buy the same item repeatedly) (Lawton IADL Scale: 46/56).
Staging and clinical rating	Results suggest a Global Deterioration Scale stage 4, indicating early dementia. She showed decreased knowledge of current and recent events; exhibited some deficits in remembering her personal history and a deficit in concentration elicited on serial subtractions; she was also noted to have a decreased ability to travel and handle finances. She denied having these deficits.

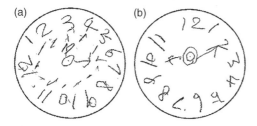

Figure 2.25 Findings from Mrs Lai's Clock Drawing Test. (a) Clock Drawing (3 o'clock). (b) Clock Copying (10 past 10)

History Taken with Carer by Primary Care Physician

Mrs Lai's son reported noticing memory problems in his mother that had concerned him for about one to two years. Delusional ideations were reported. Compared to two years ago, using the GPCOG Informant Interview, the following areas were noted to show more difficulties (✗) or were preserved (○) compared to about two years ago:

✗ Remembering recent events

✗ Recalling recent conversations

× Word finding
× Managing money and finances
× Managing medication independently
× Using transport

There were no additional clinical features to consider for non-Alzheimer's dementia. Mrs Lai has hypertension, bilateral cataract (right eye operated), hysterectomy, lumbar spinal degeneration, and osteoarthritis of the knee. No family history of psychiatric disorders or dementia was reported. There is no clear information about her education level, although she probably has received more than two years of education. Mrs Lai lives alone.

Investigations

CBP, ESR, R/LFT, calcium, VDRL, vitamin B_{12}, folate, fasting sugar, fasting lipids, CXR, and ECG were ordered. CT brain (plain) scan revealed cerebral atrophy, changes in small vessel ischemia, a GCA score of 2, and an MTA score of 1.

Diagnosis

Early Alzheimer's disease.

Management

Aspirin 80 mg daily, famotidine 20 mg daily, and donepezil 5 mg daily were prescribed. She was recommended to join a centre-based programme with cognitively stimulating activities for 18 months for the maintenance of cognitive functions and quality of life.

Suggestions for the Primary Care Team

This is a case with a typical presentation of early Alzheimer's disease. The primary care physician should note that, although small vessel disease was present on the CT scan, it does not automatically equate with mixed dementia. Considering her typical age of presentation, her MMSE score was lower than expected; this could be due to the small vessel disease accelerating or intensifying Alzheimer's disease. Cholinesterase inhibitors can be prescribed in the event of declining cognition in subsequent follow-ups. The primary care team can also investigate further the detailed results and recommendations from the assessment done one year ago and explore the motivation for the current repeated assessment. The motivation would suggest key areas of concern and thus possible priorities in management and care planning.

Mrs Lai's community living ability appeared to be much higher than expected given her poor cognitive performance. It is a strength that, at present, her functional level can be maintained at a satisfactory level. Her premorbid lifestyle may be a factor contributing to her current high daily functioning. However, considering that Mrs Lai is living alone with cognitive impairment, which will worsen further, safety precautions are important while supporting Mrs Lai to continue performing the existing ADL and IADL tasks. Supportive tools or devices such as location-tracking devices, audio cues, and reminders (e.g., for turning off a fire/water tap) should be used. Carers may also provide reminders by phone calls and seek help from shopkeepers in the neighbourhood to manage her behaviour of repeatedly buying the same items.

Case 035 Comorbid Depression

Mrs So, a 73-year-old lady, presented with concerns raised by her daughter over her memory problems. Her daughter complained of Mrs So's poor memory (e.g., with money frequently going missing) and decline in other cognitive functions; distressed behaviours and neuropsychiatric symptoms of dementia were reported: she was noted to be suspicious about her children stealing her money. Mrs So was also noted to appear depressed.

Findings from Screening Assessments by Allied Healthcare and Social Care Team

Cognitive functioning	Scored 17/30 on MMSE: results indicated cognitive impairment, adjusted for education level. Mrs So's performance was impaired in delayed recall (0/3), visuospatial relationships (0/1), calculation (1/5), and three-step commands (1/3); she was slightly impaired in orientation to time (3/5) and language (4/5). Her performance was, however, normal in place orientation (5/5) and registration (3/3). Her Clock Drawing Test results were positive, with little improvement in the copying task compared with the drawing task (Figure 2.26).
ADL/IADL	Mrs So needed moderate help with urinary continence and a little help in stair climbing; she was independent in other ADLs (Barthel Index 93/100). She needed assistance in taking medications, meal preparation, community access, handling finances, and grocery shopping; she required supervision in external communication (Lawton IADL Scale 34/56).
Depressive symptoms	Scored 11/15 on GDS-15, results indicating significant depressive mood.
Staging and clinical rating	Results suggested a Global Deterioration Scale stage 4, indicating mild dementia. She showed decreased knowledge of current and recent events; a decreased ability to travel and handle finances; and an inability to perform complex tasks.

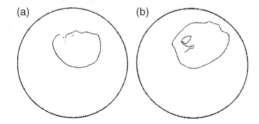

Figure 2.26 Findings from Mrs So's Clock Drawing Test. (a) Clock Drawing (3 o'clock). (b) Clock Copying (10 past 10)

History Taken with Carer by Primary Care Physician

Mrs So's daughter reported noticing memory problems in her mother that had concerned her for over a year. Delusional ideations were reported. Distressed behaviours and neuropsychiatric symptoms of dementia were reported: Mrs So was frequently suspicious about her children stealing her money, and she appeared to have a depressive mood. Using the GPCOG Informant Interview, the following areas were noted to show more difficulties (✗) or were preserved (○) compared to about two years ago:

× Remembering recent events
× Recalling recent conversations
○ Word finding
× Managing money and finances
× Managing medication independently
× Using transport

There were no additional clinical features to consider for non-Alzheimer's dementia. Mrs So has diabetes and hyperlipidaemia. No family history of psychiatric disorders or dementia was reported. There was no clear information on her education level, although it is likely that she received less than six months of education.

Investigations
ECG and CT brain (plain) scan were ordered.

Diagnosis
Mild dementia with irritability, anxiety, and depression.

Management
No medication was prescribed while awaiting the work-up results. Mrs So was recommended to join a centre-based programme with cognitively stimulating activities for 18 months to maintain cognitive, quality of life, and self-care functions; she was encouraged to have regular exercise, a healthy diet, and mental stimulation, and maintain an active social life.

Suggestions for the Primary Care Team
This is a case of mild Alzheimer's disease with depression. Primary care physicians should consider treating both conditions, using a cholinesterase inhibitor and a selective serotonin reuptake inhibitor. Mrs So's cognition, general functioning, and mood should be monitored. A multidisciplinary team can help in this difficult scenario with a relatively more complex disease profile. Mrs So's social background, especially her relationship with family members, should be further explored. This should include her family's reaction to her suspicion about them stealing her money and whether any psychosocial factors contributing to her depressive mood can be identified. The temporal sequence between dementia and depression is to be elucidated, which will inform treatment focus.

The younger-than-usual age of presentation in this case should also be noted. Mrs So presented with distressed behaviours and neuropsychiatric symptoms of dementia, delusion, and depression. The MMSE score is low, although a typical impairment pattern in keeping with Alzheimer's disease was noted. Visuospatial relationships is also impaired as shown in both MMSE (interlocking pentagon) and the Clock Drawing Test. These significant impairments may be a result of the complex interplay between Alzheimer's disease pathology, depression, and the content of the delusion. For example, the depressive mood and delusional ideation may be interrelated, with the possibility of the delusion about children stealing money from her triggering the depressive mood. If the primary care team could identify a root cause of the depressive mood and/or the delusional ideation, interventions to address the underlying cause may be possible (e.g., strategies to ensure a sense of security with her money), which could potentially lead to improvement in Mrs So's general functional performance. If non-pharmacological intervention and strategies targeting the root cause are not effective, physicians may consider the use of neuroleptics and referral for specialist attention.

Case 036 Diabetes, Depression, and Dementia

Mrs Lam, a 75-year-old lady, presented with concerns raised by her son over her memory problems. She was noted to have poor memory: she would misplace items and forget about important information or details of a conversation, had difficulty in word finding and way-finding, and showed slowness in processing information.

Findings from Screening Assessments by Allied Healthcare and Social Care Team

Cognitive functioning	Scored 17/30 on MMSE, indicating cognitive impairment, adjusted for education level. Mrs Lam's performance was impaired in delayed recall (0/3), orientation to time (2/5) and place (2/5), and calculation (2/5); she had slight problems in three-step commands (2/3). Her performance was, however, normal in registration (3/3), language (5/5), and visuospatial relationships (1/1). The Clock Drawing Test showed slight errors in time denotation and the placement of clock arms (Figure 2.27).
ADL/IADL	Mrs Lam was independent in ADLs (Barthel Index 100/100). She was dependent in taking medication; needed assistance in meal preparation; and required supervision in external communication, community access, handling finances, and grocery shopping; she was modified independent in housekeeping (Lawton IADL Scale 37/56).
Depressive symptoms	Scored 2/15 on GDS-15, results showed no indication of depression. However, depression, irritability, and recent bereavement were reported by her son.
Staging and clinical rating	Results suggested a Global Deterioration Scale stage 4, indicating mild dementia. She showed a decreased ability to handle finances and perform complex tasks; a concentration deficit was elicited on serial subtractions.

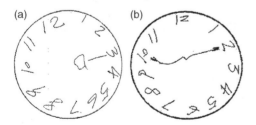

Figure 2.27 Findings from Mrs Lam's Clock Drawing Test. (a) Clock Drawing (3 o'clock). (b) Clock Copying (10 past 10)

History Taken with Carer by Primary Care Physician

Mrs Lam's son reported noticing memory problems in his mother that had concerned him for a few years. No delusional ideations were reported. According to her son, she loses her temper easily and becomes suspicious of others. Her mild depression could possibly be linked to her recent bereavement. Using the GPCOG Informant Interview, the following areas were noted to show more difficulties (✗) or were preserved (○) compared to about two years ago:

✗ Remembering recent events
✗ Recalling recent conversations
✗ Word finding

✗ Managing money and finances
○ Managing medication independently
○ Using transport

There were no additional clinical features to consider for non-Alzheimer's dementia. Mrs Lam has received diagnoses of diabetes and depression. She is currently on a daily dosage of metformin. No family history of psychiatric disorders or dementia was reported. She has never received any formal education.

Investigations

CBP, ESR, R/LFT, calcium, vitamin B_{12}, folate, and TSH were ordered. Results showed ESR 67 and normal in CBP, R/LFT, Ca/P, TSH, and vitamin B_{12}. MRI revealed MTL R = 0.67, L = 0.59, Scheltens R = 2 L = 3, ARWMC 1/3, and right frontal/occipital microhaemorrhage.

Diagnosis

Mild Alzheimer's disease with small vessel disease and mild depression.

Management

Rivastigmine transdermal system 5 mg daily was prescribed. Mrs Lam was encouraged to engage in physical, social, and cognitively stimulating activities. She was also recommended to join a centre-based programme with cognitively stimulating activities for 18 months to maintain cognitive functions and quality of life, although she refused the offer.

Suggestions for the Primary Care Team

This is a case presenting at a relatively younger age with a low MMSE score, with an impairment pattern typical of early Alzheimer's disease. The intact visuospatial ability shown in the interlocking pentagon task in MMSE versus impairment elicited on the Clock Drawing Test provided clues to a diagnosis of Alzheimer's disease. Depression and diabetes are both risk factors for dementia (4). Their treatment should be optimised, on top of a prescribing cholinesterase inhibitor, as part of her management. In view of Mrs Lam's mild depression, attention should be given to psychosocial factors contributing to it, while both the cognitive impairment and depression should be treated. Bereavement counselling and psychotherapy may be appropriate, even in the context of dementia and cognitive impairment.

Mrs Lam's cognitive assessment results showed that her cognitive impairment is still in its early stages. The primary care team can investigate further regarding the timing of the onset of the signs and symptoms of cognitive impairment in relation to her grieving. Possible relationships may include apparent cognitive deterioration due to depressive mood and low motivation; dementia triggered by a depressive episode; and depressive mood as a reaction to the delusional ideation caused by dementia. Her refusal of the centre-based service may also be reflective of her depressive mood, and the primary care team should consider ways to lower this resistance or barrier. By understanding the nature of their relations, an individualised intervention approach could be developed.

In Mrs Lam's case, it is also of note that the GDS-15 failed to pick up her depressive mood, which is not uncommon: the person may be unwilling to express their moods and feelings to a professional in a cognitive/memory clinic setting with little pre-existing rapport. For the early assessment team, the lesson here is to be sensitive and observant during the interview/assessment process, gather collateral information as far as possible, and ensure alliance and rapport during the session, while using standardised assessments as a tool to facilitate but not determine clinical judgement and discretion.

Case 037 Cholinesterase Inhibitors in an Atrial Fibrillation Patient

Ms Law, a 90-year-old lady, presented by her daughter with concerns about her memory problems, such as disorientation of time, repeated questioning, and poor sleep. These problems have lasted for about a year.

Findings from Screening Assessments by Allied Healthcare and Social Care Team

Cognitive functioning	Scored 11/30 on MMSE, indicating cognitive impairment, adjusted for education level. Ms Law's performance was impaired in orientation to time (1/5) and place (1/5), delayed recall (0/3), and calculation skills (0/3); she was unable to recall the number after computing minus seven and had slight difficulties in calculation, three-step commands (1/3), and visuospatial relationships (0/1). Her performance was, however, good in registration (3/3) and language (5/5). The Clock Drawing Test showed omission of time denotation in both drawing and copying parts, suggesting deficits in both executive function and visuospatial skills. She was, however, receptive to the test, considering her lack of formal education and inexperience with drawing (Figure 2.28).
ADL/IADL	She was semi-independent in ADLs (Barthel Index 76/100). She was mostly independent in IADLs but needed assistance due to lower limb weakness. She needed assistance in money management, outdoor activity, and meal preparation (Lawton IADL Scale 14/56).
Depressive symptoms	Scored 0/15 on GDS-15, no obvious depressive mood was noted.
Staging and clinical rating	Scored 1/3 on Clinical Dementia Rating, indicating mild dementia. She showed mild impairment in memory, orientation, and judgement and problem-solving.

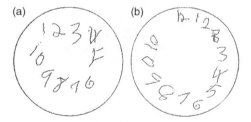

(a) (b)

Figure 2.28 Findings from Ms Law's Clock Drawing Test. (a) Clock Drawing (3 o'clock). (b) Clock Copying (10 past 10)

History Taken with Carer by Primary Care Physician

Ms Law's daughter reported noticing memory problems in her mother that had concerned her for about one year, although no delusional ideations were reported. Using the GPCOG Informant Interview, the following areas were noted to show more difficulties (×) or were preserved (○) compared to about two years ago:

× Remembering recent events
× Recalling recent conversations
× Word finding
× Managing money and finances
× Managing medication independently
× Using transport

There were no additional clinical features to consider for non-Alzheimer's dementia. Ms Law has atrial fibrillation, bilateral varicose veins, and a total knee replacement. She was noted to have lower limb weakness and is an outdoor wheelchair user. She was currently on digoxin 0.0625 mg daily, triamterene-hydrochlorothiazide daily, pantoprazole 20 mg daily, and apixaban 2.5 mg twice a day. No family history of psychiatric disorders was reported, although it is reported that Ms Law's sister has been diagnosed with dementia. She did not receive any education.

Physical Examination Findings

General examination revealed no affect or hygiene problem. In CVS examination, atrial fibrillation was found. No CNS findings.

Investigations

CBP, R/LFT, calcium, VDRL, vitamin B_{12}, fasting sugar, and fasting lipids were ordered. MRI investigation revealed severe global cortical atrophy.

Diagnosis

Alzheimer's disease.

Management

Donepezil 2.5 mg daily was prescribed. Ms Law was recommended to join a specialised day care service for two days per week to receive a structured and tailored intervention programme and cognitively stimulating activities to delay deterioration and to maintain quality of life.

Suggestions for the Primary Care Team

Considering that Ms Law has atrial fibrillation on digoxin, starting cholinesterase inhibitors at a low dose, such as donepezil 2.5 mg daily, is advisable, while observing the potential side effects of cholinesterase inhibitors. The most common side effects of cholinesterase inhibitors are gastrointestinal upset (such as reduced appetite) and - bradycardia. Physicians should be aware of the patient's baseline heart rate before prescribing cholinesterase inhibitors. Extra precaution is warranted in patients who are taking rate-controlling agents, such as digoxin, beta-blockers, and calcium channel blockers.

Ms Law presented at the age of 90 years, which is slightly older than the most common age of presentation. While her symptom pattern was compatible with Alzheimer's disease, hippocampal sclerosis (versus amyloid) pathology may be involved. Age-related cognitive frailty may play an important part in her cognitive impairment, although management as in Alzheimer's disease would be appropriate. The physical weakness and old age in this case should be considered in the care plan, including the assessment of physical discomfort, such as pain and soreness, to avoid further complications. Given the interaction between physical health and cognition, addressing physical discomfort and problems would often also have an effect on cognitive performance. The primary care team may also work with Ms Law and her family to target optimising moods and physical health, such as by encouraging participation in social gatherings, reminiscences, and other group activities that focus not only on cognitive enhancement, but are also enjoyable and promote positive experiences. Increased daytime engagement may also improve Ms Law's sleep.

Case 038 Alzheimer's Disease in a Stroke Patient

Mr Ho, a 78-year-old gentleman, presented with concerns raised by his daughter about his memory problems for about 12 months, including confusion over day and night, disorientation to place (he had got lost twice), constant searching for personal items, and craving for sweet food. Mr Ho was aware of his own memory decline.

Findings from Screening Assessments by Allied Healthcare and Social Care Team

Cognitive functioning	Scored 14/30 on MMSE, indicating cognitive impairment, adjusted for education level. Mr Ho's performance was impaired in orientation to time (1/5) and place (1/5), calculation (1/5), delayed recall (1/3), and three-step commands (1/3); his performance was, however, normal in registration (3/3), language (5/5), and visuospatial relationships (1/1). The Clock Drawing Test showed impairment in time denotation in both the drawing and copying parts (Figure 2.29).
ADL/IADL	Mr Ho was independent in most ADLs, although he needed to walk with a stick (Barthel Index 92/100). He was dependent in meal preparation, laundry, community access, handling finances, and grocery shopping. He needed supervision or assistance in taking medication and external communication (Lawton IADL Scale 15/56).
Depressive symptoms	Scored 1/15 on GDS-15, no obvious depressive mood was noted.
Staging and clinical rating	Scored 0.5/3 on Clinical Dementia Rating, indicating questionable dementia. He showed mild impairment in memory, orientation, and housework and hobbies.

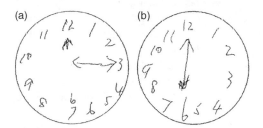

Figure 2.29 Findings from Mr Ho's Clock Drawing Test. (a) Clock Drawing (3 o'clock). (b) Clock Copying (10 past 10)

History Taken with Carer by Primary Care Physician

Mr Ho's daughter reported noticing memory problems in Mr Ho that had concerned her for about 12 months, although no delusional ideations were reported. Using the GPCOG Informant Interview, the following areas were noted to show more difficulties (×) or were preserved (○) compared to about two years ago:

× Remembering recent events
× Recalling recent conversations
× Word finding
× Managing money and finances
× Managing medication independently
× Using transport

There was an additional clinical feature to consider for non-Alzheimer's dementia: Mr Ho has early speech problems (which could potentially suggest primary progressive aphasia or frontotemporal dementia), without history of stroke or space-occupying lesions (SOLs). Mr Ho has hypertension, atrial fibrillation, an old cardiovascular accident, chronic obstructive pulmonary disease, and chronic kidney disease. He is currently on digoxin, warfarin, isosorbide dinitrate, prazosin, oxybutynin hydrochloride, and enalapril maleate. No family history of psychiatric disorders or dementia was reported. He has received primary education to P.4 (approximately four years of education).

Physical Examination Findings

General examination revealed a hygiene problem with a urine smell, although no affect problem was noted. Atrial fibrillation was found on CVS. No CNS findings.

Investigations

CBP, ESR, R/LFT, calcium, VDR, vitamin B_{12}, fasting sugar, fasting lipids, MSU × R/M & culture test, ECG, folate, and TSH were ordered. CBP, ESR, calcium, fasting sugar, MSU × R/M and culture test, folate, and TSH were normal. LFT creatinine 174. Fasting lipids: TCHL 6.0, TG 1.2, HDL-C 1.6, and LDL-C 3.88. CT brain (plain) scan revealed old infarct and chronic ischaemia.

Diagnosis

Mixed dementia (Alzheimer's disease and vascular dementia) with comorbid urinary tract infection, renal impairment, and aortic regurgitation.

Management

Donepezil 5 mg daily was prescribed. Mr Ho was recommended to join a specialised day care service for two days per week, to receive a structured and tailored intervention programme and cognitively stimulating activities to delay deterioration, and to maintain quality of life.

Suggestions for the Primary Care Team

Mr Ho has post-stroke cognitive impairment, with early speech problems. Considering that Mr Ho has got lost twice with an MMSE score of 14/30 and IADL dependency, there appeared to be some inconsistency with results in the Clinical Dementia Rating, the latter of which suggested only questionable dementia. The primary care team should pay attention to potential inconsistencies between the informant report and other findings, especially as the Clinical Dementia Rating depends heavily on the informant report, and physicians should exercise clinical discretion. In this case, it is less likely that Mr Ho's current level of deterioration has only begun within 12 months, and the possibility that some early signs and symptoms might have gone unnoticed should be revisited in subsequent follow-ups. Should this be the case, the relatively short duration of symptom onset could be an artefact, due to low awareness in the carer, which would also explain the findings from the Clinical Dementia Rating as it relies heavily on the carers' subjective report.

Physicians should pay attention to Mr Ho's response to donepezil. Mr Ho is on oxybutynin, which is an anticholinergic agent. The most common indication of anticholinergic agents in older people is an overactive bladder. Physicians should watch out for urinary symptoms after prescribing cholinesterase inhibitors and review the indication for oxybutynin.

Although the assessment results did not suggest depression, considering the fact that Mr Ho had had a stroke, the primary care team should pay attention to possible depressive symptoms that may arise/manifest in future follow-ups. For care planning, one area to focus on is to equip carers with knowledge and skills, particularly in terms of awareness and understanding of the foreseeable disease progression. Safety precautions, such as a sensor and alarm to prevent Mr Ho from leaving home unaccompanied, and a location-tracking device should be in place, and physical strength training to prevent falls is recommended.

Case 039 History of Severe Traumatic Brain Injury

Mr Yue, an 84-year-old gentleman, presented with concerns raised by his children about his memory problems. His daughter noted a deterioration in his memory over the last three years. He was unable to recognise his wife; he was also reported to have a frequent need to search for personal belongings and to be forgetful about details in a conversation.

Findings from Screening Assessments by Allied Healthcare and Social Care Team

Cognitive functioning	Scored 14/30 on MMSE, indicating cognitive impairment, adjusted for education level. Mr Yue was impaired in orientation to time (0/5), orientation to place (2/5), and calculation (1/5); he had slight impairment in three-step commands (2/3) and delayed recall (2/3). His performance was, however, normal in registration (3/3), language (5/5), and visuospatial relationships (1/1). The Clock Drawing Test showed incorrect time denotation, suggestive of deficits in executive function. Performance improved slightly on clock copying. He was able to read the clock (Figure 2.30).
ADL/IADL	Mr Yue was semi-independent in ADLs (Barthel Index 86/100): he needed company when going out, had occasional bladder incontinence, and needed to use an incontinence pad when going out. He was assisted in IADLs: he needed supervision in taking medication; he was dependent in cooking, community access, and handling finances. He was able to use a mobile phone (in a modified way) and do simple housekeeping tasks. He was unable to shop, although he was able to help pick up items when his wife went shopping with him (Lawton IADL Scale 27/56).
Depressive symptoms	Scored on GDS 15 3/15, no significant depressive mood was noted.
Staging and clinical rating	Scored 2/3 on Clinical Dementia Rating, indicating moderate dementia. He showed moderate impairment in orientation, judgement and problem-solving, and community affairs and mild impairment in memory, home and hobbies, and personal care.

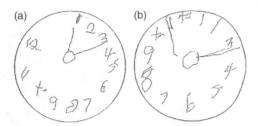

Figure 2.30 Findings from Mr Yue's Clock Drawing Test. (a) Clock Drawing (3 o'clock). (b) Clock Copying (10 past 10)

History Taken with Carer by Primary Care Physician

Mr Yue's daughter reported noticing memory problems in her father that had concerned her for about three years, although no delusional ideations were reported. Using the GPCOG Informant Interview, the following areas were noted to show more difficulties (✗) or were preserved (○) compared to about two years ago:

✗ Remembering recent events
✗ Recalling recent conversations
✗ Word finding
✗ Managing money and finances
✗ Managing medication independently
✗ Using transport

There were no additional clinical features to consider for non-Alzheimer's dementia. Mr Yue has diabetes, hypertension, old myocardial infarction/ischaemic heart disease (MI/IHD), dyslipidaemia, and a history of severe head injury with fractured left occipital bone, acute subdural haemorrhage bilateral, and bilateral frontal contusion three years ago. He is currently on enalapril 15 mg daily, gliclazide 160 mg twice a day, metformin 500 mg twice a day, vildagliptin 50 mg in the morning, simvastatin 20 mg nocte, aspirin 80 mg daily, pantoprazole 40 mg daily, and nitroglycerin sublingual PRN. No family history of psychiatric disorders or dementia was reported. He did not receive any education.

Physical Examination Findings

General examination revealed no affect or hygiene problem. No CVS or CNS findings.

Investigations

CBP, R/LFT, vitamin B_{12}, and fasting lipids were ordered. CBP, R/LFT, and fasting lipids were normal. Result of vitamin B_{12} was pending. CT brain scan would be repeated.

Diagnosis

Alzheimer's disease and traumatic brain injury.

Management

Rivastigmine transdermal system 5 mg daily was prescribed. Mr Yue was also recommended to join a specialised day care service for two days per week to receive a structured and tailored intervention programme and cognitively stimulating activities to delay deterioration and maintain quality of life.

Suggestions for the Primary Care Team

Mr Yue's case is a good illustration of Alzheimer's disease. He has several known risk factors for Alzheimer's disease, including diabetes, hypertension, and traumatic head injury (4). He presented at a common age of symptom onset for Alzheimer's disease, with an impairment pattern compatible with Alzheimer's disease: his visuospatial ability was intact on the MMSE interlocking pentagon test, with a positive Clock Drawing Test (which was worse in the drawing part but improved on the copying part). His MMSE score was lower than expected, which may be related to the history of severe head injury aggravating his symptoms and accelerating the disease progression. Physicians are advised to check his vitamin B_{12} on metformin and monitor his improvement on rivastigmine.

Although Mr Yue's general functions are at a moderate stage of dementia, his performance in delayed recall on MMSE was satisfactory. This suggests that he is still able to encode and store information, with difficulties mainly arising from the retrieval of information. This ability in information encoding and storage can be used as his strength, by encouraging Mr Yue to participate regularly in cognitively stimulating activities, as well as social activities, to maintain his good verbal communications.

Case 040 Declining Brain Imaging

Ms Yeung, an 86-year-old lady, presented with concerns raised by her daughter over her memory problems that have worsened in the past few months, such as repeated questioning, forgetting about appointments, and mistaking names of her children. Ms Yeung was aware of her own memory decline.

Findings from Screening Assessments by Allied Healthcare and Social Care Team

Cognitive functioning	Scored 18/30 on MMSE, indicating cognitive impairment, after adjusting for education level. Ms Yeung's performance was impaired in orientation to time (2/5) and place (3/5), three-step commands (1/3), calculation (3/5), and delayed recall (0/3). Her performance was, however, normal in registration (3/3), language (5/5), and visuospatial relationships (1/1). The Clock Drawing Test was normal.
ADL/IADL	Ms Yeung was independent in most ADLs (Barthel Index 92/100), although she has lower limb weakness. She was semi-dependent in IADLs (Lawton IADL Scale 49/56): she would forget to take medications and forget occasionally to turn off the stove. Her daughter reported that she would misplace money, which would be later found at her home. She was able to travel within her community and take transportation, although recently she seldom goes out.
Depressive symptoms	Scored on GDS-15 1/15, no obvious depressive mood was noted.
Staging and clinical rating	Scored 0.5/3 on Clinical Dementia Rating, indicating questionable dementia. She showed mild impairment in judgement and problem-solving, and in home and hobbies.

History Taken with Carer by Primary Care Physician

Ms Yeung's daughter reported noticing memory problems in her mother that had concerned her for about two to three years, which had worsened in the past few months, although no delusional ideations were reported. Using the GPCOG Informant Interview, the following areas were noted to show more difficulties (✗) or were preserved (○) compared to about two years ago:

   ✗ Remembering recent events
   ✗ Recalling recent conversations
   ○ Word finding
   ✗ Managing money and finances
   ○ Managing medication independently
   ○ Using transport

There were no additional clinical features to consider for non-Alzheimer's dementia. No family history of psychiatric disorders or dementia was reported. Ms Yeung has received primary education of P.6 (approximately six years of education). Ms Yeung lives alone; she used to go to a community centre for older people but has stopped going recently.

Physical Examination Findings

General examination revealed no affect or hygiene problem. Ms Yeung had a blood pressure reading of 159/78 mm Hg. No other CVS or CNS findings.

Investigations

Vitamin B_{12} and TSH were ordered. Ms Yeung declined to have any brain imaging procedures.

Diagnosis

Alzheimer's disease.

Management

Donepezil 2.5 mg daily was prescribed. Ms Yeung was recommended to join a specialised day care service for two days per week to receive a structured and tailored intervention programme and cognitively stimulating activities to delay deterioration and maintain quality of life.

Suggestions for the Primary Care Team

This is a typical case of early Alzheimer's disease. Ms Yeung's Clock Drawing Test was positive while her performance on the visuospatial part of MMSE (interlocking pentagon) was intact; this is compatible as the Clock Drawing Test is more sensitive in picking up milder impairment. Although Ms Yeung has declined brain imaging, physicians may note that brain imaging is not mandatory for the work-up of Alzheimer's disease based on current diagnostic criteria that are clinically oriented, although there are various views and guidelines surrounding this issue (see Section 1.3). The primary care team should nevertheless watch out for any deterioration in speech and language, and change in mood and personality, in subsequent follow-ups.

Ms Yue's performance in ADL/IADL was generally satisfactory, and her cognitive functions were fair, except in short-term memory. The primary care team may investigate further her decreased motivation to go out and explore the underlying reasons, such as experience and fear of getting lost. As Ms Yue is living alone, community support services and ongoing care should be discussed with Ms Yue and her family; safety precautions, such as a location-tracking device, and home modifications with monitoring/remote control by the carer, should be considered.

Case 041   Suicidal Ideation about Jumping from a Height

Ms Szeto, an 81-year-old lady, presented with concerns raised by her daughter over her memory problems. She was noted to have forgotten the home address of her son who was living on the same estate, forgotten to take a blood pressure drug for five days in a row, and forgotten her own recent activities and the telephone numbers of others. She was self-aware of her memory decline and felt bad about the deterioration.

Findings from Screening Assessments by Allied Healthcare and Social Care Team

Cognitive functioning	Scored 15/30 on MMSE, indicating cognitive impairment, adjusted for education level. Ms Szeto's performance was impaired in orientation to time (3/5) and place (0/5), delayed recall (0/3), and calculation (1/5) and slightly impaired in three-step commands (2/3). Her performance was, however, normal in registration (3/3), language (5/5), and visuospatial relationships (1/1). The Clock Drawing Test was positive (Figure 2.31).
ADL/IADL	Ms Szeto was independent in all ADLs (Barthel Index 100/100). She was independent in community living and meal preparation, although she needed reminders to check the fridge before going out to shop for food (to prevent repeated buying). She needed supervision to take medicine (Lawton IADL Scale 53/56).
Depressive symptoms	Scored 7/15 on GDS-15, indicating a significant depressive mood. She had suicidal thoughts about jumping from a height.
Staging and clinical rating	Scored 1/3 on Clinical Dementia Rating, indicating mild dementia. She showed moderate impairment in judgement and problem-solving; mild impairment in memory, orientation, and personal care; questionable impairment in community affairs; and no impairment in home and hobbies.

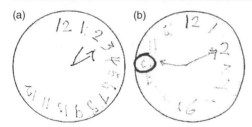

Figure 2.31 Findings from Ms Szeto's Clock Drawing Test. (a) Clock Drawing (3 o'clock). (b) Clock Copying (10 past 10)

History Taken with Carer by Primary Care Physician

Ms Szeto's daughter reported noticing memory problems in her mother that had concerned her for about a year, although no delusional ideations were reported. Using the GPCOG Informant Interview, the following areas were noted to show more difficulties (✗) or were preserved (○) compared to about two years ago:

✗ Remembering recent events
✗ Recalling recent conversations
○ Word finding

* ✗ Managing money and finances
* ✗ Managing medication independently
* ○ Using transport

There were no additional clinical features to consider for non-Alzheimer's dementia. Ms Szeto has hypertension. She is currently on losartan 50 mg daily, pantoprazole 40 mg daily, amlodipine 2 mg daily, and simvastatin 20 mg. No family history of psychiatric disorders or dementia was reported. Ms Szeto walks unaided. She has received primary education.

Physical Examination Findings

General examination revealed no affect or hygiene problem. No CVS or CNS findings.

Diagnosis

Alzheimer's disease with a significant depressive mood and suicidal ideation.

Management

Sertraline 25 mg daily and donepezil 2.5 mg daily were prescribed. Ms Szeto was recommended to join a specialised day care service for two days per week to receive a structured and tailored intervention programme and cognitively stimulating activities to delay deterioration and promote quality of life.

Suggestions for the Primary Care Team

Ms Szeto has a suicidal idea of jumping from a height, for which urgent referral to a psychiatrist and secondary care is indicated. This should be followed up with the management of depression and Alzheimer's disease after stabilisation of any imminent suicide risk. For her depression, clinical consultation on her depressive mood is needed, and physicians should check if SSRIs should be prescribed.

Her presentations of cognitive and ADL/IADL impairments are typical of Alzheimer's disease with a significant depressive mood, including typical Clock Drawing Test results, with performance improving on the copying part. While MMSE showed significant impairment in her orientation to place, interpretation should take into consideration the possibility of underscoring due to her unfamiliarity with the assessment venue. Physicians may note in this case that, despite the presence of vascular burden, a diagnosis of mixed dementia (Alzheimer's disease and vascular dementia) is not always indicated.

Despite significant deterioration in short-term memory and related functional performance as shown in the cognitive assessment, Ms Szeto remained relatively independent in her ADLs and IADLs with satisfactory performance, suggesting that her self-care and community living have yet to be severely affected by the cognitive impairments at this moment. This should be a strength to consider utilising and maximising in her care plan. This contrasted with her self-evaluation: Ms Szeto reported feeling bad about her memory problems, despite her good ADL/IADL functioning. The primary care team should explore any other factors affecting her self-evaluation. While it could potentially be explained by her significant depressive mood, which could also contribute to the cognitive deterioration, in some cases carer factors (e.g., negative comments and blaming of poor memory) may also contribute to poor self-image and stress, which should be explored. The family can be provided with psychoeducation on the impact of dementia as appropriate.

Case 042 Pain and Unilateral Rigidity

Ms Leung, an 82-year-old lady, presented with concerns raised by her daughter over her memory and functional problems, which were first observed about four to five years ago but became more obvious in the past year. She was noted to have a poor orientation to place and time, difficulties in cooking, and a poor short-term memory with repeated buying behaviour. Ms Leung was aware of her own memory decline.

Findings from Screening Assessments by Allied Healthcare and Social Care Team

Cognitive functioning	Scored 11/30 on MMSE, indicating cognitive impairment, adjusted for education level. Ms Leung's performance was impaired in orientation to time (1/5) and place (0/5), delayed recall (0/3), calculation (1/5), three-step commands (1/3), and visuospatial relationships (0/1). Her performance was, however, normal in registration (3/3) and language (5/5). The Clock Drawing Test showed impairment with numbers and omission of time denotation on the drawing part, which was improved on the copying part. She was able to read a clock (Figure 2.32).
ADL/IADL	Ms Leung was independent in most ADLs, except that some tasks would take longer due to her knee pain (Barthel Index 92/100). She was semi-independent in IADLs (Lawton IADL Scale 42/56): she needed assistance in taking medicine; she would forget to turn off the stove, buy the same item repeatedly, and get off trains at the wrong station; she also needed assistance in finance management.
Depressive symptoms	Scored 1/15 on GDS-15, no obvious depressive mood was noted.
Staging and clinical rating	Scored 1/3 on Clinical Dementia Rating, indicating mild dementia. She showed mild impairment in memory and orientation, judgement and problem-solving, home and hobbies, and community affairs.

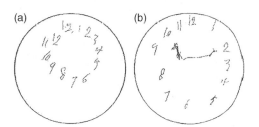

Figure 2.32 Findings from Ms Leung's Clock Drawing Test. (a) Clock Drawing (3 o'clock). (b) Clock Copying (10 past 10)

History Taken with Carer by Primary Care Physician

Ms Leung's daughter reported noticing memory problems in her mother that had become more obvious in the past year, although no delusional ideations were reported. Using the GPCOG Informant Interview, the following areas were noted to show more difficulties (✗) or were preserved (○) compared to about two years ago:

✗ Remembering recent events
✗ Recalling recent conversations
✗ Word finding
? Managing money and finances
? Managing medication independently
? Using transport

Ms Leung's daughter was unable to judge about her ability regarding managing money, managing medication independently, and using transportation: a domestic helper would help with money and medication management, and Ms Leung seldom goes out or uses transportation. She would nevertheless go to a centre for older people and a park nearby.

There is an additional feature to consider for non-Alzheimer's dementia, namely pain and rigidity on one side. Ms Leung has hypertension, right macular degeneration, breast cancer, a total knee replacement, and a prolapsed uterus. She is currently on hypertension medication prescribed to her at a geriatric outpatient clinic. No family history of psychiatric disorders or dementia was reported. She has received primary education to P.3 (approximately three years of education).

Physical Examination Findings

General examination revealed no affect or hygiene problem. A heart murmur was noted. No other CVS or CNS findings.

Investigations

TSH and free T4 were ordered.

Diagnosis

Alzheimer's disease (tentative diagnosis).

Management

Donepezil 5 mg daily was prescribed. Ms Leung was recommended to join a specialised day care service for two days per week to receive a structured and tailored intervention programme and cognitively stimulating activities to delay deterioration and to maintain quality of life.

Suggestions for the Primary Care Team

In Ms Leung's case, while her presentation is compatible with a diagnosis of early Alzheimer's disease, the presence of rigidity needs to be followed up and referred for secondary care. Physicians should observe Ms Leung's response to donepezil over time. Both pharmacological and non-pharmacological interventions and her care plan might need to be adjusted depending on the confirmation of the diagnosis.

Ms Leung's performance in ADL/IADL matches with her cognitive functioning as shown in the assessment; for example, her repeated buying can be attributed to her impairment in short-term memory. While Ms Leung's performance in orientation to place appeared to be severely impaired, interpretation should take into consideration the possibility of underscoring due to unfamiliarity with the assessment venue. Also of note is the long duration of untreated illness – with symptoms first occurring four to five years ago and her family seeking help only recently; in many cases, the delay would mean significant progression of dementia, missing the best time for intervention. This could indicate a low level of awareness of the family carers about the interventions and services for dementia. The primary care team should equip Ms Leung's family with knowledge of the disease, proper caring skills, and available resources (see Section 5.2), as well as preparing them for the later stages of dementia that will follow.

Case 043 Rapid Onset with Awareness

Ms Wai, an 83-year-old lady, presented with concerns raised by her son about her memory problems, which was noted for three months. She was reported to occasionally not recognise where she was, get off the bus at the wrong stop, and exit the lift at the wrong floor in her home building. She was aware of her own memory decline and that she would forget about her conversations with others.

Findings from Screening Assessments by Allied Healthcare and Social Care Team

Cognitive functioning	Scored 20/30 on MMSE, indicating no cognitive impairment, adjusted for education level. Ms Wai's performance was impaired in delayed recall (0/3), slightly impaired in orientation to time (2/5), place (3/5), and in calculation (3/5); her performance was, however, normal in three-step commands (3/3), registration (3/3), language (5/5), and visuospatial relationships (1/1). The Clock Drawing Test showed impaired executive function, with misplacement of numbers and no time denotation, which was slightly improved on the copying part. She was able to read the clock (Figure 2.33).
ADL/IADL	Ms Wai was independent in most ADLs (Barthel Index 98/100), except for a slight difficulty when using the stairs. She was independent in most IADLs (Lawton IADL Scale 55/56): the only exception being shopping, when she would sometimes forget to buy certain items that she intended to buy.
Depressive symptoms	Scored 2/15 on GDS-15, no obvious depressive mood was noted.
Staging and clinical rating	Scored 0.5/3 on Clinical Dementia Rating, indicating questionable dementia. She showed mild impairment in orientation and community affairs; her performance was fair in memory, judgement and problem-solving, home and hobbies, and normal in personal care.

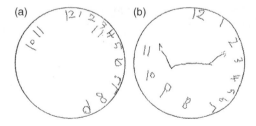

Figure 2.33 Findings from Ms Wai's Clock Drawing Test. (a) Clock Drawing (3 o'clock). (b) Clock Copying (10 past 10)

History Taken with Carer by Primary Care Physician

Ms Wai's son reported noticing memory problems in his mother that had concerned him for about two to three months. No delusional ideations were reported. Using the GPCOG Informant Interview, the following areas were noted to show more difficulties (✗) or were preserved (○) compared to about two years ago:

✗ Remembering recent events
✗ Recalling recent conversations

○ Word finding
○ Managing money and finances
○ Managing medication independently
○ Using transport

There were no additional clinical features to consider for non-Alzheimer's dementia. Ms Wai has dyslipidaemia. She is currently taking medication for asthma. No family history of psychiatric disorders or dementia was reported. She did not receive any education. Ms Wai walks unaided and attends church every week.

Physical Examination Findings

General examination revealed no affect or hygiene problem. No significant CVS or CNS findings.

Investigations

Vitamin B_{12} and TSH were ordered. MRI revealed no evidence of vascular dementia but cerebral atrophy.

Diagnosis

Alzheimer's disease, with rapid onset of memory decline and poor orientation noted.

Management

Donepezil 2.5 mg daily was prescribed. Ms Wai was recommended to join a specialised day care service for two days per week to receive a structured and tailored intervention programme and cognitively stimulating activities to delay deterioration and maintain her quality of life.

Suggestions for the Primary Care Team

In Ms Wai's case, acute stroke and vascular dementia were the differential diagnoses, but have been ruled out by the MRI brain results, which showed no evidence of vascular dementia. Her presentation was compatible with Alzheimer's disease, in terms of a typical age of presentation, impairment pattern shown on MMSE (delayed recall being the first domain affected), and Clock Drawing Test results (positive findings in the clock drawing part, with performance improved in the copying part), although her onset was rather rapid, with significant deterioration over a few months and intact self-awareness. An MRI was therefore indicated to rule out additional brain pathology. Physicians should pay attention to any mood problems and continue to monitor her progress and treatment response to donepezil in subsequent follow-ups. In similar cases, monitoring cognitive change without prescribing a cholinesterase inhibitor can also be considered.

Ms Wai's acute onset of cognitive decline has resulted in obvious impacts on her daily living within a few months. A strength to consider is that her cognitive, physical, and ADL/IADL functions were satisfactory with good performance, which can be utilised and optimised in her care plan. Another strength is her son's high level of awareness, which has contributed to the early help-seeking. The primary care team can focus on working with both Ms Wai and her son for psychoeducation, explaining the diagnosis and the need to monitor cognitive and treatment response changes over time, which would inform further care planning. Meanwhile, general advice for maintaining a healthy lifestyle for brain health from a primary care perspective can be provided.

Case 044 Feelings of Uselessness

Ms Wong, an 83-year-old lady, presented with concerns raised by her daughter over her memory problems that had started approximately two years previously. She was noted to be forgetful, such as forgetting about appointments very quickly after being told, asking the same questions repeatedly, and saying the same thing over and over again. Her ability to do housework and cooking has also deteriorated. Ms Wong was aware of her own memory decline.

Findings from Screening Assessments by Allied Healthcare and Social Care Team

Cognitive functioning	Scored 17/30 on MMSE, indicating cognitive impairment, adjusted for education level. Ms Wong's performance was impaired in delayed recall (0/3), calculation (3/5), orientation to time (2/5) and place (3/5), and visuospatial relationships (0/1); her performance was, however, normal in registration (3/3) and language (5/5). The Clock Drawing Test showed mild impairment, with incorrect time denotation on both the drawing and copying part (Figure 2.34).
ADL/IADL	Ms Wong was mostly independent in ADLs (Barthel Index 96/100). She was partly dependent in IADLs (Lawton IADL Scale 47/56): she needed assistance in community access and heavy-duty household chores.
Depressive symptoms	Scored 9/15 on GDS-15, a depressive mood was noted. She expressed that she always feels useless and was annoyed about it.
Staging and clinical rating	Scored 1/3 on Clinical Dementia Rating, indicating mild dementia. She showed questionable impairment in community affairs and mild impairment in orientation, memory, judgement and problem-solving, and home and hobbies.

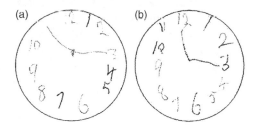

Figure 2.34 Findings from Ms Wong's Clock Drawing Test. (a) Clock Drawing (3 o'clock). (b) Clock Copying (10 past 10)

History Taken with Carer by Primary Care Physician

Ms Wong's daughter reported noticing memory problems in her mother that had concerned her for two years. No delusional ideations were reported. Using the GPCOG Informant Interview, the following areas were noted to show more difficulties (✗) or were preserved (○) compared to about two years ago:

✗ Remembering recent events
✗ Recalling recent conversations
○ Word finding
○ Managing money and finances
○ Managing medication independently
○ Using transport

There were no additional clinical features to consider for non-Alzheimer's dementia. Ms Wong has hypertension and varicose veins. She had a fall a year ago. She is currently on amlodipine 5 mg daily and losartan 50 mg daily. No family history of psychiatric disorders or dementia was reported. She has received primary education to P.3 (approximately three years of education).

Physical Examination Findings

General examination revealed no affect or hygiene problems. No significant CVS or CNS findings.

Investigations

CBP, R/LFT, VDRL, vitamin B_{12}, fasting sugar, and TFT were ordered. Result showed Hb 10.7 in CBP; vitamin B_{12} and TFT were normal. CT brain (plain) scan revealed mild cerebral atrophy.

Diagnosis

Alzheimer's disease with mild depression.

Management

Rivastigmine transdermal system 5 mg daily, fluoxetine 20 mg daily, and Calcichew one tablet twice a day were prescribed. Ms Wong was recommended to join a specialised day care service for two days per week to receive a structured and tailored intervention programme and cognitively stimulating activities to delay deterioration and improve her mood and quality of life.

Suggestions for the Primary Care Team

Ms Wong's presentation is typical of early Alzheimer's disease with depression. At this stage, ADL/IADL and cognitive functions are generally good, with only short-term memory, executive function, and other higher-level cognitive functions showing more obvious deterioration. Depression is a concern in Ms Wong's case, which will further worsen her overall functions. Physicians should monitor Ms Wong's response to cholinesterase inhibitors and SSRIs; in subsequent follow-ups, they should observe and titrate rivastigmine and fluoxetine according to her clinical condition.

Given the importance of depression in her management, the primary care team should figure out if any psychosocial factors triggering her depressive mood can be identified. While multiple possibilities exist in the relationship between dementia and depression, in this case it is likely that Ms Wong's depression may be a reaction to her awareness of the cognitive impairment. In early dementia with self-awareness, the person may be worried about the future, and it is not uncommon for carers, relatives, or friends to emphasise or blame the person for his/her weaknesses and memory problems. If this is the case, education for the family will help. The primary care team should also engage Ms Wong in meaningful leisure and failure-free activities, which could be more appropriate than emphasising the potential benefits of activities (e.g., 'memory training' and 'cognitive improvement'), as the latter may be refused or rejected as useless because of Ms Wong's prevailing mood. Motivation and improved mood are of higher priority at this moment.

Case 045 Bilateral Cataract

Ms Choi, a 90-year-old lady, presented with concerns raised by her daughter about her memory problems and delusions. She was noted to have memory problems that started about three years ago, with progressive decline in her short-term memory: she was disoriented to time, had low motivation in social interaction or participating in social activities, and showed problems in word finding (she was only able to find the right word upon seeing the actual object, for example).

Findings from Screening Assessments by Allied Healthcare and Social Care Team

Cognitive functioning	Scored 10/30 on MMSE, indicating cognitive impairment, adjusted for education level. Ms Choi was disoriented to time (0/5) and severely impaired in orientation to place (1/5); she was unable to recall her home address even with prompting, although she was able to go home from nearby places independently; her performance was severely impaired in delayed recall (0/3), calculation (0/5), three-step commands (1/3), and visuospatial relationships (0/1); her performance was, however, normal in registration (3/3) and language (5/5). The Clock Drawing Test showed severe impairment in executive function, with some evidence that a clock face was drawn; her performance was not improved in the copying task (Figure 2.35).
ADL/IADL	Ms Choi was independent in ADLs (Barthel Index 100/100). She was mostly independent in IADLs (Lawton IADL Scale 47/56), with occasional support or assistance needed in community access, handling finances, and grocery shopping.
Depressive symptoms	Scored 5/15 on GDS-15, no significant depressive mood was noted.
Staging and clinical rating	Scored 1/3 on Clinical Dementia Rating, indicating mild impairment. She showed moderate impairment in memory and orientation; mild impairment in judgement and problem-solving, and home and hobbies, and questionable impairment in community affairs.

(a)   (b)

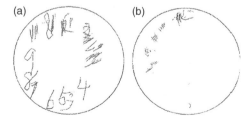

Figure 2.35 Findings from Clock Ms Choi's Drawing Test. (a) Clock Drawing (3 o'clock). (b) Clock Copying (10 past 10)

History Taken with Carer by Primary Care Physician

Ms Choi's daughter reported noticing memory problems in her mother that concerned her for about three years. Delusional ideations were reported. Using the GPCOG Informant Interview, the following areas were noted to show more difficulties (✖) or were preserved (○) compared to about two years ago:

- ✘ Remembering recent events
- ✘ Recalling recent conversations
- ✘ Word finding
- ✘ Managing money and finances
- ○ Managing medication independently
- ○ Using transport

There were no additional clinical features to consider for non-Alzheimer's dementia. Ms Choi has hypertension and blurry vision due to bilateral cataracts (not operated). No family history of psychiatric disorders or dementia was reported. She has received primary education to P.3 (approximately three years of education). She is widowed, currently lives alone, and has good support from her one daughter.

Physical Examination Findings

General examination revealed no affect or hygiene problem. No significant CVS or CNS findings.

Investigations

CBP, ESR, R/LFT, calcium, VDRL, vitamin B_{12}, fasting sugar, folate, and TSH/FT4 were ordered. CBP result: Hb 10.3 NcNc. ESR 28, VDRL negative, and vitamin B_{12} 198 (low). Folate and TSH/FT4 were normal. CT brain (plain) scan revealed meningioma at the left frontal lobe (1.9 cm × 1.6 cm × 1.3 cm), cerebral atrophy of mild temporal lobe, lacunar infarcts in both basal ganglia, and small vessel disease.

Diagnosis

Moderate Alzheimer's disease and mild vitamin B_{12} deficiency.

Management

Donepezil 5 mg daily, vitamin B-complex supplement one tablet daily, aspirin EC 100 mg daily, and pantoprazole 40 mg daily were prescribed. Ms Choi was recommended to join a specialised day care service for two days per week to receive a structured and tailored intervention programme and cognitively stimulating activities to delay deterioration and to maintain her quality of life.

Suggestions for the Primary Care Team

Delusion is not uncommon in moderate Alzheimer's disease. When it is reported, the content of the delusion and its associated mood should be explored. Delusions of theft, especially those related to money or personal belongings, are very frequently encountered by family members and carers, which can be distressing for both the person and others.

Although Ms Choi's poor eyesight and age-related frailty might have contributed to a lower score of MMSE and given her old age, there may be hippocampal sclerosis involvement in the pathology, the management should follow that of Alzheimer's disease pathology. Ms Choi's deterioration shows that she is progressing into a moderate stage of dementia. Considering that her signs and symptoms have been observed for three years already, there is a delay in help-seeking, missing the best time for intervention at an earlier stage of dementia. This could be due to a masking of her memory problems because of her independence in ADL/IADL: depending on the person's premorbid level of functioning and the requirement of independence in the person's daily living, ADL/IADL performance may not always be immediately affected by cognitive impairment (IADL, but not ADL, impairment is a diagnostic criterion for dementia, see Section 1.3), and/or it can be related to limited awareness and understanding in the person and her carers about dementia, in which case carer education would be particularly indicated.

Case 046 Treatment Response

Ms Ng, a 77-year-old lady, presented with concerns raised by her husband about her memory problems over about a year. Her husband complained of her forgetfulness, such as misplacing her personal items (she was said to be always looking for her spectacles) and asking the same questions repeatedly (a problem that was observed by both her husband and her son). Ms Ng was aware of her own memory decline.

Findings from Screening Assessments by Allied Healthcare and Social Care Team

Cognitive functioning	Scored 23/30 on MMSE, no indication of cognitive impairment, adjusted for education level. Ms Ng's performance was impaired in delayed recall (0/3; she was unable to recall any items) and orientation to time (2/5). She had slight difficulties in orientation to place (4/5). She nevertheless showed good calculation skills (5/5) but showed slight difficulties in recalling the remaining sum after each subtraction, normal performance in registration (3/3), three-step commands (3/3), language (5/5), and visuospatial relationships (1/1). Her Clock Drawing Test was negative.
ADL/IADL	She was independent in all ADLs (Barthel Index 100/100). She was independent in most IADLs, although she was noted to be highly dependent on her husband (Lawton IADL Scale 54/56).
Depressive symptoms	Scored 1/15 on GDS-15, no obvious depressive mood was noted.
Staging and clinical rating	Scored 0.5/3 on Clinical Dementia Rating, indicating questionable dementia. She showed questionable impairment in memory, orientation, and judgement and problem-solving.

History Taken with Carer by Primary Care Physician

Ms Ng's husband reported noticing memory problems in his wife that had concerned him for about a year. No delusional ideations were reported. Using the GPCOG Informant Interview, the following areas were noted to show more difficulties (×) or were preserved (○) compared to about two years ago:

× Remembering recent events
× Recalling recent conversations
× Word finding
○ Managing money and finances
× Managing medication independently
○ Using transport

There were no additional clinical features to consider for non-Alzheimer's dementia. Family history of dementia was noted: Ms Ng's mother was reported to have had dementia. No family history of other psychiatric illness was reported. She has received tertiary education and had trained as a teacher. Ms Ng has good social support and plays Mahjong with her sister every week.

Physical Examination Findings

General examination revealed a hygiene problem but no affect problem. Ms Ng has a blood pressure reading of 141/91 mm Hg. No significant CVS or CNS findings.

Investigations

CBP, ESR, R/LFT, calcium, VDRL, vitamin B_{12}, fasting sugar, fasting lipids, MSU × R/M and culture test, CXR, and ECG were ordered. All investigations were normal except high fasting lipids. MRI revealed decreased medial temporal thickness.

Diagnosis

Early Alzheimer's disease.

Management

Donepezil 5 mg daily was prescribed. Ms Ng was recommended to join a specialised day care service for two days per week to receive a structured and tailored intervention programme and cognitively stimulating activities to delay deterioration.

Suggestions for the Primary Care Team

This is a case of very early Alzheimer's disease, with mild cognitive impairment and cognitive frailty as the differential diagnoses. Some unusual features were noted, including a relatively younger age of presentation (which could suggest an aggressive amyloid load) and a negative Clock Drawing Test finding. Ms Ng's response to donepezil should be monitored in terms of changes in her clinical symptoms and functioning. A case conference with specialists is recommended for Ms Ng's case to review differential diagnoses and the evolution of atypical/typical features for Alzheimer's disease in response to donepezil and non-pharmacological interventions. Closer observation of her treatment response will provide information about the diagnosis and guide further interventions as needed.

The fact that Ms Ng's cognitive deterioration was picked up by her carer at this very early stage of dementia, with only mild impairment demonstrated upon assessment, could indicate good awareness and support from the family, which is a strength in Ms Ng's case. The primary care team should nevertheless remind her family to avoid 'over-caring' and putting too much emphasis on providing direct care at this stage: Ms Ng was noted to be quite dependent on her husband for IADL tasks, although according to the assessment results her functioning should be good at this moment. The priority now would be to motivate her to participate in daily activities, comply with drug treatment, and engage in non-pharmacological interventions and activities.

2.4 Complaints about Behaviours

Case 047 Delusions

Mrs Lau, a 69-year-old lady, presented with concerns raised by her husband about her delusions (she was suspicious of her husband stealing her personal belongings). She was also noted to be forgetful of recent events and was said to have 'declined cognitive functions'.

Findings from Screening Assessments by Allied Healthcare and Social Care Team

Cognitive functioning	Scored 19/30 on MMSE, indicating cognitive impairment, adjusted for education level. Mrs Lau's performance was impaired in orientation to

	time (2/5), delayed recall (0/3), and calculation (1/5). She was slightly impaired in orientation to place (4/5). Her performance was, however, normal in registration (3/3) and language (5/5).
ADL/IADL	She needed assistance in most IADLs tasks, including taking medications, meal preparation, community access, and handling finances due to her cognitive impairments.
Staging and clinical rating	Results suggested a Global Deterioration Scale stage 4, indicating mild dementia. She showed decreased knowledge of current and recent events, a decreased ability to travel and handle finances, and an inability to perform complex tasks.

History Taken with Carer by Primary Care Physician

Mrs Lau's husband reported noticing memory problems in his wife that had concerned him for about two years. Delusional ideations were reported, with Mrs Lau suspecting him of stealing her personal belongings. Using the GPCOG Informant Interview, the following areas were noted to show more difficulties (×) or were preserved (○) compared to about two years ago:

× Remembering recent events
× Recalling recent conversations
○ Word finding
× Managing money and finances
× Managing medication independently
× Using transport

There were no additional clinical features to consider for non-Alzheimer's dementia. Mrs Lau has hypertension and hypercholesterolaemia. She has received primary education (approximately six years of education).

Investigations

CBP, ESR, R/LFT, calcium, vitamin $B_{12,}$ and folate were ordered. MRI revealed MTL not atrophic, ARWMC 1.

Diagnosis

Mild Alzheimer's disease (hippocampal-sparing type).

Management

Donepezil 5 mg every alternate night was prescribed. Mrs Lau was recommended to join a centre-based programme with cognitively stimulating activities to maintain her cognitive and self-care functioning. She was also encouraged to have regular exercise, a healthy diet and mental stimulation, and maintain an active social life. Non-pharmacological intervention to manage the distressed behaviours and neuropsychiatric symptoms of dementia was also recommended.

Suggestions for the Primary Care Team

The relatively young age of onset of Alzheimer's disease in Mrs Lau's case highlighted several areas the primary care team should pay attention to. First is the need for further investigations, with an MRI to investigate hippocampus atrophy and other pathology, and

PiB PET amyloid imaging can be recommended. Her treatment response to donepezil should also be monitored. Another consideration is the educational background; the low education level in this case may contribute to a lower cognitive reserve and thus an earlier presentation of symptoms. Finally, as hypertension is a risk factor for Alzheimer's disease, Mrs Lau's case with an onset age of 69 years should remind primary care physicians of the importance of good control of hypertension and other cardiovascular risk factors, as well as drug compliance.

While the impairment pattern and symptoms in Ms Ng's case are compatible with Alzheimer's disease, the early presentation of delusions mandates further assessment of their causes other than memory problems. For example, the primary care team could observe her home setting during home visits to identify any environmental factors that can be modified, or if any clues are available to suggest further investigation (e.g., is her home cluttered and disorganised? Is there any space for her to keep her important personal belongings?). The team should also try to find out more about Ms Ng's relationship with her husband. On the other hand, given the delusional content, carer stress will be a concern in the care plan for Ms Ng. The primary care team can work with the family to identify needs and the possibility of sharing/shifting part of the caring role from Ms Ng's husband to other family members to prevent burnout and other negative psychological impacts on her husband.

Case 048 Getting Lost

Mrs Cheung, a 78-year-old lady, presented with concerns raised by her daughter about her memory problems; she was noted to have cognitive function decline with problems in wayfinding and orientation.

Findings from Screening Assessments by Allied Healthcare and Social Care Team

Cognitive functioning	Scored 24/30 on MMSE, no indication of cognitive impairment. Mrs Cheung's performance was impaired in delayed recall (1/3); she had slight problems in orientation to time (4/5), to place (4/5), and calculation (3/5); her performance was, however, normal in registration (3/3), language (5/5), three-step commands (3/3), and visuospatial relationships (1/1). Scored 15/30 on MoCA, indicating mild cognitive impairment. She was impaired in visuospatial/executive performance (2/5), attention (1/2), abstraction (0/2), and delayed recall (0/5).
ADL/IADL	Mrs Cheung's ADL performance was intact. She had a mild decline in IADL performance.
Depressive symptoms	Scored 4/15 on GDS-15, no indication of significant depressive symptoms.
Staging and clinical rating	Results suggested a Global Deterioration Scale stage 3, indicating mild cognitive impairment. Mrs Cheung would sometimes get lost when travelling to an unfamiliar location. She retains little information after reading a passage. She showed decreased ability in remembering names upon introduction to new acquaintances. She also showed a concentration deficit during testing.

History Taken with Carer by Primary Care Physician

Mrs Cheung's daughter reported noticing memory problems in her mother that had concerned her for about two years. No delusional ideations were reported. Using the

GPCOG Informant Interview, the following areas were noted to show more difficulties (✗) or were preserved (○) compared to about two years ago:

✗ Remembering recent events
✗ Recalling recent conversations
○ Word finding
✗ Managing money and finances
✗ Managing medication independently
✗ Using transport

There were no additional clinical features to consider for non-Alzheimer's dementia. Mrs Cheung has hypertension, diabetes, hypercholesterolaemia, and mild depression. Her education level was unclear, although it is likely that she has received more than six months but less than two years of education.

Investigations

CBP, ESR, R/LFT, calcium, vitamin $B_{12,}$ and folate were ordered. MRI revealed MTLA R = 6.9, L = 7.0, with Scheltens score R = L = 2; ARWMC 3/3, and empty sella.

Diagnosis

Early Alzheimer's disease with small vessel disease.

Management

Donepezil 5 mg daily and esomeprazole 20 mg daily were prescribed. She was recommended to join a centre-based programme with cognitively stimulating activities to maintain cognitive functions and quality of life. She was also encouraged to have regular exercise, a healthy diet and mental stimulation, manage stress, and maintain an active social life.

Suggestions for the Primary Care Team

This is a typical case of Alzheimer's disease with small vessel disease. Diabetes is a known risk factor for Alzheimer's disease, with insulin resistance being a core feature of type 2 diabetes mellitus and an important feature of Alzheimer's disease (the 'brain insulin resistance' concept) (5,6). Mrs Cheung's case highlighted the need to optimise the treatment of cardiovascular risk factors. Given her low education level and likely low cognitive reserve to mask neuropathology, Alzheimer's disease should still be in its early stages. Her ADL/IADL performance was also satisfactory, which should be considered a strength. However, the primary care team should note a discrepancy between the apparent good performance in orientation to place on MMSE and the reported history of Mrs Cheung getting lost in unfamiliar places. Further investigation into Mrs Cheung's ability to navigate in the community and a detailed history of the previous episodes when she was unable to find her way will be needed to facilitate the care plan in terms of safety precautions. Whether it indicates a decline in ability, or whether it was linked to lifestyle habits (e.g., unfamiliarity with certain transportation) unrelated to a change in cognitive ability, should be investigated. In any case, a location-tracking device when going out would be advisable to ensure safety.

Case 049 They Took My Money

Mrs Choi, a 78-year-old lady, presented with concerns raised by her son over her memory problems. She was noted to have poor short-term memory (e.g., repeated questioning and misplacing her ID card) and problems in wayfinding in familiar locations. She would also accuse her family members of taking her money from time to time and has had an incident of going to the bank three days in a row to allege money being taken away by the bank.

Findings from Screening Assessments by Allied Healthcare and Social Care Team

Cognitive functioning	Scored 16/30 on MMSE, indicating cognitive impairment, adjusted for education level. Mrs Choi's performance was impaired in delayed recall (0/3), orientation to time (1/5), place (2/5), and in calculation (1/5). Her performance was, however, normal in registration (3/3), language (5/5), three-step commands (3/3), and visuospatial relationships (1/1). Her Clock Drawing Test finding was negative.
ADL/IADL	Mrs Choi was independent in ADLs (Barthel Index 100/100). She was independent in laundry and modified independent in grocery shopping (she was able to buy a few simple items, such as bread and oranges); she needed assistance in taking medications (needed to be reminded with a phone call), meal preparation, and housekeeping; she also needed supervision in community access (she stayed on her own estate most of the time) and handling finances (pocket money given by son). For external communication, she had a problem remembering phone numbers (Lawton IADL Scale 32/56).
Staging and clinical rating	Results suggested a Global Deterioration Scale stage 4, indicating mild dementia. She showed clear deficits during the clinical interview, with decreased knowledge of current and recent events, a decreased ability to travel and handle finances, and a concentration deficit on serial subtractions.

History Taken with Carer by Primary Care Physician

Mrs Choi's son reported noticing memory problems in his mother that had concerned him for about a year. Delusional ideations were reported: she would accuse family members of taking her money from time to time. Using the GPCOG Informant Interview, the following areas were noted to show more difficulties (✗) or were preserved (○) compared to about two years ago:

- ✗ Remembering recent events
- ✗ Recalling recent conversations
- ○ Word finding
- ✗ Managing money and finances
- ✗ Managing medication independently
- ✗ Using transport

There were no additional clinical features to consider for non-Alzheimer's dementia. Mrs Choi has hypertension, hypercholesterolaemia, and coronary artery disease. No family history of psychiatric disorders or dementia was reported. Her education level was unclear, although it is likely that she has received more than two years of education.

Diagnosis

Early Alzheimer's disease.

Management

Donepezil 5 mg every alternate night was prescribed. She was recommended to join a centre-based programme with cognitively stimulating activities, for the maintenance of cognitive functions and quality of life.

Suggestions for the Primary Care Team

This is a case of very early Alzheimer's disease with a typical pattern of impairment shown on assessment. Mrs Choi's performance in the Clock Drawing Test was better than other cognitive tests, suggesting a good response to donepezil. Her MMSE score, however, was slightly lower than expected for her dementia stage. The distressed behaviours and neuropsychiatric symptoms of dementia, such as the delusion observed in this case, may aggravate the cognitive symptoms of Alzheimer's disease and affect a person's community functioning.

Considering that there was significant impairment in Mrs Choi's general functional performance in most IADL domains, which will further deteriorate if her delusional ideations are not managed, the current management focus would be to identify strategies for preventing/minimising the occurrence of these ideations and/or their consequences. The primary care team may equip carers with appropriate caring and communication skills for working with delusions, such as avoiding direct confrontation (e.g., defending or arguing when being suspected as a thief in this case), providing locked drawers, cupboards, or even a room for the person to store his/her own belongings (while keeping spare keys in a safe place in case of loss of keys), housekeeping, and organising personal belongings only when she is away to avoid being suspected while at the same time keeping the items in their original place. Potential carers' stress and strain in family relationships caused by the delusion should also be explored and addressed.

Case 050 How Did I Spend That Money?

Mr Hui, an 81-year-old man, presented with concerns raised by a social worker from a home care team about his memory problems. He was noted to have poor short-term memory: forgetting appointments and meal delivery dates and showing a decreased ability to handle finances (he was noted to have withdrawn large sums of money but was unable to report how the money was spent).

Findings from Screening Assessments by Allied Healthcare and Social Care Team

Cognitive functioning	Scored 13/30 on MMSE, indicating cognitive impairment, adjusted for education level. Mr Hui's performance was impaired in calculation (0/5) and visuospatial relationships (0/1), delayed recall (1/3), and language (2/5); he was slightly impaired in orientation to time (3/5) and place (3/5), registration (2/3), and three-step commands (2/3). The Clock Drawing Test was positive: he was unable to construct a clock according to the instruction given (Figure 2.36); when given a clock face with numbers and asked to indicate the time, he wrote the time on the clock instead of using clock arms to indicate time, suggestive of conceptual deficits.
ADL/IADL	Mr Hui was independent in ADL performance (Barthel Index 100/100). For IADL, he was independent in external communication and laundry and modified independent in housekeeping (a bad smell was reported by staff); he needed assistance in meal preparation (required meal delivery service; he was able to boil water), handling finances, and grocery shopping; he needed supervision on taking medication (with help from a community nurse) and community access (to nearby area only) (Lawton IADL Score 39/56).

Staging and clinical rating	Results suggested a Global Deterioration Scale stage of 4, indicating mild dementia. He showed decreased knowledge of current and recent events and a decreased ability to travel and handle finances. He has maintained general orientation to time and place and the ability to travel to familiar locations.

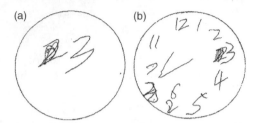

Figure 2.36 Findings from Mr Hui's Clock Drawing Test. (a) Clock Drawing (3 o'clock). (b) Clock Copying (10 past 10)

History Taken with Carer by Primary Care Physician

Mr Hui's social worker reported noticing memory problems in him for a few months. No delusional ideations were reported. Using the GPCOG Informant Interview, the following areas were noted to show more difficulties (×) or were preserved (O) compared to about two years ago:

× Remembering recent events
× Recalling recent conversations
O Word finding
× Managing money and finances
× Managing medication independently
O Using transport

There were no additional clinical features to consider for non-Alzheimer's dementia. Mr Hui has hypertension and benign prostatic hyperplasia. No family history of psychiatric disorders or dementia was reported. His education level was unclear, although it is likely that he has received less than six months of education.

Investigations

CBP, ESR, R/LFT, calcium, vitamin B_{12}, folate, fasting sugar, fasting lipids, and T4 were ordered.

Diagnosis

Early Alzheimer's disease.

Management

Mr Hui was recommended to join a centre-based programme with cognitively stimulating activities, for the maintenance of cognitive functions and quality of life.

Suggestions for the Primary Care Team

This is a typical case of early Alzheimer's disease. The positive finding on the Clock Drawing Test, which was worse in the drawing part and improved in the copying part, is compatible with a typical presentation of Alzheimer's disease. While Mr Hui's MMSE score was lower than expected for this stage of Alzheimer's disease, this should be interpreted in the context of a low education level and therefore the relatively low cognitive reserve that would be available to compensate for or mask the impact of Alzheimer's disease neuropathology. The primary care physician may consider the use of cholinesterase inhibitors to maintain Mr Hui's cognition and enhance the effects of the non-pharmacological interventions.

With Mr Hui's typical presentation of Alzheimer's disease, it is foreseeable that his memory and other cognitive problems will continue to affect his daily functions as he progresses along the disease stages. Advance care planning is needed at this stage, taking into consideration whether support from family carers may be identified; for example, an appointed carer will be needed to handle his finances and to support Mr Hui's future care planning. As Mr Hui's informant who prompted the help-seeking was his social worker, some information about Mr Hui's family situation and current care arrangements could be available through service liaison. The primary care team should pay attention to the likelihood that Mr Hui may become dependent shortly and will be in need of companions for living in the community; carers (if any) have to prepare for better arrangements and planning.

Case 051 Midnight Meal

Mrs Mok, a 90-year-old lady, presented with concerns raised by her friend about her memory problems. She was reported to have problems with short-term memory (such as repeated questioning and misplacing valuable items), disorientation in time (for example, she was calling her friend in the middle of night to ask if she had eaten yet), and problems in wayfinding.

Findings from Screening Assessments by Allied Healthcare and Social Care Team

Cognitive functioning	Scored 8/30 on MMSE, indicating cognitive impairment, adjusted for education level. Mrs Mok's performance was impaired in orientation to time (0/5) and place (0/5), delayed recall (0/3), calculation (0/5), and visuospatial relationships (0/1); her performance was slightly impaired in three-step commands (2/3), registration (2/3), and language (4/5). The Clock Drawing Test showed no reasonable or understandable attempt at drawing a clock face. She was educated but was unable to write numbers independently. Her performance improved slightly on the copying part, although she was still unable to complete the clock, with difficulties in copying numbers (Figure 2.37).
ADL/IADL	She required some help in hygiene (there was an incident of her placing toilet paper on the bed), bathing (questionable), stair climbing, and dressing (unwilling to change her clothes); she was independent in other ADLs (Barthel Index 94/100). She was dependent in laundry and housekeeping; she required assistance in taking medications, meal preparation (she uses a meal delivery service), community access (with a history of getting lost), handling finances (needed assistance to go to the bank and misplacing money frequently), and grocery shopping (she may forget to pay and will go out to buy dessert frequently; the shop owner

was aware and would only do business with her once a day) (Lawton IADL Scale 24/56).

Staging and clinical rating	Results suggested a Global Deterioration Scale stage 5, indicating moderate dementia. During the interview, she was unable to recall a major relevant aspect of her current life, such as her full address and telephone number, or to recall the name of her husband who had passed away five years ago. She was usually disoriented in time and place and had difficulty counting backwards from 40 by 4s or 20 by 2s. She required no assistance with toileting or eating, but might have difficulty choosing proper clothing to wear; personal hygiene was also impaired, with her friend reporting that she would wear the same outfit over a long period despite having a large collection of clothes.

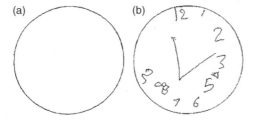

Figure 2.37 Findings from Mrs Mok's Clock Drawing Test. (a) Clock Drawing (3 o'clock). (b) Clock Copying (10 past 10)

History Taken with Carer by Primary Care Physician

Mrs Mok's friend reported noticing Mrs Mok's memory problems that had concerned her for about three years. No delusional ideations were reported. Using the GPCOG Informant Interview, the following areas were noted to show more difficulties (×) or were preserved (○) compared to about two years ago:

× Remembering recent events
× Recalling recent conversations
× Word finding
× Managing money and finances
× Managing medication independently
× Using transport

It was unclear whether Mrs Mok's tendency to shop repeatedly for desserts was related to overeating and craving sweet food. There were no additional clinical features to consider for non-Alzheimer's dementia. Mrs Mok has hypertension. No family history of psychiatric disorders or dementia was reported. Her education level was unclear, although it was reported that she had probably received more than two years of education. She lives alone.

Investigations

CT brain (plain) scan was ordered.

Diagnosis

Moderate Alzheimer's disease.

Management

No medication was prescribed at the time of the report, when Mrs Mok's drug record was being retrieved from a hospital. She was recommended to join a centre-based programme with cognitively stimulating activities, for the maintenance of cognitive functions and quality of life.

Suggestions for the Primary Care Team

Mrs Mok presented at a slightly older age for Alzheimer's disease symptom onset. Her MMSE score was lower than expected for her disease stage, which may be related to the additional effect of age-related cognitive frailty on top of Alzheimer's disease. Given that her condition is compatible with moderate Alzheimer's disease, it is recommended that Mrs Mok be treated accordingly. A cholinesterase inhibitor is indicated.

Based on the symptoms reported and overall clinical picture, Mrs Mok's ADL/IADL functioning as assessed from her friend's report may not be entirely accurate: she lives alone and her friend may not be fully aware of her daily self-care ability. To derive an appropriate care plan, the primary care team is recommended to conduct a home visit and gather further information from multiple sources about Mrs Mok's daily functioning, with direct tests/assessments where appropriate. While Mrs Mok's communication ability remained intact (language and attention), considering her severe deterioration in other cognitive functions, full-time caring would be recommended to ensure safety and quality of life.

Case 052   Reporting a 10-Year-Old Traffic Accident

Mr Yip, a 74-year-old gentleman, presented with concerns raised by his son about his memory problems that had been noted for about two years: Mr Yip was observed to misplace his personal belongings, be unable to find his way home after returning from a trip, and mix up the dates of past events (e.g., he has mistaken events that happened 20 years ago as something that happened a few days ago; there was a recent incident when he went to the police station to report a traffic accident, which happened more than 10 years ago with the file closed).

Findings from Screening Assessments by Allied Healthcare and Social Care Team

Cognitive functioning	Scored 13/30 on MMSE, indicating cognitive impairment, adjusted for education level. Mr Yip's performance was impaired in orientation to time (2/5) and place (2/5), three-step commands (1/3), calculation (1/5), delayed recall (0/3), and visuospatial relationships (0/1); he had slight difficulties in language (4/5); his performance was normal in registration (3/3). The Clock Drawing Test showed misplaced numbers on the clock face, with half of the numbers in clockwise and another half in anticlockwise order. His performance was significantly improved on the copying task. He was able to read the clock (Figure 2.38).
ADL/IADL	He was independent in all ADLs (Barthel Index 100/100) and independent in most IADLs (Lawton IADL Scale 50/56), except that he was unable to use the phone.

| Depressive symptoms | Scored 3/15 on GDS-15, no obvious depressive mood was noted. |
| Staging and clinical rating | Scored 0.5/3 on Clinical Dementia Rating, indicating questionable dementia. He showed mild impairment in memory, orientation, judgement, and problem-solving; he was fair in community affairs and home and hobbies, and normal in personal care. |

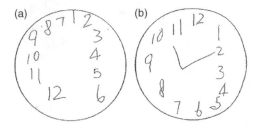

Figure 2.38 Findings from Mr Yip's Clock Drawing Test. (a) Clock Drawing (3 o'clock). (b) Clock Copying (10 past 10)

History Taken with Carer by Primary Care Physician

Mr Yip's son reported noticing memory problems in his father that had concerned him for about two years. No delusional ideations were reported. Using the GPCOG Informant Interview, the following areas were noted to show more difficulties (×) or were preserved (○) compared to about two years ago:

× Remembering recent events
× Recalling recent conversations
○ Word finding
○ Managing money and finances
× Managing medication independently
× Using transport

There were no additional clinical features to consider for non-Alzheimer's dementia. No family history of psychiatric disorders or dementia was reported. Mr Yip walks unaided. He has received an education to P.6 (approximately eight years of education).

Physical Examination Findings

General examination revealed no affect or hygiene problem. No significant CVS or CNS findings.

Investigations

CBP, R/LFT, vitamin B_{12}, fasting sugar, fasting lipids, and TFT were ordered. The result showed 5.7 in the fasting sugar test. CT brain (plain) scan revealed cerebral atrophy.

Diagnosis

Probable Alzheimer's disease.

Management

Rivastigmine transdermal system 5 mg daily was prescribed. Mr Yip was recommended to join a specialised day care service for two days per week to receive a structured and tailored intervention programme and cognitively stimulating activities to delay deterioration and maintain his quality of life.

Suggestions for the Primary Care Team

This is a probable case of Alzheimer's disease with a positive Clock Drawing Test. Mr Yip's impairment pattern is typical of Alzheimer's disease, although his MMSE score was slightly lower than expected for his relatively young age, which could suggest a high amyloid pathology load. His poor performance in orientation to place should be interpreted with caution, taking into account that he might have been taken to the assessment site by the carer without being informed. The provisional diagnosis will require observation of his cognition over time for confirmation. Meanwhile, a cholinesterase inhibitor can be started in the event of deteriorating cognition.

Confusion of long-term and short-term memories may be more common in moderate and later stages of dementia, which is consistent with Mr Yip's cognitive assessment result, showing moderate impairment in cognition. The primary care team should note that his ADL and IADL appeared better than expected, given his moderate cognitive impairment, which should be considered as his strengths. Carers should, however, be cautious about risks and avoid underestimating Mr Yip's deterioration, as he would need more care and verbal reminders and would need to be accompanied in situations of potential safety concerns. Considering his confusion over time, the primary care team can give him a trial of intensive reality orientation or even incorporate reality orientation into his 24-hour living schedule.

Case 053 Pushing Wife to the Ground

Mr Au, an 83-year-old gentleman, presented with concerns raised by his son about his memory problems, poor temper, and problems in his social life. His son complained of Mr Au's forgetfulness (e.g., repeatedly paying for the administration cost of his wife's residential care), losing his temper and becoming easily agitated, and poor judgement: there was an incidence when he fought with his wife (who was diagnosed as having dementia) in her care home, pushing her to the ground and squeezing her neck, because he took his wife's hallucinations as real, according to a witness (daughter-in-law).

Findings from Screening Assessments by Allied Healthcare and Social Care Team

Cognitive functioning	Scored 21/30 on MMSE, indicating cognitive impairment, adjusted for education level. Mr Au's performance was impaired in orientation to place (1/5), calculation (3/5; even when cues were given, he was not able to recall the remainder), delayed recall (2/3), three-step commands (2/3), and visuospatial relationships (0/1). The Clock Drawing Test showed slight impairments in executive function and visuospatial relationships, with deviation in spacing between numbers on the clock face.
ADL /IADL	Mr Au was moderately dependent in ADLs (Barthel Index 87/100). He required supervision in toileting, bathing, transfers, ambulation, and walking up and down stairs due to lower limb weakness and unsteady gait. He had occasional functional incontinence (1–2 times per year) if travelling for a long distance. He required regular support from family for community living tasks; needed supervision on community access due to unsteady gait; and required assistance in handling finances (unable to handle residential administration costs of his wife, but able to draw money from the bank). He was dependent in meal preparation and housekeeping (mainly due to physical decline) (Lawton IADL Scale 38/56).

| Depressive symptoms | Scored 6/15 on GDS-15, no clinically significant depressive symptoms were suggested. However, he was observed to be worrying a lot about his wife and thought of himself as being useless. He would feel tired easily. |
| Staging and clinical rating | Scored 0.5/3 on Clinical Dementia Rating, indicating questionable dementia. He showed questionable impairment in memory, judgement and problem-solving, and community affairs and mild impairment in orientation and home and hobbies. |

History Taken with Carer by Primary Care Physician

Mr Au's son reported noticing memory problems in his father that had concerned him for about one year. Delusional ideations were reported. He started to present with tremor about two years ago, about the same time that his wife was admitted to the care home. He was noted to always blame himself as the major cause of the cognitive decline of his wife, and he worried a lot about her. He has given up almost all of his social life, staying in the care home with his wife most of the day. He has avoided travelling far due to his worries about his wife in the care home. Using the GPCOG Informant Interview, the following areas were noted to show more difficulties (✗) or were preserved (○) compared to about two years ago:

✗ Remembering recent events
✗ Recalling recent conversations
○ Word finding
○ Managing money and finances
○ Managing medication independently
○ Using transport

There were no additional clinical features to consider for non-Alzheimer's dementia. Mr Au has diabetes, hypertension, old myocardial infarction/ischaemic heart disease, dyslipidaemia, chronic obstructive pulmonary disease, gout, benign prostatic hyperplasia with transurethral resection of the prostate, and possible cervical myelopathy. He is currently on amlodipine 5 mg daily, metoprolol 25 mg twice a day, metformin 1 g twice a day, simvastatin 5 mg nocte, allopurinol 200 mg daily, isosorbide mononitrate 20 mg three times daily, aspirin 100 mg daily, beclomethasone two puffs twice a day, salbutamol four puffs four times per day, ipratropium bromide four puff four times per day, crotamiton cream PRN, and nitroglycerin PRN. No family history of psychiatric disorders or dementia was reported. He has received a secondary education of Form 2 (approximately eight years of education). Mr Au walks with a stick.

Physical Examination Findings

General examination revealed no affect or hygiene problem. No significant CVS or CNS findings.

Investigations

CBP, R/LFT, vitamin B_{12}, fasting sugar, fasting lipids, and TSH/FT4 were ordered. TSH/FT4 was normal. CT brain (plain) scan revealed mild cerebral atrophy; no significant medial temporal lobe atrophy or small vessel disease was found.

Diagnosis

Early Alzheimer's disease.

Management

Rivastigmine transdermal system 4.6 mg daily was prescribed. He was recommended to join a specialised day care service for two days per week to receive a structured and tailored intervention programme and cognitively stimulating activities to delay deterioration and maintain his quality of life.

Suggestions for the Primary Care Team

Mr Au has Alzheimer's disease with a typical presentation pattern of impairment and positive Clock Drawing Test results, although his poor performance in orientation to place on MMSE should be interpreted with caution, taking into account that he might have been taken to the assessment site by the carer without being informed. Physicians should look for clinical features of parkinsonism, consider cortical Lewy body disease, and ask about a history of hallucinations and rapid eye movement behaviour disorder (REMBD). The primary care team should also pay attention to Mr Au's irritability and self-blaming, with possible depression. Starting rivastigmine transdermal system treatment is appropriate, while an atypical antipsychotic, such as quetiapine, should be considered if behavioural problems do not improve with rivastigmine.

Mr Au's cognitive function shown in the assessment was good, and therefore his ADL and IADL appeared to be worse than expected for his cognitive performance. The primary care team should explore whether the impairments in ADL/IADL were more related to older age and physical frailty or to distressed behaviours and neuropsychiatric symptoms of dementia. Although no problems with managing medication were reported, with the polypharmacy and as his cognition continues to deteriorate, some safety precautions would be needed. Mr Au has more prominent psychiatric symptoms than cognitive impairment; the team is recommended to rule out the impact of these symptoms and reassess after symptom stabilisation.

Case 054 Smelly Clothes

Mr Lau, an 80-year-old gentleman, presented with concerns raised by his spouse about his memory problems. His wife complained of his memory deterioration over about 12 months. He was noted to be forgetting frequently about conversations with others, misplacing his money, and forgetting that he had already eaten.

Findings from Screening Assessments by Allied Healthcare and Social Care Team

Cognitive functioning	Scored 11/30 on MMSE, indicating cognitive impairment, adjusted for education level. Mr Lau's performance was impaired in orientation to time (2/5), three-step commands (0/3), and calculation (1/5), delayed recall (0/3), and visuospatial relationships (0/1); he was also impaired in orientation to place (3/5). His performance was, however, normal in registration (3/3) and language (5/5). The Clock Drawing Test showed some problems in the placement of numbers, with impaired executive function observed. He was able to read the clock (Figure 2.39).

ADL/IADL	Mr Lau was assisted in ADLs (Barthel Index 69/100); he has lower limb weakness after a stroke. He needed assistance in personal hygiene, toileting, and ambulation. He has bladder incontinence. He was dependent in IADLs (Lawton IADL Scale 10/56) including requiring help in taking medications, meal preparation, laundry, housekeeping, handling finances, and grocery shopping; he needed company for community access. He was not able to use phones.
Depressive symptoms	Scored on GDS-15 3/15, no obvious depressive mood was noted.
Staging and clinical rating	Scored 2/3 on Clinical Dementia Rating, indicating moderate impairment. He showed moderate impairment in memory, orientation, judgement and problem-solving, community affairs, personal care, and severe impairment in home and hobbies.

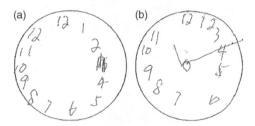

Figure 2.39 Findings from Mr Lau's Clock Drawing Test. (a) Clock Drawing (3 o'clock). (b) Clock Copying (10 past 10)

History Taken with Carer by Primary Care Physician

Mr Lau's wife reported noticing memory problems in her husband that had concerned her for about two years. No delusional ideations were reported. Using the GPCOG Informant Interview, the following areas were noted to show more difficulties (×) or were preserved (○) compared to about two years ago:

× Remembering recent events
× Recalling recent conversations
× Word finding
× Managing money and finances
× Managing medication independently
× Using transport

Mr Lau had a stroke two years ago. He walks with a quadripod. There is an additional feature to consider for non-Alzheimer's disease: Mr Lau has apraxia in self-care and was unable to dress himself and use feeding utensils, for which corticobasal degeneration may be considered. Mr Lau has diabetes, atrial fibrillation, an old cerebrovascular accident, and dyslipidaemia. He is on warfarin 3 mg daily, pantoprazole 40 mg daily, metformin 500 mg twice a day, simvastatin 20 mg, paracetamol 500 mg qid, tramadol 50 mg twice a day PRN, and insulin lispro. No family history of psychiatric disorders or dementia was reported. He has received primary education to P.6 (approximately six years of education). He has limited social activities.

Physical Examination Findings

General examination revealed a hygiene problem (smelly clothes) but not an affect problem. Mr Lau was found to have atrial fibrillation during CVS examination. No significant CNS findings.

Investigations

CBP, R/LFT, fasting sugar, fasting lipids, chest X-ray, and ECG were ordered. CT brain (plain) scan revealed an old infarct at the parieto-occipital region.

Diagnosis

Mixed dementia (Alzheimer's disease and vascular dementia).

Management

Rivastigmine transdermal system was prescribed. He was recommended to join a specialised day care service for two days per week to receive a structured and tailored intervention programme and cognitively stimulating activities to delay deterioration and maintain quality of life.

Suggestions for the Primary Care Team

Mr Lau had early Alzheimer's disease, and it was appropriate to start with cholinesterase inhibitors. The history of stroke and physical frailty has contributed to Mr Lau's cognitive impairment, which has also affected his self-care ability; it is therefore appropriate to interpret his apraxia in self-care as part of the symptomatology of mixed dementia instead of corticobasal degeneration. The primary care physician is advised to gradually titrate up the dose of the cholinesterase inhibitor in the event of deteriorating cognition.

The primary care team is recommended to figure out whether the apraxia and inability to perform the self-care tasks is because of post-stroke physical dysfunctions. Physical maintenance will be of higher priority than cognitive enhancement at this stage. Another focus of the care plan is to prevent complications when Mr Lau progresses to a later stage of dementia. Carer support services and preparation for long-term care should be planned together with Mr Lau's family.

Case 055   Fire Hazards

Ms Chu, an 85-year-old lady, presented with concerns raised by her daughter over her memory problems. She had been self-aware of her memory decline for about two years, noting that she would often forget about her conversations with others and appointments. Her daughter noted the memory deterioration of Ms Chu over about six months, citing that she often forgets to switch off the stove after cooking and gets lost and cannot find her way home.

Findings from Screening Assessments by Allied Healthcare and Social Care Team

Cognitive functioning	Scored 10/30 on MMSE, indicating cognitive impairment, adjusted for education level. Ms Chu's performance was impaired in orientation to time (1/5) and place (1/5), three-step commands (1/3), calculation (0/5), delayed recall (0/3), and visuospatial relationships (0/1); her performance was, however, fair in language (4/5) and normal in registration (3/3). The Clock Drawing Test was not completed as Ms Chu refused to draw because she has never received any education. She was not able to read the clock.
ADL/IADL	Ms Chu was independent in most ADLs (Barthel Index 92/100); she has lower limb weakness and slight difficulties in using stairs. She

	needed supervision and occasional assistance for IADLs (Lawton IADL Scale 43/56): she needed reminders for medications and assistance for laundry, housekeeping, and community access. She can manage simple cooking only. She was able to answer phone calls but not able to dial. She was able to shop but would forget items and repeatedly buy the same items.
Depressive symptoms	Scored 7/15 on GDS-15, no clinically significant depressive mood was evidenced. She nevertheless showed some difficulties in understanding the questions; she appeared frustrated about the fact that she had never received any education.
Staging and clinical rating	Scored 2/3 on Clinical Dementia Rating, indicating moderate dementia. She showed moderate impairment in memory, orientation, and community affairs and mild impairment in judgement and problem-solving, home and hobbies. She rated fair in personal care.

History Taken with Carer by Primary Care Physician

Ms Chu's daughter reported noticing memory problems in her mother that had concerned her for about two years. No delusional ideations were reported. Using the GPCOG Informant Interview, the following areas were noted to show more difficulties (×) or were preserved (○) compared to about two years ago:

× Remembering recent events
× Recalling recent conversations
○ Word finding
× Managing money and finances
× Managing medication independently
× Using transport

There were no additional clinical features to consider for non-Alzheimer's dementia. Ms Chu has hypertension. No family history of psychiatric disorders or dementia was reported. She did not receive any education. She walked unaided.

Physical Examination Findings

General examination revealed no affect or hygiene problem. Ms Chu had normal blood pressure. No significant CVS or CNS findings.

Investigations

CT brain (plain) imaging was ordered.

Diagnosis

Alzheimer's disease.

Management

Rivastigmine transdermal system 4.6 mg daily was prescribed. She was recommended to join a specialised day care service for two days per week to receive a structured and tailored intervention programme and cognitively stimulating activities to delay deterioration and maintain her quality of life.

Suggestions for the Primary Care Team

This is a typical presentation of Alzheimer's disease in an older person who has not received any formal education. For staging, the primary care team could use the Functional Assessment Staging Test (FAST) method, paying attention to whether Ms Chu was unable to choose appropriate clothing: an indicator of her entering into the moderate stage of dementia. Starting treatment with cholinesterase inhibitors would be appropriate, while primary care physicians may consider memantine in the event of deteriorating cognition.

Ms Chu's assessment results on GDS-15 showed marginally significant depressive symptoms. Depression in older age and Alzheimer's disease have multiple pathways of relationships, with some shared neurosubstrates; managing the depressive symptoms at the same time is therefore an important aspect of her treatment plan.

While Ms Chu's current profile suggests a moderate to severe stage of dementia already, she was still able to maintain community living and able to go out by herself, which should be considered her strength; carers will, however, need to be reminded about her risk of getting lost and other safety concerns. Her level of signs and symptoms suggested an onset earlier than the reported two years, which might have been missed by carers. Carers' awareness and education may be needed if this is the case. Home assessment for safety measures, adaptive aids with reminders, a stove with an automatic shut-off, and other safety appliances may help, as well as home security IP cameras.

Case 056 Forgetting to Pick up Grandchildren

Mr Cheung, a 78-year-old gentleman, presented with concerns raised by his son about his memory problems. Mr Cheung was self-aware of his own memory decline for about a year, noting that he would forget his conversations with others. His son had noted his memory deterioration for about a year: he would occasionally forget to pick up his grandchildren from kindergarten, have difficulties with orientation even in familiar places, and forget the names of some family members.

Findings from Screening Assessments by Allied Healthcare and Social Care Team

Cognitive functioning	Scored 15/30 on MMSE, indicating cognitive impairment, adjusted for education level. Mr Cheung's performance was impaired in orientation to time (1/5), three-step commands (1/3), calculation (2/5), delayed recall (0/3), and visuospatial relationships (0/1); he was slightly impaired in orientation to place (3/5); his performance was normal in registration (3/3) and language (5/5). The Clock Drawing Test showed a normal executive function, but with slight impairment in number spacing. He was able to read the clock and was aware of his poor placement of some numbers.
ADL/IADL	Mr Cheung was semi-dependent in ADLs (Barthel Index 95/100). He was unaware that the weather was getting cold and of the need for putting on more clothes. He wore the same outfit for more than 10 days without washing it. He has modified independence in IADLs (Lawton IADL Scale 47/56). He needed assistance in handling finances (e.g., he was only able to handle change while shopping); he can only do simple housework, and his home was noted to be messy; he was able to do laundry and use

	the phone with a modified method. He can shop but would sometimes forget items and bought the same items repeatedly.
Depressive symptoms	Scored 4/15 on GDS-15, no obvious depressive mood was noted.
Staging and clinical rating	Scored 1/3 on Clinical Dementia Rating, indicating mild dementia. He showed mild impairment in memory, orientation, judgement and problem-solving, community affairs, home and hobbies, and personal care.

History Taken with Carer by Primary Care Physician

Mr Cheung's son reported noticing memory problems in his father that had concerned him for about a year. No delusional ideations were reported. Using the GPCOG Informant Interview, the following areas were noted to show more difficulties (×) or were preserved (○) compared to about two years ago:

× Remembering recent events
× Recalling recent conversations
× Word finding
× Managing money and finances
× Managing medication independently
× Using transport

There were no additional clinical features to consider for non-Alzheimer's dementia. Mr Cheung has hypertension and a right inguinal hernia (repaired). He was currently on terazosin 2 mg daily and hypromellose eyedrops. No family history of psychiatric disorders or dementia was reported. He has received primary education to P.3 (approximately three years of education). He walks unaided.

Physical Examination Findings

General examination revealed no depressive-looking mood/affect problem and no affect or hygiene problem. Mr Cheung had no atrial fibrillation, heart murmur, or carotid bruit problem, with normal cardiac impulse on CVS examination. CNS examination revealed no focal pyramidal sign, extra-pyramidal sign, gait abnormalities, or speech problems.

Investigations

CT brain (plain) scan was ordered.

Diagnosis

Alzheimer's disease.

Management

Donepezil 2.5 mg daily was prescribed. He was recommended to join a specialised day care service for two days per week to receive a structured and tailored intervention programme and cognitively stimulating activities to delay deterioration and to maintain quality of life.

Suggestions for the Primary Care Team

In view of the relatively young age of onset, Mr Cheung's education level and occupational history should be considered to help interpret the level of impairment taking into account the level of premorbid cognitive reserve. In this case, while the impairment pattern was typical of Alzheimer's disease, Mr Cheung's MMSE score was lower than expected for the early stage of dementia. There is no other obvious comorbidity in his history, so a more aggressive amyloid load may be possible, although the primary care team should note a low level of education (about three years) that suggests a low cognitive reserve.

It is likely that Mr Cheung's onset was earlier than one year before, as his signs and symptoms might have been masked by a high level of independence in ADLs and IADLs. It could also be because Mr Cheung's carers were not able to observe his performance in these tasks, missing the signs of decline and impairment, or because the person has already adapted to the dysfunctions by himself, given his high functioning level, which could result in a phenomenon of 'sudden' deterioration from the informants' point of view. The primary care team should try to investigate Mr Cheung's actual and potential self-care ability to determine if discrepancies – or excess disability – exist, in which case strategies to close the gap and support the best possible functioning would be appropriate until Mr Cheung reaches a later stage of disease.

Case 057 Living Alone and Getting Lost

Ms Soo, an 86-year-old lady, presented with concerns raised by her daughter about her memory problems. She was aware of her own memory decline, noting that she had got lost in the community once and could not find her way home. A social worker on her housing estate also noticed Ms Soo's recent memory deterioration. She was noted to have poor short-term memory, being forgetful about appointments, as well as having problems with calculation.

Findings from Screening Assessments by Allied Healthcare and Social Care Team

Cognitive functioning	Scored 12/30 on MoCA and 17/30 on MMSE. She was impaired in orientation to time (1/5), three-step commands (1/3), calculation (0/5), and visuospatial relationships (0/1); she showed slight difficulties in language (4/5); her performance was, however, normal in orientation to place (5/5), registration (3/3), and delayed recall (3/3). The Clock Drawing Test was not completed: she refused to complete the clock drawing task as she had not received any education and maintained that she does not know how to draw. When persuaded to complete the copying part of the task, she showed some impairment (Figure 2.40).
ADL/IADL	She was independent in most ADLs (Barthel Index 92/100), except that she may take longer to complete some tasks due to lower limb weakness. She was independent in all IADLs (Lawton IADL Scale 56/56): she was able to use the phone and a microwave to reheat meals.
Depressive symptoms	Scored 0/15 on GDS-15, no obvious depressive mood was found.
Staging and clinical rating	Clinical Dementia Rating or other staging assessment results were not available as Ms Soo was seen unaccompanied by a family member/informant.

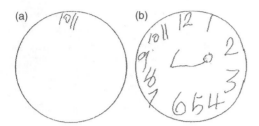

Figure 2.40 Findings from Ms Soo's Clock Drawing Test. (a) Clock Drawing (3 o'clock). (b) Clock Copying (10 past 10)

History Taken with Carer by Primary Care Physician

Ms Soo's daughter reported noticing memory problems in her mother that had concerned her for several years. No delusional ideations were reported. Using the GPCOG Informant Interview, the following areas were noted to show more difficulties (✗) or were preserved (○) compared to about two years ago:

- ✗ Remembering recent events
- ✗ Recalling recent conversations
- ✗ Word finding
- ○ Managing money and finances
- ✗ Managing medication independently
- ✗ Using transport

Ms Soo was reported to have no problem managing money as her relatives would help her with her finances.

There were no additional clinical features to consider for non-Alzheimer's dementia. Ms Soo was not on any medication. She has not received any education. Ms Soo has limited social activity, except that her daughter visits her sometimes. She stays at home most of the time; she lived alone and seldom goes out or attends any activities in community centres for older people.

Physical Examination Findings

General examination revealed no affect or hygiene problem. Ms Soo had no atrial fibrillation, heart murmur, or carotid bruit problem, with normal cardiac impulse on CVS examination. On CNS examination, no focal pyramidal sign, extra-pyramidal sign, gait abnormalities, or speech problems were found.

Investigations

Vitamin B_{12}, T4, and CT brain (plain) scan were ordered.

Diagnosis

Alzheimer's disease.

Management

Donepezil 2.5 mg daily for the first two weeks and donepezil 5 mg thereafter were prescribed. She was recommended to join a specialised day care service for two days per week to receive a structured and tailored intervention programme and cognitively stimulating activities to delay deterioration, promote social connection, and enhance her quality of life.

Suggestions for the Primary Care Team

This is a case of typical early Alzheimer's disease, and starting treatment with donepezil is acceptable. The primary care physician should consider titrating up the dose of donepezil in the event of worsening cognition. In addition, given the general lack of activity and social life, it is likely that her cognition can be enhanced with stimulation provided regularly at the day care service. The primary care team is advised to identify the causes for her disengagement from the community (e.g., personality, low motivation); addressing them would potentially help to re-engage Ms Soo for a more enriched way of life.

Ms Soo's assessment suggested a good orientation to place, with a high level of ADL and IADL functioning; these suggested that she should still be able to live well in the community with support. The cause of her episodes of getting lost should be further explored: from her profile, it appears that her functional level should allow her to look for cues in the environment or seek help from others on the street to find her way. It would be worth investigating and observing her performance when going out to find out her actual dysfunctions or difficulties. Advance care planning is indicated to prepare Ms Soo and her carers for when she may no longer be able to live alone safely.

Case 058 Repeated Bathing

Ms Siu, a 76-year-old lady, presented with concerns raised by her daughter about her memory and functional problems. Ms Siu was aware of her own memory and functional decline. Her daughter had noticed her memory decline over about 20 months, with decreased short-term memory and repetitive behaviour. Her husband also reported that she would sometimes make up stories in conversation.

Findings from Screening Assessments by Allied Healthcare and Social Care Team

Cognitive functioning	Scored 24/30 on MMSE, no evidence of cognitive impairment. Ms Siu's performance was impaired in visuospatial relationships (0/1) and calculation (2/5); she had slight difficulties with language (4/5) and orienting to time (4/5); her performance was, however, normal in orientation to place (5/5; able to recall her address), three-step commands (3/3), registration (3/3), and delayed recall (3/3). The Clock Drawing Test showed abnormalities, with one set of numbers placed clockwise whereas another set was placed anticlockwise. Clock copying was also impaired. She was able to read the clock (Figure 2.41).
ADL/IADL	Ms Siu was slightly dependent in ADLs (Barthel Index 99/100), with repeated bathing noted. She needed occasional support in IADLs (Lawton IADL Scale 41/56): she was able to handle medication and use the phone with modified methods. She would forget about her washed clothes and would leave them in the washing machine. She was able to draw money from the bank, although her financial decisions were assisted by her son. She claimed that she was able to cook, but has decreased motivation in cooking. She can shop but would frequently forget items.
Depressive symptoms	Scored 10/15 on GDS-15, clinically significant depressive mood was noted.

Staging and clinical rating	Scored 1/3 on Clinical Dementia Rating, indicating mild dementia. She showed mild impairment in memory, judgement and problem-solving, community affairs, home and hobbies, and personal care; she has questionable impairment in orientation.

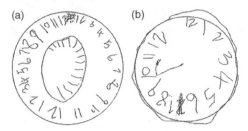

Figure 2.41 Findings from Ms Siu's Clock Drawing Test. (a) Clock Drawing (3 o'clock). (b) Clock Copying (10 past 10)

History Taken with Carer by Primary Care Physician

Ms Siu's daughter reported noticing memory problems in her mother that had concerned her for about 20 months. No delusional ideations were reported. Using the GPCOG Informant Interview, the following areas were noted to show more difficulties (✗) or were preserved (○) compared to about two years ago:

✗ Remembering recent events
✗ Recalling recent conversations
○ Word finding
○ Managing money and finances
○ Managing medication independently
○ Using transport

There were no additional clinical features to consider for non-Alzheimer's dementia. Ms Siu has hypertension. She is currently on amlodipine 5 mg daily, clopidogrel 75 mg daily, and enalapril 5 mg daily. No family history of psychiatric disorders or dementia was reported. Ms Siu did not receive any education. She lives with her husband and their youngest daughter. A poor relationship with her husband was noted. She also reported poor sleep quality. Ms Siu walked unaided, with satisfactory balance.

Physical Examination Findings

General examination revealed no affect or hygiene problem. Ms Siu was found to have hypertension on blood pressure check. No other significant CVS or CNS findings.

Investigations

CBP, R/LFT, calcium. VDRL, vitamin B_{12}, fasting sugar, MSU × R/M and culture test, chest X-ray, ECG, and CT brain (plain) scan were ordered.

Diagnosis

Alzheimer's disease.

Management

Rivastigmine transdermal system 9.5 mg daily was prescribed. She was recommended to join a specialised day care service for two days per week to receive a structured and tailored intervention programme and cognitively stimulating activities to delay deterioration and promote quality of life.

Suggestions for the Primary Care Team

This is a case of typical Alzheimer's disease with strong depressive elements. Treatment for her chronic depression with a selective serotonin reuptake inhibitor, such as escitalopram, may be considered. Ms Siu was noted to have repetitive bathing, a behaviour that can be linked to her depressive symptoms and other mental health issues such as obsession and anxiety not related to her cognitive impairment; the primary care team should clarify the premorbid personality of Ms Siu and rule out other psychological or psychiatric causes such as depression, mixed anxiety and depressive disorder, and obsessive compulsive disorder.

Ms Siu's cognitive functions, including short-term memory as shown in delayed recall, were well maintained at this moment, except for a more obvious deterioration in executive functions and other higher cognitive functions. Her ADL and IADL were still generally preserved, except for slight 'clumsiness' reported because of memory impairment. These should be regarded as her strengths, and the primary care team should try to educate her carers to encourage her participation for the maintenance of functioning as far as possible. When engaging her family in developing a care plan, the primary care team should explore family support, including the poor relationship between Ms Siu and her husband, which would be potentially relevant also for the management of her depressive symptoms.

Case 059 Denial of Functional Decline and Dementia

Ms Tse, an 80-year-old lady, presented with concerns raised by her daughter about her memory problems. Ms Tse was aware of her memory decline, although she denied any functional decline and dementia. She also complained about difficulty falling asleep. Her daughter noted her memory decline had first begun about two years ago and noted a decline in short-term memory with Ms Tse mixing up events that had happened in the past.

Findings from Screening Assessments by Allied Healthcare and Social Care Team

Cognitive functioning	Scored 14/30 on MMSE, indicating cognitive impairment, adjusted for education level. Ms Tse was disoriented in time (1/5) and partially oriented in place (3/5); she was able to recall her home address with prompting and was able to partially recognise the place where the assessment was conducted. She was able to follow simple instructions, which was affected by attention deficits. Her performance was impaired in calculation (1/5), delayed recall (1/3), three-step commands (1/3), and visuospatial relationships (0/1); she had slight difficulties in registration (2/3) but was normal in language (5/5). The Clock Drawing Test showed number misplacement impaired ability in time denotation. Her performance improved on the copying task. She was able to read the clock: she mistakenly placed the clock arms at 10:15 on the first attempt and corrected them to show 10:10 on the second attempt (Figure 2.42).

ADL/IADL	Ms Tse was independent in all ADLs (Barthel Index 100/100). She was independent in community living with occasional support needed (Lawton IADL Scale 46/56): she was able to travel to familiar places, cook, and handle housework. She would occasionally forget about taking medications and needed supervision.
Depressive symptoms	Scored on GDS-15 2/15, no obvious depressive mood was found.
Staging and clinical rating	Scored 1/3 on Clinical Dementia Rating, indicating mild dementia. She showed mild impairment in memory, orientation, judgement and problem-solving, and questionable impairment in community affairs and home and hobbies.

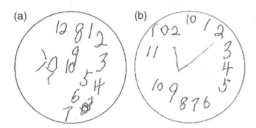

Figure 2.42 Findings from Ms Tse's Clock Drawing Test. (a) Clock Drawing (3 o'clock). (b) Clock Copying (10 past 10)

History Taken with Carer by Primary Care Physician by Primary Care Physician

Ms Tse's daughter reported noticing memory problems in her mother that had concerned her for about two years. No delusional ideations were reported. Using the GPCOG Informant Interview, the following areas were noted to show more difficulties (×) or were preserved (○) compared to about two years ago:

× Remembering recent events
× Recalling recent conversations
○ Word finding
× Managing money and finances
× Managing medication independently
○ Using transport

There were no additional clinical features to consider for non-Alzheimer's dementia. Ms Tse has hypertension. She is currently on nifedipine retard 20 mg twice a day. Worsened vision and anxiety were noted. No family history of psychiatric disorders or dementia was reported. She had not received any education. Ms Tse lives with her husband and a son. She walks unaided with satisfactory balance.

Physical Examination Findings

General examination revealed no affect or hygiene problem. Ms Tse had a high blood pressure of 130/80 mm Hg. No significant CVS or CNS findings.

Investigations

CT brain (plain) scan was ordered.

Diagnosis

Alzheimer's disease.

Management

Donepezil 5 mg daily was prescribed. She was recommended to join a specialised day care service for two days per week to receive a structured and tailored intervention programme and cognitively stimulating activities to delay deterioration and maintain her quality of life.

Suggestions for the Primary Care Team

In this case of mild Alzheimer's disease, an unusually low MMSE score was noted. While this may suggest a high amyloid load, considering the fact that Ms Tse has never received any formal education, her low cognitive reserve may also explain the low score. Ms Tse has difficulty sleeping. Primary care physicians should clarify the duration of insomnia and any mood changes.

Denial of dementia, cognitive impairment, and functional decline are common in people living with dementia, and in some otherwise healthy older people. The primary care team should equip carers with suitable caring and communication skills, such as avoiding an emphasis or focus on Ms Tse's weaknesses, dysfunctions, or poor memory; instead, appearing to be supervising, instructing, or coaching the person, carers could participate directly in the task together with Ms Tse. The primary care team may remind the carers that there is no need to confront Ms Tse for the mistakes she has made in completing the task, although mistakes (and thus failures) should be avoided as much as possible to ensure motivation, for example, by providing reminders in advance, preparing the environment well to facilitate her independence, and simplifying tasks to maximise success. Ways to minimise Ms Tse's denial are important for ensuring compliance with the medication and non-pharmacological interventions.

Case 060 What Was My Previous Job?

Ms Tang, an 82-year-old lady, presented with concerns raised by her daughter about her memory and orientation. Her daughter noted frequent episodes of forgetfulness, such as asking the same questions repeatedly and constantly looking for her belongings; she has forgotten about the last job she did before her retirement; obvious disorientation to time and place was also observed. Ms Tang was aware of her memory decline.

Findings from Screening Assessments by Allied Healthcare and Social Care Team

Cognitive functioning	Scored 18/30 on MMSE, indicating cognitive impairment, adjusted for education level. Ms Tang showed slight impairment in delayed recall (2/3) and calculation (3/5). She was disoriented to time (0/5) and impaired in orientation to place (3/5). She had slight difficulties in three-step commands (2/3); her performance was, however, normal in registration (3/3), language (5/5), and visuospatial relationships (1/1). The Clock Drawing Test showed slight impairment in spacing of numbers only.
ADL/IADL	Ms Tang needed reminders/assistance in most ADL tasks such as dressing, bathing, and toileting (Barthel Index 73/100) and most IADL tasks such as meal preparation, drug management, community access, housekeeping, and handling finances (Lawton IADL Scale 18/56).

Depressive symptoms	Scored 5/15 on GDS-15. She has limited social activities, but no obvious depressed mood was observed.
Staging and clinical rating	Scored 1/3 on Clinical Dementia Rating, indicating mild dementia. She showed mild impairment in memory, community affairs, home and hobbies, and personal care and moderate impairment in orientation and judgement and problem-solving.

History Taken with Carer by Primary Care Physician

Ms Tang's daughter reported noticing memory problems in her mother that had concerned her for about two years. No delusional ideations were reported. Using the GPCOG Informant Interview, the following areas were noted to show more difficulties (✖) or were preserved (○) compared to about two years ago:

- ✖ Remembering recent events
- ✖ Recalling recent conversations
- ✖ Word finding
- ✖ Managing money and finances
- ✖ Managing medication independently
- ✖ Using transport

There were no additional clinical features to consider for non-Alzheimer's dementia. Ms Tang had hypertension, an old cerebrovascular accident, and old myocardial infarction/ischaemic heart disease. She had hearing loss but was not wearing a hearing aid. She was on aspirin 100 mg daily, pantoprazole 40 mg daily, isosorbide mononitrate 10 mg twice a day, vitamin B complex daily, enalapril 40 mg daily, betahistine 6 mg three times a day, PRN, nitroglycerin, and trimetazidine modified release 35 mg at night. No family history of psychiatric disorders or dementia was reported. She has received secondary education of Form 3 (approximately nine years of education). She walked assisted by a helper, refused to use a stick indoors, and used a wheelchair outdoors. Ms Tang lived with her daughter, with good family support.

Physical Examination Findings

General examination revealed no affect or hygiene problem. Ms Tang had normal blood pressure of 110/70 mm Hg. Heart murmur was noted. No CNS findings.

Investigations

CBP, ESR, R/LFT, calcium, vitamin B_{12}, fasting sugar, MSU × R/M and culture test, chest X-ray, and ECG were ordered. Results were normal in CBP, calcium, vitamin B_{12}, and fasting sugar; ESR 52, ALT 54, MSU × R/M, and culture test were negative. Chest X-ray showed wide mediastinum, and ECG showed SR. CT brain (plain) scan revealed small vessel disease and lacunar infarcts at external capsule.

Diagnosis

Mild neurocognitive disorder (possible Alzheimer's disease and vascular cause), left shoulder tendonitis, and low back pain scoliotic spine with possible underlying osteoporosis.

Management

Rivastigmine transdermal system 5 mg daily, Calcichew 500 mg twice a day, and morphine patch daily in the afternoon were prescribed. Ms Tang was recommended to join a specialised day care service for two days per week to receive a structured and tailored intervention programme and cognitively stimulating activities to delay deterioration and maintain her quality of life.

Suggestions for the Primary Care Team

This is a typical case of early Alzheimer's disease with hearing issues, with an expected good treatment response to transdermal rivastigmine. Hearing impairment is a known key risk factor for dementia, contributing to a significant 8 per cent of the population attributable fraction of potentially modifiable risk factors for dementia (4). Considering Ms Tang's cognitive functioning level as shown in the MMSE assessment, her ADL/IADL performance was worse than expected, which might have been affected by her hearing problem. The primary care team should identify possible ways of improving Ms Tang's hearing, while at the same time preparing the family for the potential occurrence of distressed behaviours and neuropsychiatric symptoms of dementia: with the confusion about or lack of sensory input, it is not uncommon for people living with dementia to misinterpret others' gestures, facial expressions, or behaviours. Family carer education on better ways to communicate and handle such situations would be helpful to minimise their negative impact (when they occur) and even prevent them from arising.

Case 061 Worsening Hygiene

Mr Cheng, an 83-year-old gentleman, presented with concerns raised by his daughter over his memory and hygiene problems. Mr Cheng was aware of his own memory decline. His daughter noted that his memory decline could be traced back about 12 months, becoming more obvious in the last six months. He was noted to be forgetful about conversation content, misplacing personal items, asking the same questions repeatedly, and buying the same items over and over again. His hygiene also appeared to have declined, and he would sometimes forget to brush his teeth.

Findings from Screening Assessments by Allied Healthcare and Social Care Team

Cognitive functioning	Scored 17/30 on MMSE, indicating cognitive impairment, adjusted for education level. Mr Cheng's performance was impaired in orientation to time (2/5), place (1/5), and delayed recall (0/3); he was unable to complete three-step commands (1/3). He was able to perform calculation (4/5), and his performance was normal in registration (3/3), language (5/5), and visuospatial relationships (1/1). The Clock Drawing Test showed good number spacing and time denotation.
ADL/IADL	Mr Cheng was independent in all ADLs (Barthel Index 100/100) and semi-independent in IADLs (Lawton IADL Scale 54/56). He was not able to use the microwave. He would misplace his personal items and money.
Depressive symptoms	Scored 3/15 on GDS-15, no obvious depressive mood was found. However, he was noted to be upset about his memory decline.
Staging and clinical rating	Scored 0.5/3 on Clinical Dementia Rating, indicating questionable dementia, he showed mild impairment in memory, orientation, and judgement and problem-solving.

History Taken with Carer by Primary Care Physician

Mr Cheng's daughter reported noticing memory problems in her father that had concerned her for about one year. No delusional ideations were reported. Using the GPCOG Informant Interview, the following areas were noted to show more difficulties (✗) or were preserved (○) compared to about two years ago:

✗   Remembering recent events
✗   Recalling recent conversations
○   Word finding
○   Managing money and finances
○   Managing medication independently
○   Using transport

There were no additional clinical features to consider for non-Alzheimer's dementia. No family history of psychiatric disorders or dementia was reported. Mr Cheng received tertiary education at university.

Physical Examination Findings

General examination revealed no affect or hygiene problem. Mr Cheng had a blood pressure reading of 122/67 mm Hg. No significant CVS or CNS findings.

Investigations

CBP, R/LFT, VDRL, vitamin B_{12}, fasting sugar and MSU × R/M, and culture test were ordered. All investigations were normal but the results of MSU × R/M and culture test were pending. Chest X-ray and ECG were conducted. MRI was ordered.

Diagnosis

Mild Alzheimer's disease.

Management

Donepezil 5 mg daily was prescribed. Mr Cheng was recommended to join a specialised day care service for two days per week to receive a structured and tailored intervention programme and cognitively stimulating activities to delay deterioration and to maintain his quality of life.

Suggestions for the Primary Care Team

This is a case of early Alzheimer's disease with typical presentations, including greater impairment in delayed recall and orientation, while other cognitive domains were relatively spared. The help-seeking behaviour of the family, namely noticing a problem for 12 months and taking action when triggered by a more recent significant decline, is also typical. Although the performance in orientation to place was unexpectedly poor in comparison with orientation to time, this should be interpreted with caution, taking into account that he might have been taken to the assessment site by the carer without being informed. An MRI scan is needed to investigate medial lateral temporal atrophy. With the tertiary level of education, which suggests a higher cognitive reserve, it is possible that there is significant brain pathology despite a questionable dementia rating as shown in the Clinical Dementia Rating. Mr Cheng is expected to have good clinical response to donepezil.

Mr Cheng's performance was impaired in higher cognitive functions and memory, which are typical at this stage; his strengths are well-maintained ADL/IADL and active participation in community activities. This is a good time to receive intensive cognitively stimulating activities, while he should continue to be empowered in participating in ADL and IADL activities. Family carers, however, need to be reminded to closely observe Mr Cheng's changes in cognitive functioning and prepare for later stages of dementia.

Case 062 Subjective Cognitive Decline in a Carer

Ms Chung, an 80-year-old lady, presented with concerns raised by her son about her memory problems and poor social life. She was noted to have memory decline that can be traced back about 12 months, becoming more obvious in the last six months. She would forget about conversation content and misplace personal items. She was aware of her own memory decline.

Findings from Screening Assessments by Allied Healthcare and Social Care Team

Cognitive functioning	Scored 15/30 on MMSE, indicating cognitive impairment, adjusted for education level. Ms Chung had difficulties in orientation to time (1/5) and place (3/5); her performance was impaired in delayed recall (0/3) and calculation (1/5); she had difficulties in recalling the remaining sum after subtraction. She had difficulties in three-step commands (2/3) and visuospatial relationships (0/1). Her performance was, however, normal in registration (3/3) and language (5/5). The Clock Drawing Test showed slight errors in time denotation in the drawing part, though she was able to complete the copying part without problem.
ADL/IADL	Ms Chung was independent in all ADLs (Barthel Index 100/100) and mostly independent in IADLs (Lawton IADL Scale 55/56), except that she would forget to turn off the stove occasionally after cooking.
Depressive symptoms	Scored 3/15 on GDS-15, no obvious depressive mood was noted. One of Ms Chung's sons has a mental illness, and she expressed a high level of caring stress.
Staging and clinical rating	Scored 0.5/3 on Clinical Dementia Rating, indicating questionable dementia. She showed mild impairment in memory, orientation, and judgement and problem-solving.

History Taken with Carer by Primary Care Physician

Ms Chung's son reported noticing memory problems in his mother that had concerned him for about 12 months. No delusional ideations were reported. Using the GPCOG Informant Interview, the following areas were noted to show more difficulties (×) or were preserved (○) compared to about two years ago:

× Remembering recent events
× Recalling recent conversations
○ Word finding
○ Managing money and finances
○ Managing medication independently
○ Using transport

There were no additional clinical features to consider for non-Alzheimer's dementia. No family history of dementia was reported. A family history of depression was reported, with one of her sons diagnosed with depression. She had not received any education. She has limited social activities and was not attending any activities organised by community centres for older people.

Physical Examination Findings

General examination revealed no affect or hygiene problem. No significant CVS or CNS findings.

Investigations

CBP, R/LFT, VDRL, vitamin B_{12}, RBS, folate test, and TSH/FT4 were ordered. Vitamin B_{12}, RBS, folate and TSH/FT4 were normal. VDRL was negative. CT brain (plain) scan revealed no evidence of disease.

Diagnosis

Alzheimer's disease and overactive bladder.

Management

Rivastigmine transdermal system 5 mg daily and solifenacin were prescribed. Ms Chung was recommended to join a specialised day care service for two days per week to receive a structured and tailored intervention programme and cognitively stimulating activities to delay deterioration and maintain her quality of life.

Suggestions for the Primary Care Team

This is a typical case of early Alzheimer's disease. Medications and non-pharmacological interventions for early Alzheimer's disease are therefore appropriate. Primary care physicians should, however, watch out for symptoms of an overactive bladder after commencing rivastigmine.

While Ms Chung's deterioration in cognitive functions was obvious, her ADL and IADL performance was better than one would otherwise expect for her level of cognitive impairment. Considering that she has been taking care of a son with mental illness for many years, it is possible that Ms Chung has good premorbid independence and ADL/IADL functions, which have now become a protective factor delaying the presentation of impairments in her daily living.

Although her GDS-15 results did not suggest a significant depressive mood, a high level of carer stress is a strong risk factor for depression, and the primary care team should explore her mood further. With Ms Chung being aware of her own cognitive decline, breaking the news about her dementia diagnosis may trigger worries over the future care of her son with mental illness, which may further worsen her depressive mood. The primary care team should also pay attention to Ms Chung's future mood changes that may occur as the dementia affects her role or ability as a carer. It is advisable to engage Ms Chung and her family in discussing care arrangements, for both herself and the son she is caring for, while Ms Chung still has the mental capacity to make and communicate more complex decisions, to provide reassurance for her.

2.5 Normal Ageing, Mild Cognitive Impairment, or Mild Dementia?

Case 063 Intact Registration

Mrs Fan, a 71-year-old lady, presented with concerns raised by her younger sister about her memory problems. She was reported to show worsening memory with episodes where she has forgotten to switch off the stove, repeatedly purchased the same grocery item, and lost everyday items such as her keys.

Findings from Screening Assessments by Allied Healthcare and Social Care Team

Cognitive functioning	Score 20/30 on MMSE, indicative of cognitive impairment after adjusting for education level. Mrs Fan had impaired performance in delayed recall (0/3) and calculation (2/5) and slight problems in orientation to time (3/5) and place (4/5) and language (4/5). Her performance was, however, normal in registration (3/3), three-step commands (3/3), and visuospatial relationships (1/1). The Clock Drawing Test result was normal.
ADL/IADL	Mrs Fan was independent in all ADLs (Barthel Index 100/100). For IADLs, she required supervision in meal preparation (she would sometimes forget to switch off the stove), and she was modified independent in taking medication, community access (she showed problems in finding her way), handling finances, and grocery shopping (repeated buying of the same products and forgetting to pay and get change) (Lawton IADL Scale 50/56).
Depressive symptoms	Scored 2/15 on GDS-15, suggesting no indication of depression. She had a good appetite and maintained her hobbies (dancing).
Staging and clinical rating	Results suggested a Global Deterioration Scale stage 4, indicating moderate dementia. She showed decreased knowledge of current and recent events and a decreased ability to travel and handle finances.

History Taken with Carer by Primary Care Physician

Mrs Fan's daughter reported noticing memory problems in her mother that had concerned her for about two years, although no delusional ideations were reported. Using the GPCOG Informant Interview, the following areas were noted to show more difficulties (✗) or were preserved (○) compared to about two years ago:

✗ Remembering recent events
✗ Recalling recent conversations
✗ Word finding
○ Managing money and finances
○ Managing medication independently
○ Using transport

There were no additional clinical features to consider for non-Alzheimer's dementia. Mrs Fan had had her uterus removed, and she is currently being followed up at a medicine outpatient clinic for sphincter problems. No family history of psychiatric disorders or dementia was reported. She has received more than 10 years of education.

Investigations

Calcium, VDRL, vitamin B_{12}, folate, ECG, and TSH were ordered. CT brain (plain) scan revealed no significant atrophy, a GCA score of 0, and MTA score of 0.

Diagnosis

Mild cognitive impairment/very early Alzheimer's disease.

Management

Mrs Fan was encouraged to have regular exercise, a healthy diet, and mental stimulation, and maintain an active social life. She was recommended to join a centre-based programme with cognitively stimulating activities to maintain cognitive and self-care functions and promote quality of life.

Suggestions for the Primary Care Team

Mrs Fan presented with an impairment pattern that borders on mild cognitive impairment and very mild Alzheimer's disease. Her MMSE results showed delayed recall impairment in other cognitive domains, and ADL/IADL appeared largely intact. Considering her relatively young age of presentation and more than 10 years of education, however, the occurrence of mild impairment may nevertheless imply a more aggressive amyloid load, which is no longer being masked despite her high cognitive reserve. The recommendation for the primary care physician is therefore to treat Mrs Fan as having early Alzheimer's disease. A cholinesterase inhibitor can be trialled and observed for any improvement. A case conference with specialists would be appropriate in this case.

Mrs Fan has an active social life, and she is maintaining her hobbies, which should be considered her strengths. She also seems to be enjoying relatively good physical health and basic self-care abilities. The primary care team may make use of these strengths in maximising her community engagement and independence, while also paying attention to safety and risks, such as her risks of getting lost due to problems in finding her way, and home hazards due to poor short-term memory when using the stove. The use of anti-lost or location-tracking devices and stoves with an automatic safety switch, for example, would be helpful.

Case 064   Cognitive Frailty

Mr Lee, a 91-year-old gentleman, presented with concerns raised by his wife and daughter about his memory problem. His wife complained of his decline in short-term memory, citing that he would misplace items, forget what he/others had said, and have difficulty finding appropriate words or finding his way.

Assessments from Occupational Therapist/Social Worker

| Cognitive functioning | Scored 22/30 on MMSE, indicating cognitive impairment, adjusted for education level. Mr Lee's performance was impaired in orientation to time (2/5) and place (2/5), and visuospatial relationships (0/1) and was fair in delayed recall (2/3). His performance was, however, normal in registration (3/3), calculation (5/5), language (5/5), and visuospatial |

	relationships (1/1). Scored 18/30 on MoCA, indicating cognitive impairment, adjusted for education level. His performance was impaired in delayed recall (0/5) and slightly impaired in visuospatial/executive (3/5), naming (2/3), language (2/3), abstraction (1/2), and orientation (3/6). The Clock Drawing Test was negative, with correct denotation of time and normal spacing of numbers on the clock face.
ADL/IADL	Mr Lee needed moderate help in bathing and getting dressed because of physical limitations; he also needed some minimal help in stair climbing; he was independent in other ADLs (Barthel Index 81/100). He was dependent in meal preparation, laundry, and housekeeping; he needed supervision in community access (he was able to go to nearby places and would usually take a taxi if he needed to go to other places), handling finances (he would forget where his money was), and grocery shopping (able to buy simple items only); he was independent in other IADLs (Lawton IADL Scale 32/56).
Staging and clinical rating	Results suggested a Global Deterioration Scale stage 4, indicating mild dementia. His wife and daughter noted Mr Lee's poor cognitive performance; for example, he would read a passage or book and retain little information; he also showed a decreased ability to travel and handle finances; he showed a flattening of affect and withdrawal from challenging situations.

History Taken with Carer

Mr Lee's wife and daughter reported noticing memory problems in their husband/father that had concerned them for about two years. No delusional ideations were reported. Using the GPCOG Informant Interview, the following areas were noted to show more difficulties (✗) or were preserved (○) compared to about two years ago:

✗ Remembering recent events
✗ Recalling recent conversations
✗ Word finding
✗ Managing money and finances
✗ Managing medication independently
✗ Using transport

No additional clinical features of non-Alzheimer's dementia were noted. Comorbidities of hypercholesterolaemia, cataract (operated on), and glaucoma were reported. No family history of psychiatric disorders or dementia was reported. Mr Lee's education level was unclear, although he was suggested to have probably received more than two years of education.

Diagnosis

Alzheimer's disease, with no distressed behaviours and neuropsychiatric symptoms of dementia, and decline in memory, executive function, and language ability.

Management

No medication was prescribed due to pending blood results. Mr Lee was recommended to join a centre-based programme with cognitively stimulating activities, for the maintenance of cognitive functions and quality of life.

Comments

This is a good case to illustrate mild Alzheimer's disease in old age (over 90 years), when cognitive frailty should also be considered. While there were some features that were less compatible with a stage of mild dementia, with an intact Clock Drawing Test and the ability to manage medication by himself, Mr Lee's deterioration in ADL/IADL was more concerning. Primary care physicians may try a low dose of cholinesterase inhibitors, such as donepezil 2.5 mg, and observe if there is any improvement.

The primary care team is also recommended to find out more about Mr Lee's biography, interests, and reasons for withdrawing from challenging situations, for tailoring suitable activities in the centre. It is not uncommon for older people who have a higher level of education and some insight into his/her cognitive decline to feel ashamed of showing others their impairment. If this is the case for Mr Lee, activities should be framed as more intellectually challenging yet failure free: many arts and crafts activities may serve this purpose, and it is important to identify activities that align with Mr Lee's interests and role identity, to give him a sense of meaning and preserve his dignity. From a 'use it or lose it' perspective, Mr Lee's previous avoidance of challenges could have contributed further to his cognitive decline; by reintroducing cognitively stimulating activities in a safe setting (in terms of failures and potential humiliation) in his everyday life, there is good potential that Mr Lee's cognitive functioning can be maintained or even enhanced.

Case 065 Memory Problems Post-Discharge

Mrs Chau, an 85-year-old lady, presented with concerns raised by her daughter-in-law about her memory problems. She complained of her poor memory after a three-month hospitalisation, when she was noted to have a decline in short-term memory, such as asking the same questions repeatedly and forgetting about the stove after switching it on.

Findings from Screening Assessments by Allied Healthcare and Social Care Team

Cognitive functioning	Scored 26/30 on MMSE, no indication of cognitive impairment, adjusted for education level. Scored 17/30 on MoCA, indicating cognitive impairment, adjusted for education level. Mrs Chau did not score in naming, abstraction, and delayed recall. She showed impairment in visuospatial/executive function (2/5) and had slight problems in language (2/3). The Clock Drawing Test showed slight impairment in spacing of lines or numbers.
ADL/IADL	Mrs Chau was independent in ADLs (Barthel Index 100/100). She had modified independence in taking medication (able to remember her own medications, with medication box prepared by daughter-in-law); she needed supervision in meal preparation (reheating meals and cooking noodles), community access (to nearby areas), handling finances (can handle daily transactions), and grocery shopping (simple items). She needed assistance in housekeeping. Her IADL performance was affected by cognitive impairment; for example, she did not know how much water is needed for rice cooking, and her community access was limited to the nearby environment (Lawton IADL Scale 43/56).

| Staging and clinical rating | Results suggested a Global Deterioration Scale stage 4, indicating mild dementia. For example, she was reported to have a decreased ability to travel and handle finances. |

History Taken with Carer by Primary Care Physician

Mrs Chau's daughter-in-law reported noticing memory problems in her mother-in-law that had concerned her for about two years. Slow yet progressive decline in cognitive functions was noted; however, significant impairment was evident after a three-month hospitalisation early last year. No delusional ideations were reported. Using the GPCOG Informant Interview, the following areas were noted to show more difficulties (×) or were preserved (○) compared to about two years ago:

× Remembering recent events
× Recalling recent conversations
○ Word finding
× Managing money and finances
× Managing medication independently
× Using transport

There were no additional clinical features to consider for non-Alzheimer's dementia. Mrs Chau had hypertension and a biliary stone in the common bile duct. No family history of psychiatric disorders or dementia was reported. Her education level was unclear, although it is likely that she has received more than six months but less than two years of education.

Investigations

VDRL, vitamin B_{12}, folate, fasting sugar, and fasting lipids were ordered. CT scan was ordered.

Diagnosis

Probable early Alzheimer's disease.

Management

Mrs Chau was recommended to join a centre-based programme with cognitively stimulating activities for the maintenance of cognitive functions and quality of life.

Suggestions for the Primary Care Team

This is a case of very early Alzheimer's disease, while post-hospitalisation delirium is a differential diagnosis the primary care physician should consider. It is common for older people to develop delirium and/or dementia after hospitalisation. The primary care team should explore the signs and symptoms of delirium in Mrs Chau during her hospitalisation, as half of the post-hospitalisation delirium has its symptom onset during hospitalisation. Hospitalisation can cause disorientation; together with Mrs Chau's health condition (including physical and mental health), she may need time to recover.

Mrs Chau's cognitive screening assessment borders on cognitively intact (results from MMSE and Clock Drawing Test) and impairment (from MoCA). As these cognitive screening assessments are not definitive indicators of impairment, with cut-off scores obtained from a one-off assessment reflecting population norms instead of within-person absolute decline, they should be used as a reference to support clinical judgement only. The primary care team is therefore recommended to reassess Mrs Chau's condition in six months, after her condition has stabilised and recovered. A cholinesterase inhibitor is indicated in the event of worsening cognition in subsequent follow-ups. Meanwhile, engaging Mrs Chau in cognitively stimulating activities that are enjoyable and meaningful would be appropriate, which could support rehabilitation in the event of cognitive impairment as a result of hospitalisation, and maintain/enhance cognition in the case of early Alzheimer's disease. The primary care team may also identify ways to support Mrs Chau's reorientation by establishing healthy daily routines, including going regularly to a centre, which would be beneficial whether or not the Alzheimer's disease diagnosis is eventually confirmed.

Case 066   Intact Activities of Daily Living

Mr Lee, an 83-year-old gentleman, presented with concerns raised by his son over his memory problems. His son complained about Mr Lee's poor memory (forgetting about recent events) and declined cognitive functions.

Findings from Screening Assessments by Allied Healthcare and Social Care Team

Cognitive functioning	Scored 17/30 on MMSE, indicating cognitive impairment, adjusted for education level. Mr Lee's performance was impaired in delayed recall (0/3), visuospatial relationships (0/1), orientation to time (2/5), and calculation (1/5); he was slightly impaired in orientation to place (3/5). His performance was, however, normal in registration (3/3), language (5/5), and three-step commands (3/3). The Clock Drawing Test was positive: he was unable to complete the drawing part, with performance improving on the copying part (Figure 2.43).
ADL/IADL	Mr Lee was independent in ADLs (Barthel Index 100/100). Mr Lee was dependent in meal preparation; needed assistance in housekeeping, community access, and grocery shopping; and needed supervision in taking medications and handling finances (Lawton IADLs Scale: 34/56).
Depressive symptoms	Scored 5/15 on GDS-15, with no indication of clinically significant depressive symptoms.
Staging and clinical rating	Results suggested a Global Deterioration Scale stage 4, indicating mild dementia. He showed decreased knowledge of current and recent events; some deficits in memory of personal history; a decreased ability to travel and handle finances; and an inability to perform complex tasks.

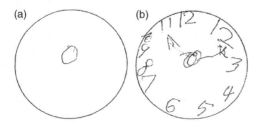

Figure 2.43 Findings from Mr Lee's Clock Drawing Test. (a) Clock Drawing (3 o'clock). (b) Clock Copying (10 past 10)

History Taken with Carer by Primary Care Physician

Mr Lee's son reported noticing memory problems in his father that had concerned him for about two years. No delusional ideations were reported. Using the GPCOG Informant Interview, the following areas were noted to show more difficulties (✗) or were preserved (○) compared to about two years ago:

- ✗ Remembering recent events
- ✗ Recalling recent conversations
- ○ Word finding
- ✗ Managing money and finances
- ✗ Managing medication independently
- ✗ Using transport

There were no additional clinical features to consider for non-Alzheimer's dementia. Mr Lee had hypertension, diabetes with neuropathy, benign prostatic hyperplasia, hypercholesterolaemia, glaucoma, and cataract. No family history of psychiatric disorders or dementia was reported. His education level was unclear, although it is likely that he has received more than two years of education.

Investigations

CBP, ESR, R/LFT, calcium, vitamin B_{12}, folate, and TSH were ordered. Results: Hb10 in CBP; 41 in ESR; urea 13.3, creatinine 161, and eGFR 38 in RFT; vitamin B_{12} 134 on 100 mg BD; and normal in LFT and TSH. MRI revealed mild age-related atrophy/multiple small foci of bilateral cerebral small vessel ischaemic changes.

Diagnosis

Mild dementia and probable Alzheimer's disease.

Management

Donepezil 2.5 mg every alternate night was prescribed. Mr Lee was recommended to a centre-based programme with cognitively stimulating activities to maintain his cognitive functioning, self-care functioning, and quality of life; he was encouraged to have regular exercise, a healthy diet and mental stimulation, and maintain an active social life.

Suggestions for the Primary Care Team

This is a typical case of early Alzheimer's disease, with a compatible impairment pattern showing delayed recall being most obviously affected compared with other cognitive domains and a positive Clock Drawing Test with worse performance in the drawing part and improvement in the copying part. Medication and non-pharmacological interventions for early Alzheimer's disease are appropriate in Mr Lee's case.

Although Mr Lee's depressive mood on assessment did not reach a clinically significant level, the primary care team can explore more about factors that would contribute to improved mood and quality of life. From a biopsychosocial perspective, psychological factors such as mood, social psychology, and personality are factors that would affect a person's dementia presentation; by optimising these factors – possibly through positive social interactions at the centre and other strategies – it is possible for Mr Lee's cognitive performance and functioning to be enhanced.

Case 067 Severe Hearing Impairment

Mrs Ma, a 77-year-old lady, presented with concerns raised by her friend about her memory problems. Her friend noted Mrs Ma to have poor memory (especially short-term memory) and declined cognitive functions.

Findings from Screening Assessments by Allied Healthcare and Social Care Team

Cognitive functioning	Scored 9/30 on MMSE, indicating cognitive impairment, adjusted for education level. Mrs Ma's performance was impaired in orientation to time (0/5), delayed recall (0/3), calculation (0/5), three-step commands (0/3), and visuospatial relationships (0/1); she was slightly impaired in orientation to place (3/5) and language (3/5). Her performance was, however, normal in registration (3/3). The Clock Drawing Test was not completed and assessment was not possible due to Mrs Ma's hearing problems. Her cognitive assessment scores on MMSE might also have been affected by her severe hearing impairment.
ADL/IADL	Mrs Ma was independent in ADLs (Barthel Index 100/100). She was dependent in external communication and laundry and needed supervision in taking medication, meal preparation, community access, handling finances, and grocery shopping (Lawton IADL Scale 29/56).
Depressive symptoms	GDS-15 was not conducted. She was noted to have a stable mood, without signs or symptoms of depression.
Staging and clinical rating	Results suggested a Global Deterioration Scale stage 5, indicating moderate dementia. She was unable to recall major relevant aspects of her current life, such as her phone number of many years and the names of her grandchildren; she had impaired IADLs due to cognitive impairment and needed assistance in choosing proper clothing to wear.

History Taken with Carer by Primary Care Physician

Mrs Ma's friend reported noticing memory problems in her friend that had concerned her for about a year. No delusional ideations were reported. Using the GPCOG Informant Interview, the following areas were noted to show more difficulties (×) or were preserved (○) compared to about two years ago:

× Remembering recent events
× Recalling recent conversations
○ Word finding
× Managing money and finances
× Managing medication independently
○ Using transport

There were no additional clinical features to consider for non-Alzheimer's dementia. Mrs Ma has hypertension and was receiving follow-up consultations for this at a geriatric medicine outpatient clinic. No family history of psychiatric disorders or dementia was reported. She has received six years of education.

Investigations

Calcium, VDRL, vitamin B_{12}, folate, ECG, and TSH were ordered. CT brain (plain) scan revealed prominent cerebral sulci/ventricles that are age-related changes.

Diagnosis

Moderate Alzheimer's disease.

Management

Mrs Ma was recommended to join a centre-based programme with cognitively stimulating activities, for the maintenance of cognitive functioning, self-care functioning, and quality of life; she was encouraged to have regular exercise, a healthy diet and mental stimulation, and maintain an active social life.

Suggestions for the Primary Care Team

Mrs Ma presented with a typical impairment pattern compatible with Alzheimer's disease. For staging, the primary care team can refer to the FAST method for guidance and explore whether she can dress herself properly or not. If help is needed, it would suggest a moderate stage of dementia. The primary care team should pay attention to her severe hearing deficit for a number of reasons: hearing deprivation can lead to social isolation and limited sensory and mental stimulation and aggravate cognitive decline; hearing problems would also significantly affect performance in daily living and the accuracy of cognitive assessment. At the same time, hearing problems can be corrected, with proper assessment and management. Bedside otoscopic examination, the use of hearing aids and/ or referral to otolaryngologists should be considered. The correction of hearing disability is equally important as the pharmacological management of dementia. The primary care team is recommended to manage Mrs Ma's hearing problem first, observe her response to intervention, and reassess her to find out more accurately about her strengths and weaknesses, so as to suggest suitable care planning and caring strategies.

Case 068 Observe? Or Start Treatment?

Mrs Cheng, an 84-year-old lady, presented with concerns raised by her daughter about her memory problems. She complained of Mrs Cheng's poor memory, noting repeated questioning and forgetfulness of recent events, and suspiciousness about strangers stealing her money.

Findings from Screening Assessments by Allied Healthcare and Social Care Team

Cognitive functioning	Scored 19/30 on MMSE, indicating cognitive impairment, adjusted for education level. Mrs Cheng's performance was impaired in delayed recall (0/3), and she could not complete the visuospatial relationships test (0/1); she was also impaired in calculation (1/5) and had slight problems in orientation to time (4/5), and place (4/5), and three-step commands (2/3). Her performance was, however, normal in registration (3/3) and language (5/5). The Clock Drawing Test showed obvious errors in time denotation, with clock arms grossly misplaced and numbers drawn in the wrong place, suggesting an impaired executive function. The copying part of the test was not completed, as Mrs Cheng refused to continue with the test (Figure 2.44).
ADL/IADL	Mrs Cheng was independent in ADLs (Barthel Index 100/100). She required supervision in meal preparation, community access, handling

	finances, and grocery shopping; she was independent in other IADLs (Lawton IADL Scale 44/56).
Depressive symptoms	Scored 0/15 on GDS-15, no obvious depressive mood was noted.
Staging and clinical rating	Results suggested a Global Deterioration Scale stage 4, indicating mild dementia. She showed decreased knowledge of current and recent events; a decreased ability to travel and handle finances; and an inability to perform complex tasks; she was, however, able to select proper clothing to wear.

Figure 2.44 Findings from Mrs Cheng's Clock Drawing Test – Clock Drawing (3 o'clock)

History Taken with Carer by Primary Care Physician

Mrs Cheng's daughter reported noticing memory problems in her mother that had concerned her for about six months. Delusional ideations were reported: Mrs Cheng was noted to be suspicious about strangers stealing her money. Using the GPCOG Informant Interview, the following areas were noted to show more difficulties (×) or were preserved (○) compared to about two years ago:

× Remembering recent events
× Recalling recent conversations
× Word finding
× Managing money and finances
○ Managing medication independently
○ Using transport

There were no additional clinical features to consider for non-Alzheimer's dementia. Mrs Cheng has hypertension. No family history of psychiatric disorders or dementia was reported. Her education level was unclear, although it is likely that Mrs Cheng has received more than two years of education.

Investigations

CBP, Vitamin B_{12}, and TSH were ordered.

Diagnosis

Alzheimer's disease.

Management

No medication was prescribed while waiting for blood work-up findings. Mrs Cheng was recommended to join a centre-based programme with cognitively stimulating activities to maintain cognitive and self-care functions; she was encouraged to have regular exercise, a healthy diet and mental stimulation, and maintain an active social life; non-pharmacological interventions to manage distressed behaviours and neuropsychiatric symptoms of dementia were also recommended.

Suggestions for the Primary Care Team

This is a case of amnestic mild cognitive impairment bordering on very early Alzheimer's disease. Often with public awareness and early detection efforts in the community, people in a preclinical or very early state would be more likely to get in touch with services, by themselves or with the support of a family member, as in Mrs Cheng's case. The primary care team will therefore have to differentiate and manage/triage those with dementia, amnestic mild cognitive impairment, and cognitive frailty. Cognitive frailty refers to the predisposition to cognitive impairment secondary to physical frailty (a state of vulnerability to stressors as a consequence of a cumulative decline in many physiological systems (7)). In amnestic mild cognitive impairment, impaired memory is the presenting feature, while the person is functioning well otherwise.

Based on the person's education level and previous occupation, physicians will need to use discretion to decide on the management direction. For people with higher cognitive reserve to be showing these early symptoms, there could be a higher amyloid load and starting treatment would be appropriate while observing for clinical improvement. In Mrs Cheng's case, given her lower level of education, observation for six months and starting treatment if deterioration is evident would be advisable. Giving a label of amnestic mild cognitive impairment (versus Alzheimer's disease) here is for diagnostic purposes, while clinically this can be considered a case of sub-threshold early Alzheimer's disease, with typical signs and symptoms and compatible ADL/IADL performance. The primary care team should pay attention to Mrs Cheng's delusional ideations that her belongings were being stolen by strangers, which can negatively affect her mood, increasing her tendency to develop more severe distressed behaviours and neuropsychiatric symptoms of dementia. Early intervention and prevention of the delusion and complications are needed.

Case 069 5 or 10 mg?

Mrs Fong, a 77-year-old lady, presented with concerns raised by her daughter over her memory problems. Her daughter reported a decline in her short-term memory (e.g., forgetting what she had had to eat) and ability to find her way (e.g., she could not find her daughter's home after getting off a minibus).

Findings from Screening Assessments by Allied Healthcare and Social Care Team

Cognitive functioning	Scored 18/30 on MMSE, indicating cognitive impairment, adjusted for education level. Mrs Fong's performance was impaired in delayed recall (0/3) and calculation (0/5); she was slightly impaired in orientation to time (3/5) and place (4/5) and three-step commands (2/3). Her performance was, however, normal in registration (3/3), language (5/5), and visuospatial relationships (1/1). The Clock Drawing Test showed slight impairment in the spacing of lines and numbers only.
ADL/IADL	Mrs Fong required set-up assistance in ADL, such as help to set water temperature due to poor vision, and occasional verbal reminders for showering, as she might forget that she has already showered. She was

independent in other ADLs (Barthel Index 99/100). Her laundry and housekeeping were done by her carer; she required assistance in taking medication (prepared by her daughter; she may forget that she has already taken her medications); she also needed supervision in meal preparation, community access (she goes to the nearby area only), handling finances (needed assistance in banking), and grocery shopping (Lawton IADL Scale 32/56).

Staging and clinical rating	Results suggested a Global Deterioration Scale stage 4 approaching 5, indicating mild dementia. She showed decreased knowledge of current and recent events and exhibited deficits in memory of her own personal history; a concentration deficit was elicited on serial subtractions; a decreased ability to travel and handle finances was noted; she was, however, able to maintain general orientation to time and place and able to travel to familiar locations near home; memory impairment was starting to affect her ADL performance as she may occasionally forget that she has showered.

History Taken with Carer by Primary Care Physician

Mrs Fong's daughter reported noticing memory problems in her mother that had concerned her for about two years. No delusional ideations were reported. Using the GPCOG Informant Interview, the following areas were noted to show more difficulties (✗) or were preserved (○) compared to about two years ago:

- ✗ Remembering recent events
- ✗ Recalling recent conversations
- ○ Word finding
- ✗ Managing money and finances
- ✗ Managing medication independently
- ✗ Using transport

There were no additional clinical features to consider for non-Alzheimer's dementia. Mrs Fong has left eye blindness and right eye poor night vision. No family history of psychiatric disorders or dementia was reported. Her exact education level was unclear, although it is likely that she has received more than two years of education.

Investigations

Vitamin B_{12} and TSH were ordered. All investigations were normal. Brain CT scan revealed mild cerebral atrophy.

Diagnosis

Alzheimer's disease.

Management

Rivastigmine transdermal system 5 mg alternate day was prescribed. She was recommended to join a centre-based programme with cognitively stimulating activities to maintain cognitive functions.

Suggestions for the Primary Care Team

Mrs Fong's presentation is compatible with early Alzheimer's disease, with intact visuospatial performance. Her performance in the Clock Drawing Test was excellent considering her bilateral visual impairment. The management of her visual impairment should be optimised, if she has not been under the care of the ophthalmologist. Starting treatment at a low dose is recommended, with a rivastigmine patch of 5 mg (versus 10 mg) sufficient as a starting dose, and observation of her response to medication. The dose of rivastigmine should be increased in the event of declining cognitive function. The consideration here is to balance the medication side effects and maintenance of her ADL/IADL functioning.

Mrs Fong's current impairment in ADL/IADL was mainly attributable to her memory impairment, such as forgetting whether she has taken medication or showered. She could nevertheless still be able to execute the tasks satisfactorily, such as getting around and using public transportation. The primary care team should therefore coach her family carers to use reminders, adopt a routine schedule, and modify the environment to help maintain her existing functions for as long as possible. As a safety precaution, the use of anti-lost and location-tracking devices would help support her continued active participation in the community.

Case 070 Subjective Cognitive Impairment

Mrs Tsang, an 88-year-old lady, presented with concerns raised by her nephew over her memory problems. She was noted to have poor memory (e.g., forgetting phone numbers and misplacing items) and problems in orientation. Mrs Tsang was also self-aware of her decline in memory, including her forgetfulness of conversation content, misplacing of items, and word-finding difficulties.

Findings from Screening Assessments by Allied Healthcare and Social Care Team

Cognitive functioning	Scored 19/30 on MMSE, no indication of cognitive impairment, adjusted for education level. Scored 14/30 on MoCA, indicating cognitive impairment. Results showed impairments in attention, executive function, verbal fluency, and delayed-recall tasks (free recall: 0/5; multiple choice cue: 3/5). The Clock Drawing Test showed an abnormal clock face drawing with an inaccurate time denotation (Figure 2.45).
ADL/IADL	Mrs Tsang needed a little help in ambulation and stair climbing; she was independent in other ADLs (Barthel Index 95/100). She required assistance in taking medication, meal preparation, laundry, housekeeping, handling finances, and grocery shopping; she also needed supervision in community access (Lawton IADL Scale 23/56).
Staging and clinical rating	Results suggested a Global Deterioration Scale stage 4, indicating mild dementia. A concentration deficit was elicited on serial subtractions; she was noted to have a decreased ability to travel and handle finances; there was, however, maintained general orientation to time and place and an ability to travel to familiar locations near home.

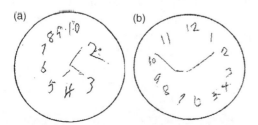

Figure 2.45 Findings from Mrs Tsang's Clock Drawing Test. (a) Clock Drawing (3 o'clock). (b) Clock Copying (10 past 10)

History Taken with Carer by Primary Care Physician

Mrs Tsang's nephew reported noticing memory problems in his aunt that had concerned him for about one to two years. No delusional ideations were reported. Using the GPCOG Informant Interview, the following areas were noted to show more difficulties (✗) or were preserved (○) compared to about two years ago:

✗ Remembering recent events
✗ Recalling recent conversations
✗ Word finding
✗ Managing money and finances
✗ Managing medication independently
✗ Using transport

There were no additional clinical features to consider for non-Alzheimer's dementia. Mrs Tsang had hypertension, heart disease, left eye cataract (operated on), gastroesophageal reflux disease, and osteoporosis. She was having pantoprazole and supplements for osteoporosis. No family history of psychiatric disorders or dementia was reported. Her education level was unclear, although it is likely that she has received less than six months of education.

Investigations

CBP, vitamin B_{12}, and TSH were ordered.

Diagnosis

Early Alzheimer's disease.

Management

No medication was prescribed while blood results were awaited. She was recommended to join a centre-based programme with cognitively stimulating activities, for the maintenance of cognitive abilities and quality of life.

Suggestions for the Primary Care Team

Mrs Tsang's presentation is typical of early Alzheimer's disease. It is sometimes the case that results from various cognitive screen assessments may differ, as in this case for the negative MMSE and positive MoCA results. Unlike detailed neuropsychological assessments that are developed to provide more precise testing of cognitive functions, both MMSE and MoCA are developed as quick screening tools to facilitate clinical judgement and triage, with varied sensitivity and specificity for different levels of cognitive impairment, as well as other pros and cons (e.g., influence of education on performance). The primary care team should therefore exercise clinical judgement and make reference to available information from multiple sources in deciding on the best course of action and management plan. In Mrs Tsang's case, her MMSE score was marginal, while the positive MoCA and Clock Drawing Test (which was worse in the drawing part and improved in the copying part), together with IADL impairment, provided evidence of deterioration. Cholinesterase inhibitors would help Mrs Tsang. Starting with a low dose of cholinesterase inhibitor, such as donepezil 2.5 mg, while observing her progress would be appropriate.

The primary care team should also note that her IADL performance appeared worse than would otherwise be expected from her cognitive assessment results, which may be attributable to her premorbid lifestyle/habits. Further exploration would be useful to inform her care plan and strategy. Another point to note is the possible involvement of age-related cognitive decline in frailty given Mrs Tsang's age. The management of frailty should be optimised while treatment and intervention for Alzheimer's disease is being arranged.

Case 071 Increasing Social Isolation

Mrs Ip, an 85-year-old lady, presented with concerns raised by her friend, who lived with her, about her memory problems. Her friend complained of her poor memory (e.g., misplacing items and forgetting conversation content) and declined cognitive functions. Mrs Ip was aware of her own poor memory (e.g., she noted that she would forget what she had in her fridge) and decreased motivation to go out.

Findings from Screening Assessments by Allied Healthcare and Social Care Team

Cognitive functioning	Scored 17/30 on MMSE, indicating cognitive impairment, adjusted for education level. Mrs Ip's performance was impaired in delayed recall (0/3); she was unable to recall even with cues; orientation to time (2/5); and calculation (1/5); she was slightly impaired in orientation to place (3/5) and three-step commands (2/3). Her performance was, however, normal in registration (3/3), language (5/5), and visuospatial relationships (1/1). The Clock Drawing Test showed an abnormal clock face drawing with an inaccurate time denotation (Figure 2.46).
ADL/IADL	Mrs Ip needed minimal help in stair climbing and was independent in other ADLs (Barthel Index 98/100). She needed assistance in housekeeping; she also required supervision in taking medication (may forget or mix up time of taking medication, although she was able to organise her own medications), laundry, community access, and handling finances; she was modified independent in meal preparation and grocery shopping (able to manage by herself but may buy more/repeatedly) (Lawton IADL Scale 39/56).
Staging and clinical rating	Results suggested a Global Deterioration Scale stage 4, indicating mild dementia. She showed a decreased ability to remember names upon introduction to new acquaintances; she showed a deficit in memory of her own personal history; a concentration deficit was elicited on serial subtractions; and she has a decreased ability to travel, handle finances, etc.

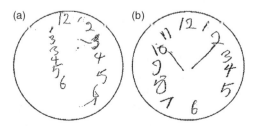

Figure 2.46 Findings from Mrs Ip's Clock Drawing Test. (a) Clock Drawing (3 o'clock). (b) Clock Copying (10 past 10)

History Taken with Carer by Primary Care Physician

Mrs Ip's friend reported noticing memory problems in her friend that had concerned her for about two years. Delusional ideations were reported: Mrs Ip was noted to be blaming her flatmate for stealing her food. Self-reported decreased motivation to go out was noted. Using the GPCOG Informant Interview, the following areas were noted to show more difficulties (✗) or were preserved (○) compared to about two years ago:

✗ Remembering recent events
✗ Recalling recent conversations
✗ Word finding
✗ Managing money and finances
○ Managing medication independently
✗ Using transport

There were no additional clinical features to consider for non-Alzheimer's dementia. Mrs Ip had hypertension and hypercholesterolaemia. No family history of psychiatric disorders or dementia was reported. Her education level was uncertain, although it is likely that she has received less than six months of education.

Investigations

CBP, ESR, R/LFT, calcium, vitamin B_{12}, folate, fasting sugar, fasting lipids, MSU × R/M and culture test, chest X-ray, ECG, and T4 were ordered. CT brain (plain + control) scan was ordered as well.

Diagnosis

Early Alzheimer's disease.

Management

No medication was prescribed due to pending investigation results. She was recommended to join a centre-based programme with cognitively stimulating activities, for the maintenance of cognitive abilities and quality of life.

Suggestions for the Primary Care Team

This is a typical case of early Alzheimer's disease, with the potential involvement of age-related cognitive frailty. Although Mrs Ip's performance appeared intact in the visuospatial test on MMSE (i.e., interlocking pentagon), her impairment was evident on the Clock Drawing Test (with worse performance on drawing and improving on the copying part). Starting treatment with low-dose cholinesterase inhibitors would be appropriate.

Care planning is needed to support Mrs Ip in maintaining her quality of life and quality of care to prepare for the foreseeable rise in care needs when she may no longer be able to take care of herself. A home assessment is needed to investigate if there is any clutter or whether her belongings are well organised. The primary care team can help identify strategies, such as adding cues and putting her belongings in more intuitive or obvious places, to ensure she can find her items easily and not suspect others of stealing things from her. Mrs Ip has limited social support as she is living with another older person in the flat. The primary care team should explore her social background and be attentive to depressive symptoms. Meanwhile, support could be solicited from Mrs Ip's friend to understand her relationship with her other flatmates, as conflict might have occurred/happened with the accusation of theft; providing information for her flatmate about dementia and/or identifying strategies to minimise Mrs Ip's chance of missing items in the flat – which could be the cause for the delusion about theft – would be helpful.

Case 072 91-Year-Old Needing Reminder for Medications

Mrs Chong, a 91-year-old lady, presented with concerns raised by her daughter over her memory problems. She was noted to have poor memory and declined cognitive functions, such as repeated questioning, misplacing items, disorientation, difficulties in finding her way even in familiar places, and problems with word finding.

Findings from Screening Assessments by Allied Healthcare and Social Care Team

Cognitive functioning	Scored 15/30 on MMSE, indicating cognitive impairment, adjusted for education level. Mrs Chong's performance was impaired in delayed recall (0/3) and visuospatial relationships (0/1), orientation to time (2/5), and calculation (1/5); she had slight impairment in orientation to place (3/5), registration (2/3), and three-step commands (2/3). Her performance was, however, normal in language (5/5). The Clock Drawing Test showed obvious errors in time denotation, such as the time shown on the clock; results suggested executive function and conceptual deficits. (Figure 2.47).
ADL/IADL	Mrs Chong was unsafe in stair climbing without assistance; she also needed some minimal help with toilet, ambulation, bowel control, and bladder control; she was independent in other ADLs (Barthel Index 83/100). She was dependent in meal preparation, laundry (able to hang and fold clothes), and housekeeping; she also needed assistance in taking medications (needed verbal reminder) and external communication; she required supervision in community access, handling finances, and grocery shopping (able to buy simple items) (Lawton IADL Scale 24/56).
Staging and clinical rating	Results suggested a Global Deterioration Scale stage 4, indicating mild dementia. She showed decreased knowledge of current and recent events; for example, she was unable to name Hong Kong's current chief executive; she showed some deficit in memory of her personal history; concentration deficit was elicited in the serial subtraction test; she also showed a decreased ability to travel and handle finances.

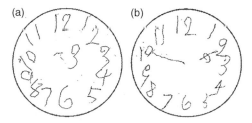

Figure 2.47 Findings from Mrs Chong's Clock Drawing Test. (a) Clock Drawing (3 o'clock). (b) Clock Copying (10 past 10)

History Taken with Carer by Primary Care Physician

Mrs Chong's daughter reported noticing memory problems in her mother that had concerned her for about two years. No delusional ideations were reported. Using the GPCOG Informant Interview, the following areas were noted to show more difficulties (✗) or were preserved (○) compared to about two years ago:

✗ Remembering recent events
✗ Recalling recent conversations
✗ Word finding
✗ Managing money and finances
✗ Managing medication independently
○ Using transport

There was an additional clinical feature to consider for non-Alzheimer's dementia: she had experienced complex visual hallucinations once or twice about a year ago. Mrs Chong had hypertension and a left hip fracture with replacement this year. No family history of psychiatric disorders or dementia was reported. Her education level was unclear, although it is possible that Mrs Chong had about three to four years of education.

Investigations

CBP, ESR, R/LFT, calcium, vitamin B_{12}, folate, fasting sugar, fasting lipids, MSU × R/M and culture test, chest X-ray, ECG, and T4 were ordered. CT brain (plain) scan was ordered.

Diagnosis

Mild cognitive impairment or mild Alzheimer's disease.

Management

No medication was prescribed at this stage. Mrs Chong was recommended to join a centre-based programme with cognitively stimulating activities, for the maintenance of cognitive abilities and quality of life.

Suggestions for the Primary Care Team

This is a case of age-related cognitive frailty on top of a slow disease process of Alzheimer's disease, with impairment in visuospatial ability (i.e., interlocking pentagon on MMSE) and positive Clock Drawing Test findings. Primary care physicians should pay attention to her complex visual hallucinations, clarify their nature, and investigate whether they are related to cortical Lewy body disease. In some cases, the so-called visual hallucination may also simply be the recollection and verbalisation of vivid memory. Starting a cholinesterase inhibitor at a low dose, such as donepezil 2.5mg, would be appropriate.

Considering Mrs Chong's older age of presentation, the primary care team would need to bear in mind her stamina when working out a care plan with Mrs Chong and her family. Instead of recommending high-intensity cognitive stimulation only, adding some social and leisure activities as part of her daily routine would be advisable to ensure some more restful periods for Mrs Chong to recover from more challenging activities. At this stage of the disease, maintaining a stable mood and avoiding confusion that could trigger distressed behaviours and neuropsychiatric symptoms of dementia would be important.

Case 073   Independent IADLs

Ms Cheng, a 75-year-old lady, presented with concerns raised by her son over her memory decline. She was self-aware of her own memory decline, such as forgetting to take medication and missing appointments (e.g., meetings and volunteer services).

Findings from Screening Assessments by Allied Healthcare and Social Care Team

Cognitive functioning	Scored 28/30 on MMSE, with no indication of cognitive impairment, after adjusting for education. Ms Cheng had slight difficulty in place orientation (4/5). Her performance was good in delayed recall (3/3; able to recall all three items), calculation (5/5), time orientation (5/5), registration (3/3), three-step commands (2/3), language (5/5), and visuospatial relationships (1/1). Scored 18/30 on MoCA, indicating mild cognitive impairment. The Clock Drawing Test showed slight difficulties, with errors in placement of numbers. Ms Cheng was aware of her problem in visuospatial performance and asked for a second trial, but was still unable to draw even though she was fully aware of the problem. Clock copying was largely normal (Figure 2.48).
ADL/IADL	Ms Cheng was independent in all ADLs (Barthel Index 100/100). She was mostly independent in IADLs, except that she would forget to take medicine occasionally, and sometimes she would have difficulty finding her way home upon leaving shopping centres (Lawton IADL Scale 55/56).
Depressive symptoms	Scored 0/15 on GDS-15, no indication of depression.
Staging and clinical rating	No Clinical Dementia Rating score was available as Ms Cheng attended the assessment session unaccompanied by a family member or informant. Impression from the assessment was that Ms Cheng had questionable dementia, with mild impairment in orientation and judgement and problem-solving noted.

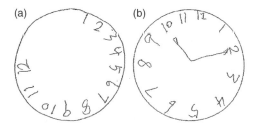

Figure 2.48 Findings from Ms Cheng's Clock Drawing Test. (a) Clock Drawing (3 o'clock). (b) Clock Copying (10 past 10)

History Taken with Carer by Primary Care Physician

Ms Cheng's son reported noticing memory problems in his mother that had concerned him for about one year. No delusional ideations were reported. Using the GPCOG Informant Interview, the following areas were noted to show more difficulties (×) or were preserved (○) compared to about two years ago:

- × Remembering recent events
- × Recalling recent conversations
- ○ Word finding
- ○ Managing money and finances
- × Managing medication independently
- ○ Using transport

There were no additional clinical features to consider for non-Alzheimer's dementia. Ms Cheng has diabetes mellitus, hypertension, dyslipidaemia, cervical cancer (treated with radiation therapy), and radiation cystitis. She was having amlodipine besylate 5 mg daily and metformin 50 mg twice a day. No family history of psychiatric disorders or dementia was reported. Ms Cheng did not receive any education. She attended a community centre for older people and participated in voluntary work.

Physical Examination Findings

General examination revealed no affect or hygiene problem. Ms Cheng had no atrial fibrillation, heart murmur, or carotid bruit problem, with a normal cardiac impulse on CVS examination. On CNS examination, no focal pyramidal sign, extra-pyramidal sign, gait abnormalities, or speech problems were found.

Investigations

CBP, ESR, R/LFT, calcium, vitamin B_{12}, and VDRL were ordered. CT brain (plain) scan revealed no evidence of disease.

Diagnosis

Mild cognitive impairment.

Management

No medication was prescribed. She was recommended to join a specialised day care service for two days per week to receive a structured and tailored intervention programme and cognitively stimulating activities to delay deterioration and maintain quality of life.

Suggestions for the Primary Care Team

This is likely a case of mild cognitive impairment of the amnestic type. Ms Cheng presented at a relatively younger age, being self-aware of her memory problems, with nearly normal performance on MMSE, but MoCA and the Clock Drawing Test showed her impairment. Considering the difference between MMSE and MoCA scores, a detailed comparison of the impaired domains to identify any inconsistencies may provide insight. At the mild cognitive impairment stage, no medication is indicated at this moment, although Ms Cheng should be followed up to observe for changes in cognitive performance and the onset of clinical Alzheimer's disease. Cholinesterase inhibitors should be started in the event of cognitive decline six months later. Mecobalamin or metformin twice a day can be prescribed to Ms Cheng.

Considering her obvious impairment in executive function as shown on the Clock Drawing Test, her intact ADL/IADL ability and good self-awareness are of note. The primary care team is recommended to also reassess this functioning after six months. At the same time, Ms Cheng and her family members can be encouraged to keep a diary or chart of the memory problems that occur in her everyday life, including their frequency and other characteristics, to inform further investigation and care planning.

Case 074 Keys Left in the Door

Ms Kwan, an 84-year-old lady, presented with concerns raised by her daughter over her memory problem, poor calculation, low motivation, and bad temper. Memory problems (e.g., leaving her keys in the door) and declined ability in calculation were noted by her daughter for about 12 months, which had become more obvious in the last six months. Ms Kwan was aware of her own memory decline.

Findings from Screening Assessments by Allied Healthcare and Social Care Team

Cognitive functioning	Scored 24/30 on MMSE, no indication of cognitive impairment, adjusted for education level. Ms Kwan's performance was impaired in orientation to place (2/5); however, she was able to complete the pentagon drawing (1/1), showing normal visuospatial relationships. Her performance in calculation was also satisfactory (4/5). She was impaired in delayed recall (1/3), although her orientation to time (5/5), registration (3/3), three-step commands (3/3), and language (5/5) were unimpaired. The Clock Drawing Test showed good number spacing and time denotation, suggesting normal executive function. Clock copying similarly showed good number spacing and time denotation.
ADL/IADL	Ms Kwan was independent in all ADLs (Barthel Index 100/100). She was semi-independent in IADLs (Lawton IADL Scale 48/56): she needed reminders for taking medicine for the last six months; she would also forget to buy items from a shopping list and would often leave her keys in the door.
Depressive symptoms	Scored on GDS-15 2/15, no obvious depressive mood was noted.
Staging and clinical rating	Scored 0.5/3 on Clinical Dementia Rating, indicating questionable dementia. She showed mild impairment in memory, orientation, and judgement and problem-solving.

History Taken with Carer by Primary Care Physician

Ms Kwan's daughter reported noticing memory problems in her mother that had concerned her for about a year. No additional delusional ideations were reported. Using the GPCOG Informant Interview, the following areas were noted to show more difficulties (✗) or were preserved (○) compared to about two years ago:

✗ Remembering recent events

✗ Recalling recent conversations

○ Word finding
✗ Managing money and finances
○ Managing medication independently
○ Using transport

There were no additional clinical features to consider for non-Alzheimer's dementia. Ms Kwan had hypertension and dyslipidaemia, for which she was receiving follow-up consultations at a geriatric medicine outpatient clinic. She was having amlodipine besylate 10 mg daily, valsartan 40 mg daily, Minipress 2 mg three times a day, pantoprazole 40 mg daily as needed, and clotrimazole cream. No family history of psychiatric disorders or dementia was reported. She had received primary education to P.6 (approximately six years of education).

Physical Examination Findings

General examination revealed no affect or hygiene problem. No CVS findings. CNS findings showed frontal lobe releasing sign in palmomental and glabellar reflexes.

Investigations

CBP, ESR, R/LFT, calcium, VDRL, vitamin B_{12}, and TFT were ordered. VDRL was negative, and other investigations were normal. CT brain (plain) scan revealed a $0.8 \times 0.7 \times 0.8$ cm nodule in the pituitary gland, which could represent a pituitary adenoma.

Diagnosis

Mild cognitive impairment/early Alzheimer's disease.

Management

Rivastigmine transdermal system 5 mg daily was prescribed. She was recommended to join a specialised day care service for two days per week for two years to receive a structured and tailored intervention programme and cognitively stimulating activities to delay deterioration.

Suggestions for the Primary Care Team

This is a case of mild cognitive impairment bordering on very early Alzheimer's disease. Ms Kwan had a relatively short disease history of around one year but has impaired IADL; starting treatment is therefore recommended. The primary care team should watch out for possible depressive symptoms, even though her GDS-15 assessment was negative. On top of the rivastigmine patch, memantine should also be considered for temper tantrums. Antidepressants may also be considered for low volition.

The performance on the cognitive assessment of Ms Kwan is consistent with her daily living performance, with ADL/IADL mainly affected by short-term memory at this moment. Cues and reminders can still be useful in this early stage of the disease. Meanwhile, identifying any psychosocial issues that might have contributed to or triggered Ms Kwan's motivation and temper issues would give clues to the possible causes (e.g., manifestation of depression) and tailor appropriate intervention strategies.

Case 075 Living Alone with Self-Reported Deficits

Ms Ng, a 78-year-old lady, presented with concerns raised by her nephew over her memory problems. She was self-aware of her own memory decline and worried about her memory.

Findings from Screening Assessments by Allied Healthcare and Social Care Team

Cognitive functioning	Scored 17/30 on MMSE, indicating cognitive impairment, adjusted for education level. Ms Ng's performance was impaired in orientation to time (2/5) and place (2/5), delayed recall (1/3), and three-step commands (1/3); she picked up the paper and then asked what to do next. She had slight difficulties in calculation and was unable to recall the remainder (3/5). Her performance was normal in registration (3/3), language (5/5), and visuospatial relationships (1/1). The Clock Drawing Test showed slight difficulties in time denotation. She drew an arm pointing to 9 instead of 12 when attempting to draw a clock showing 3 o'clock. Clock copying showed some improvement; she was able to read a clock, but she forgot to draw the arms at the beginning (Figure 2.49).
ADL/IADL	Ms Ng was independent in most ADLs (Barthel Index 92/100), except that she needed longer to finish the tasks, due to right knee pain. Ms Ng self-reported that she would forget to take medication occasionally and buy the same item repeatedly, and she had difficulties handling money.
Depressive symptoms	Scored 2/15 on GDS-15, no obvious depressive mood was noted.
Staging and clinical rating	Scored 0.5/3 on Clinical Dementia Rating, indicating questionable dementia. She showed mild impairment in memory, orientation, judgement and problem-solving.

(a) (b)

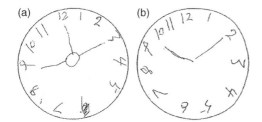

Figure 2.49 Findings from Ms Ng's Clock Drawing Test. (a) Clock Drawing (3 o'clock). (b) Clock Copying (10 past 10)

History Taken with Carer by Primary Care Physician

Ms Ng's nephew reported noticing memory problems in his aunt that had concerned him for about two to three years. No delusional ideations were reported. Using the GPCOG Informant Interview, the following areas were noted to show more difficulties (✗) or were preserved (○) compared to about two years ago:

✗ Remembering recent events
✗ Recalling recent conversations
○ Word finding
✗ Managing money and finances
✗ Managing medication independently
✗ Using transport

There were no additional clinical features to consider for non-Alzheimer's dementia. Ms Ng was on a daily dosage of glucosamine supplement. No family history of psychiatric disorders was reported. However, Ms Ng had a family history of dementia; both her father and sister were diagnosed with dementia. She did not receive any education. Ms Ng is single and lives alone.

Physical Examination Findings

General examination revealed no affect or hygiene problem. Ms Ng had a normal blood pressure. No other CVS or CNS findings.

Investigations

CBP, R/LFT, calcium, vitamin B$_{12}$, fasting sugar, fasting lipids, chest X-ray, ECG, and TFT were ordered.

Diagnosis

Alzheimer's disease.

Management

Donepezil 2.5 mg daily was prescribed. She was recommended to join a specialised day care service for two days per week to receive a structured and tailored intervention programme and cognitively stimulating activities to delay deterioration and maintain quality of life.

Suggestions for the Primary Care Team

This is a typical case of early Alzheimer's disease. With her self-awareness of her memory problems, it is a good time for intervention. For her medication treatment, primary care physicians should consider escalating the dose of donepezil in the event of deteriorating cognition. Considering her premorbid independent ADL and lifestyle habits, Ms Ng can be expected to be able to maintain her functional level for a relatively long time. Home modifications, such as automatic light switches, safety sensors to alert overheating of the stove and full water in the sink, an electric cooking device, and an IP camera for her family members to monitor her home safety can be recommended. Ms Ng's social support is another area of concern: she was living alone and appeared weak on her social support network. Social services should be introduced at this time to strengthen her support network. Although her self-awareness is a strength on the one hand as a motivation for intervention compliance, on the other hand it could also lead to a potential depressive mood and anxiety. The primary care team should pay attention to Ms Ng's mood and adjustment, and develop preventive strategies in her care plan.

Case 076 Disorientation to Place?

Ms Lam, an 81-year-old lady, presented with concerns raised by her daughter over her memory problems. Complaints from her daughter included memory deterioration for about one year: she was frequently looking for personal belongings; she would repeatedly buy loads of raw food and put it inside the fridge and would sometimes forget to switch off the water tap after use. She was aware of her memory decline.

Findings from Screening Assessments by Allied Healthcare and Social Care Team

Cognitive functioning	Scored 18/30 on MMSE, indicating cognitive impairment, adjusted for education level. Ms Lam's performance was impaired in orientation to

	time (3/5) and place (2/5), three-step commands (1/3), calculation (2/5), delayed recall (1/3), and visuospatial relationships (0/1); her performance was, however, normal in registration (3/3) and language (5/5). The Clock Drawing Test showed normal executive function.
ADL/IADL	Ms Lam was independent in all ADLs (Barthel Index 100/100). She was independent in most IADLs (Lawton IADL Scale 48/56); she was not able to cook and needed to go out for meals. For external communication, she can only call some family members whose phone numbers are preset.
Depressive symptoms	Scored 2/15 on GDS-15, no obvious depressive mood was noted.
Staging and clinical rating	Scored 1/3 on Clinical Dementia Rating, indicating early dementia. She showed mild impairment in memory, orientation, judgement and problem-solving, and home and hobbies; she was fair in community affairs and personal care.

History Taken with Carer by Primary Care Physician

Ms Lam's daughter reported noticing memory problems in her mother that had concerned her for about one year. No delusional ideations were reported. Using the GPCOG Informant Interview, the following areas were noted to show more difficulties (✗) or were preserved (○) compared to about two years ago:

- ✗ Remembering recent events
- ✗ Recalling recent conversations
- ✗ Word finding
- ✗ Managing money and finances
- ○ Managing medication independently
- ○ Using transport

There were no additional clinical features to consider for non-Alzheimer's dementia. Ms Lam had hypertension. She did not have regular medication. No family history of psychiatric disorders or dementia was reported. She had not receive any education. She was active in social activities: she would go swimming and play badminton and table tennis with her friends every week.

Physical Examination Findings

General examination revealed no affect or hygiene problem. Ms Lam had a blood pressure reading of 153/80 mm Hg. No other CVS or CNS findings.

Investigations

Vitamin B_{12}, folate test, and MRI were ordered.

Diagnosis

Mild cognitive impairment/early Alzheimer's disease.

Management

Donepezil 2.5 mg daily was prescribed. She was recommended to join a specialised day care service for two days per week to receive a structured and tailored intervention programme and cognitively stimulating activities to delay deterioration and maintain her quality of life.

Suggestions for the Primary Care Team

This is a case of either mild cognitive impairment of the amnestic type or very early Alzheimer's' disease, with a typical presentation of more obvious deterioration in executive functions and short-term memory. Given that most findings were negative, there is a heavier reliance on the lower MMSE score in determining Ms Lam's diagnosis, with the current results suggesting dementia instead of mild cognitive impairment. However, Ms Lam's performance in orientation to place should be interpreted with caution, taking into account that she might have been taken to the assessment site by the carer without being informed. In borderline cases like this, observation of change over time would be the recommended strategy, before the commencement of cholinesterase inhibitors. Meanwhile, cognitively stimulating activities in a day centre would be appropriate regardless, provided that the activities are adjusted for her higher cognitive level and grouping arranged with people of similar functioning ability; a healthy and active lifestyle could also be recommended, with some precaution regarding safety and environmental modification (e.g., cues regarding shopping items) to maximise Ms Lam's functioning.

Case 077 Training Effects?

Ms Ng, a 74-year-old lady, presented with concerns raised by her daughter-in-law about her memory problems. She was aware of her memory decline. Complaints by her daughter-in-law about her memory deterioration in the last six months included poor short-term memory (Ms Ng was noted to be unable to recall events and having confusion over date and place), with frequent incidents of forgetfulness (e.g., her son would instruct her but she would forget most of the time).

Findings from Screening Assessments by Allied Healthcare and Social Care Team

Cognitive functioning	Scored 16/30 on MoCA and 25/30 on MMSE. Her apparent high score on MMSE was suspected to be due to her daily tasks, such as writing a diary and daily activity log. Ms Ng was oriented to time (4/5) and place (3/5) and able to recall her address and follow three-step commands (3/3). Her performance was fair in calculation (3/5), registration (3/3), delayed recall (3/3), language (5/5), and visuospatial relationships (1/1). Her Clock Drawing Test showed moderate impairment, which did not match with the MMSE result. She drew most of the numbers on one side of the clock (Figure 2.50).
ADL/IADL	Ms Ng was independent in most ADLs (Barthel Index 92/100), except that she needed extra time to finish tasks. She was assisted by a helper in IADLs (Lawton IADL Scale 22/56): she needed assistance and supervision with medication; she would not count her change after paying.
Depressive symptoms	Scored 1/15 on GDS-15, no depressive mood was found.
Staging and clinical rating	Scored 0.5/3 on Clinical Dementia Rating, indicating questionable dementia. She showed mild impairment in memory, orientation, community affairs, and personal care; questionable impairment in judgement and problem-solving; and moderate impairment in home and hobbies.

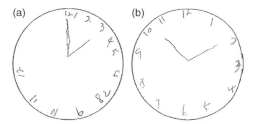

Figure 2.50 Findings from Ms Ng's Clock Drawing Test. (a) Clock Drawing (3 o'clock). (b) Clock Copying (10 past 10)

History Taken with Carer by Primary Care Physician

Ms Ng's daughter-in-law reported noticing memory problems in her mother that had concerned her for about two years. No delusional ideations were reported. Using the GPCOG Informant Interview, the following areas were noted to show more difficulties (✗) or were preserved (○) compared to about two years ago:

✗ Remembering recent events
✗ Recalling recent conversations
○ Word finding
✗ Managing money and finances
✗ Managing medication independently
✗ Using transport

There were no additional clinical features to consider for non-Alzheimer's dementia. Ms Ng had impaired fasting glucose, hypertension, an old cerebrovascular accident, old myocardial infarction/ischaemic heart disease, and dyslipidaemia. She was having aspirin 80 mg daily, metoprolol succinate 12.5 mg twice a day, pepcidine 40 mg twice a day, amlodipine besylate 5 mg daily, flupentixol 0.5 mg and melitracen 10 mg daily, chlordiazepoxide 2.5 mg daily, strontium ranelate one tablet daily, and vitamin D_1 tablet daily. No family history of dementia was reported. There is family history of psychiatric illness of insomnia. She has received secondary education. Her son would provide her with some self-developed cognitive training/learning such as giving her assignments to write a diary and activity log daily.

Physical Examination Findings

General examination revealed no affect or hygiene problem. Ms Ng had a blood pressure reading of 132/69 mm Hg. No other significant CVS or CNS findings.

Investigations

CBP done two years ago was normal, and R/LFT one year ago was normal. Fasting sugar two years ago was 5.6. CT brain (plain) scan seven years ago revealed right anterior subdural haemorrhage after a fall, and MRI six years ago revealed subdural haemorrhage in a lacunar infarct bilateral (frontal). Vitamin B_{12}, folate test, VDRL, and MRI were ordered.

Diagnosis

Likely early Alzheimer's disease and differential diagnosis mixed dementia.

Management

Donepezil 5 mg daily was prescribed. She was recommended to join a specialised day care service for two days per week to receive a structured and tailored intervention programme and cognitively stimulating activities to delay deterioration.

Suggestions for the Primary Care Team

This is a typical example of early Alzheimer's disease with a relatively younger age of onset. More obvious impairments in short-term memory and executive functions were observed, as well as in IADL functions. In this case, Ms Ng's old cerebrovascular accident has affected her brain reserve, with vascular burden possibly adding to amyloid deposition. Her engagement in cognitive training provided by her son, with repeated information input and mentally stimulating activities, might have helped to delay her deterioration. The primary care team is reminded to pay attention, however, to her son's level of carer stress and burden and to manage his expectations at a level that is realistic in Ms Ng's case.

Case 078 Comorbid Depression and Knee Pain

Ms Chan, an 88-year-old lady, presented with concerns raised by her daughter about her memory problems and delusion. Her daughter had noted her memory decline for about one year, with her short-term memory worsening progressively. She has deteriorating perform-ance in familiar tasks and is impaired in orientation to place. She was also reported to be suspicious about an affair going on between her husband and a domestic helper. Ms Chan was aware of her memory decline.

Findings from Screening Assessments by Allied Healthcare and Social Care Team

Cognitive functioning	Scored 11/30 on MoCA and 13/30 on MMSE. Ms Chan's performance was impaired in orientation to time (1/5) and place (1/5; she was unable to recall her home address without prompting), delayed recall (0/3), calculation (1/5), and visuospatial relationships (0/1); her performance was, however, normal in registration (3/3) and language (5/5). The Clock Drawing Test showed normal executive function, with slight problems in line spacing noted. She was able to read the clock.
ADL/IADL	Ms Chan was mostly dependent in ADLs, with assistance needed in toileting, bathing, transfers, ambulation, and stairs; she has urinary incontinence (Barthel Index 58/100). She was also mostly dependent in IADLs, with assistance needed in all IADL tasks (Lawton IADL Scale 12/56).
Depressive symptoms	Scored 10/15 on GDS-15, significant depressive mood was noted.
Staging and clinical rating	Scored 1/3 on Clinical Dementia Rating, indicating mild impairment. She showed mild impairment in memory, judgement and problem-solving, community affairs, and home and hobbies and moderate impairment in orientation and personal care.

History Taken with Carer by Primary Care Physician

Ms Chan's daughter reported noticing memory problems in her mother that had concerned her for about one year. Delusional ideations were reported. Using the

GPCOG Informant Interview, the following areas were noted to show more difficulties (✗) or were preserved (○) compared to about two years ago:

✗ Remembering recent events
✗ Recalling recent conversations
○ Word finding
✗ Managing money and finances
✗ Managing medication independently
✗ Using transport

There were no additional clinical features to consider for non-Alzheimer's dementia. Ms Chan had diagnosed depression and a right hip fracture with operation done. She was on tianeptine 6.25 mg twice a day, valproate 100 mg, diclofenac 25 mg three times a day, and famotidine 20 mg three times a day prescribed by a psychiatrist. No family history of psychiatric disorders or dementia was reported. She had received secondary education. She has two sons and three daughters with good family support. She walks with a walking frame with fair balance indoors.

Physical Examination Findings

General examination revealed no affect or hygiene problem. No atrial fibrillation, heart murmur, abnormal cardiac impulse, or carotid bruit were found on CVS examination. On CNS findings, no focal pyramidal sign, extra-pyramidal sign, frontal lobe releasing sign, or speech problems were found, but gait abnormalities were found after right hip fracture.

Investigations

CBP, R/LFT, calcium, VDRL, vitamin B_{12}, fasting sugar, and fasting lipids were ordered. CBP, R/LFT, calcium, vitamin B_{12}, fasting sugar, and fasting lipids were normal, whereas VDRL result was negative. CT brain (plain) scan revealed cerebral atrophy in medial temporal lobes and chronic small vessel disease.

Diagnosis

Alzheimer's disease and depression.

Management

Rivastigmine transdermal system 5 mg daily, aspirin 100 mg daily, pantoprazole 40 mg on the morning, and paracetamol 1 g twice a day PRN for knee pain were prescribed. She was recommended to join a specialised day care service for two days per week, to receive a structured and tailored intervention programme and cognitively stimulating activities to delay deterioration and maintain her quality of life.

Suggestions for the Primary Care Team

This is a typical case of Alzheimer's disease with depression, although her MMSE score was unusually low, with a high level of physical dependence that is not accounted for by Alzheimer's disease. Physicians should ask about the hip fracture and possible delirium in hospital. Hip fractures commonly occur in people aged 80 years or above, with 50 per cent of patients developing delirium and 50 per cent of patients who develop delirium showing symptom onset of Alzheimer's disease in two years.

Ms Chan has a history of depression; the primary care team should watch out for depressive elements in her dementia. Selective serotonin receptor inhibitors should be considered for her depression. The primary care physician may consider stopping the neuroleptic, and check for possible hallucinations and rapid eye movement behaviour disorder (REMBD). If present, the possibility of cortical Lewy body disease needs to be considered. A case conference with specialists is recommended.

Ms Chan's performance in daily living and cognitive assessment findings should be interpreted under the context of her depressive mood, which could significantly affect the results in the event of extremely low motivation. Her delusional ideation may require medical attention, although the primary care team should note that non-pharmacological intervention is equally important: strategies such as equipping carers with appropriate communication skills, including the avoidance of direct confrontation or a correctional approach to the delusional ideations, minimising exposure to delusional content (in Ms Chan's case, minimising the time when her husband would be seen together with the domestic helper), and a scheduled routine with regular social/cognitive failure-free activities to increase her positive emotions, would be helpful.

Case 079 Vitamin B$_{12}$ Deficiency

Ms Lau, a 74-year-old lady, presented with concerns raised by her granddaughter about her memory problems. Ms Lau was self-aware of her poor short-term memory. Her memory decline had been noted for two to three years, with a more rapid deterioration in the last year, and a progressive decline in short-term memory according to her grandson-in-law.

Findings from Screening Assessments by Allied Healthcare and Social Care Team

Cognitive functioning	Scored 22/30 on MMSE, indicating cognitive impairment, adjusted for education level. She was slightly disoriented to time (3/5) and place (3/5; she was able to recall her home address), impaired in visuospatial relationships (0/1), had slight difficulties in calculation (4/5), and three-step commands (2/3); her performance was, however, normal in registration (3/3), delayed recall (3/3), and language (5/5). The Clock Drawing Test was negative, showing normal executive function.
ADL/IADL	Ms Lau was independent in all ADLs (Barthel Index 100/100). She was mostly independent in IADLs, with occasional support or assistance needed in taking medication, external communication, housekeeping, and community access (Lawton IADL Scale 49/56).
Depressive symptoms	Scored 2/15 on GDS-15, no depressive mood was noted.
Staging and clinical rating	Scored 0.5/3 on Clinical Dementia Rating, indicating questionable dementia. She showed questionable impairment in memory and mild impairment in orientation.

History Taken with Carer by Primary Care Physician

Ms Lau's granddaughter reported noticing memory problems in her grandmother that had concerned her for about three years. No delusional ideations were reported. Using the GPCOG Informant Interview, the following areas were noted to show more difficulties (✗) or were preserved (○) compared to about two years ago:

✗ Remembering recent events
✗ Recalling recent conversations
○ Word finding

○ Managing money and finances
× Managing medication independently
○ Using transport

There were no additional clinical features to consider for non-Alzheimer's dementia. Ms Lau had diabetes, hypertension, an old cerebrovascular accident, palpitations, dyslipidaemia, vitamin B_{12} deficiency, impaired renal function, hysterectomy, and osteoarthritis of the knee. She was on metoprolol succinate 100 mg daily, hydralazine 10 mg twice a day, amlodipine besylate 10 mg daily, lisinopril 20 mg daily, gliclazide modified release 120 mg daily, vildagliptin 50 mg, metformin 750 mg twice a day, simvastatin 10 mg at night, T4 75 mg daily, vitamin B_{12} 1000 mcg daily, aspirin 100 mg daily, and zopiclone 7.5 mg N PRN. No family history of psychiatric disorders or dementia was reported. She has received secondary education. She is widowed and lives with a domestic helper. Ms Lau has a son and three daughters with good family support. She uses an umbrella as a walking aid with good balance.

Physical Examination Findings

General examination revealed no affect or hygiene problem. No significant CVS or CNS findings.

Investigations

CBP, R/LFT, calcium, fasting sugar, fasting lipids, Hb A1c, FT4, vitamin B_{12}, folate test, and TSH were ordered. Results were normal in fasting lipids and LFT; Hb 9.6 NcNc in CBP; R/LFT was normal; 5.7 in fasting sugar, vitamin B_{12} 98 (low), folate 36, Hb A1c 5–9 per cent, FTA 17.7, and TSH 0.08. CT brain (plain) scan revealed lacunar infarcts in right basal ganglia, bilateral thalami, and small vessel disease.

Diagnosis

Mild cognitive impairment of the amnestic type/early Alzheimer's disease.

Management

Rivastigmine transdermal system 5 mg daily was prescribed. She was recommended to join a specialised day care service for two days per week to receive a structured and tailored intervention programme and cognitively stimulating activities to delay deterioration and maintain her quality of life.

Suggestions for the Primary Care Team

This is a typical case of mild cognitive impairment bordering on very early Alzheimer's disease. Ms Lau showed a typical pattern of impairment presentation at a slightly younger age than usual. The vitamin B_{12} deficiency caused by metformin may have contributed to the cognitive impairment. Physicians could start with a low dose of cholinesterase inhibitors while monitoring her symptoms, correct the metformin-related vitamin B_{12} deficiency, and optimise thyroid function.

Ms Lau's cognitive performance was close to normal, with good ADL/IADL, including money management and handling other complex tasks in daily living and no impairment in short-term memory found on cognitive assessment. These findings showed some discrepancy with her subjective complaints and those of the informants. The primary care team is therefore suggested to reassess in six months to determine whether her cognitive impairment has improved with an increased vitamin B_{12} level.

Case 080 'Passing' in MMSE

Mr Kwok, an 83-year-old gentleman, presented with concerns raised by his daughter about his memory problems. She complained of his memory decline that can be traced back about 12 months, with more obvious impairments in the last six months. He was noted to appear forgetful with repeated questioning. Mr Kwok was aware of his own memory decline.

Findings from Screening Assessments by Allied Healthcare and Social Care Team

Cognitive functioning	Scored 22/30 on MMSE, results suggested no indication of cognitive impairment, adjusted for education level. Mr Kwok's performance was impaired in orientation to time (2/5) and delayed recall (0/3). He had slight difficulties in orientation to place (4/5), calculation (4/5), and three-step commands (2/3); his performance was normal in registration (3/3), language (5/5), and visuospatial relationships (1/1). The Clock Drawing Test showed normal executive function: he was able to self-correct an inaccurate time denotation and planned number placement by dividing the clock face into four quarters.
ADL/IADL	Mr Kwok was independent in all ADLs (Barthel Index 100/100). He was semi-independent in IADLs (Lawton IADL Scale 54/56): he had needed reminders to take his medication over the last six months. He would also sometimes forget that he had already eaten.
Depressive symptoms	Scored 1/15 on GDS-15, no obvious depressive mood was noted.
Staging and clinical rating	Scored 0.5/3 on Clinical Dementia Rating, indicating questionable dementia. He showed mild impairment in memory, orientation, and judgement and problem-solving.

History Taken with Carer by Primary Care Physician

Mr Kwok's daughter reported noticing memory problems in her father that had concerned her for a year. No delusional ideations were reported. Using the GPCOG Informant Interview, the following areas were noted to show more difficulties (×) or were preserved (○) compared to about two years ago:

× Remembering recent events
× Recalling recent conversations
○ Word finding
○ Managing money and finances
× Managing medication independently
○ Using transport

There were no additional clinical features to consider for non-Alzheimer's dementia. Mr Kwok had diabetes, hypertension, benign prostatic hyperplasia, and kidney cancer (left) with nephrectomy. He is currently on amlodipine besylate 2.5 mg daily, diazoxide 40 mg, and medicine for his benign prostatic hyperplasia. No family history of psychiatric disorders or dementia was reported. He had received primary education to P.2 (approximately two years of education). Mr Kwok had limited social activities and stayed at home most of the time.

Physical Examination Findings

General examination revealed no affect or hygiene problem. No significant CVS or CNS findings.

Investigations

CBP, R/LFT, VDRL, vitamin B_{12}, fasting sugar, fasting lipids, and TFT were ordered. Vitamin B_{12} and TFT were normal. VDRL was negative. CT brain (plain) scan revealed lacunar infarct in right basal ganglia.

Diagnosis

Early Alzheimer's disease.

Management

Rivastigmine transdermal system 5 mg daily, diltiazem hydrochloride extended release 100 mg daily, and omeprazole 20 mg daily were prescribed. He was recommended to join a specialised day care service for two days per week for two years to receive a structured and tailored intervention programme and cognitively stimulating activities to delay deterioration.

Suggestions for the Primary Care Team

This is a case that illustrates cognitive frailty, mild cognitive impairment of the amnestic type, and very early Alzheimer's disease. In this case, mild cognitive impairment is suggested from the assessment and clinical interview, with satisfactory cognitive and daily living functions observed, except for short-term memory and related cognitive functions (delayed recall and orientation to time). At this moment, the primary care team should observe and monitor his situation and repeat the assessment in six months. Mr Kwok nevertheless needs to be supported and treated in view of his significant symptom of forgetting meals.

References

1. Dickson DW, Davies P, Bevona C, Van Hoeven KH, Factor SM, Grober E, et al. Hippocampal sclerosis: A common pathological feature of dementia in very old (> or = 80 years of age) humans. Acta Neuropathology. 1994;88(3):212–21.

2. Barkhof F, Polvikoski TM, van Straaten EC, Kalaria RN, Sulkava R, Aronen HJ, et al. The significance of medial temporal lobe atrophy: A postmortem MRI study in the very old. Neurology. 2007;69(15):1521–27.

3. Prasad K, Wiryasaputra L, Ng A, Kandiah N. White matter disease independently predicts progression from mild cognitive impairment to Alzheimer's disease in a clinic cohort. Dementia Geriatric Cognitive Disorders. 2011;31(6):431–44.

4. Livingston G, Huntley J, Sommerlad A, et al. Dementia prevention, intervention, and care: 2020 report of the Lancet Commission [published correction appears in The Lancet. 2023 Sep 30;402(10408):1132]. The Lancet. 2020;396(10248):413–46. doi:10.1016/S0140-6736(20)30367-6

5. Arnold SE, Arvanitakis Z, Macauley-Rambach SL, et al. Brain insulin resistance in type 2 diabetes and Alzheimer disease: Concepts and conundrums. Nature Review Neurology. 2018;14(3):168–81. doi:10.1038/nrneurol.2017.185

6. Talbot K, Wang HY, Kazi H, et al. Demonstrated brain insulin resistance in Alzheimer's disease patients is associated with IGF-1 resistance, IRS-1 dysregulation, and cognitive decline. Journal of Clinical Investment. 2012;122(4):1316–38. doi:10.1172/JCI59903

7. Clegg A, Young J, Iliffe S, Rikkert MO, Rockwood K. Frailty in elderly people [published correction appears in The Lancet. 2013 Oct 19;382(9901):1328]. The Lancet. 2013;381(9868):752–762. doi:10.1016/S0140-6736(12)62167-9

Atypical Alzheimer's Disease, Other Dementias, and Differential Diagnoses

3.1 When Imaging and Further Observation Are Needed

Case 081 Could It Be Stroke?

Mr Chan, a 69-year-old gentleman, presented with concerns raised by his daughter about his memory problem. He was said to be forgetful of recent events.

Findings from Screening Assessments by Allied Healthcare and Social Care Team

Cognitive functioning	Scored 22/30 on MMSE, indicating cognitive impairment after adjusting for education level. Mr Chan's performance was significantly impaired in delayed recall (0/3) and poor in calculation (2/5), and he had slight problems in orientation to time (4/5) and place (4/5). His performance was, however, normal in registration (3/3), language (5/5), three-step commands (3/3), and visuospatial relationship (1/1). When tested using MoCA, he scored 19/30, indicating mild cognitive impairment after adjusting for education level.
ADL/IADL	Mr Chan was independent in all activities of daily living (100/100 on the Barthel Index) and instrumental activities of daily living (56/56 on the Lawton IADL Scale), except for occasional verbal cues needed when there is a change in his medication dosage.
Staging and clinical rating	Results suggested a Global Deterioration Scale stage of 3 progressing to stage 4, indicating questionable to mild dementia. Concentration deficit was evident during assessment and when asked to read a passage; he was able to retain relatively little information.

History Taken with Carer by Primary Care Physician

Mr Chan's daughter reported noticing memory problems in her father that had concerned her for a year, although no delusional ideations were reported. Using the GPCOG Informant Interview, the following areas were noted to show more trouble (✗) or were preserved (○) compared to about two years ago:

✗ Remembering recent events
✗ Recalling recent conversations
○ Word finding
○ Managing money and finances
✗ Managing medication independently
○ Using transport

There were no additional clinical features to consider for non-Alzheimer's dementia. Other medical history includes hypertension, hypercholesterolaemia, diabetes mellitus, and a previous stroke. No family history of psychiatric disorders or dementia was reported. Mr Chan had little education: according to his daughter, he probably had more than two years but less than six years of education.

Investigations
CT brain (plain) scan was ordered.

Diagnosis
Mild cognitive impairment.

Management
No medication was prescribed due to the pending investigation findings. Non-pharmacological intervention was indicated: Mr Chan was recommended to a centre-based programme with cognitive stimulation to maintain cognitive and self-care functioning and was encouraged to do regular exercise, have a healthy diet and mental stimulation, manage stress, and maintain an active social life to promote general health and quality of life.

Suggestions for the Primary Care Team
The primary care team may sometimes find it challenging to differentiate between mild vascular cognitive impairment and mild dementia of the vascular subtype. While in this case, the IADLs (basic and instrumental) suggested mild cognitive impairment only, Mr Chan's cognitive screening test scores were unusually low for mild cognitive impairment. The presence of vascular risk factors nevertheless does not equate to the diagnosis of vascular dementia. The primary care team is advised to monitor the cognitive changes over time and his response to the interventions. A CT scan could help understand the extent of the stroke, while a PET amyloid scan is suggested.

Presentation at the mild cognitive impairment stage or very early dementia is a good time for equipping the person with memory skills or adaptive strategies to enhance memory performance. Although vascular dementia is not yet evident at this moment, preventive measures to minimise vascular-related risk factors are always recommended, such as adopting a healthy diet and exercising regularly, especially in cases with high vascular risk as in Mr Chan's case. The primary care team should engage him in cognitively stimulating activities while developing a healthy lifestyle.

Case 082 A Sweet Tooth

Mrs Kwan, a 79-year-old lady, presented with concerns raised by her daughter about her memory problem. She was noted to have misplaced valuable items, getting lost, and being unable to find her way home.

Findings from Screening Assessments by Allied Healthcare and Social Care Team

Cognitive functioning	Scored 10/30 on MMSE: indication of cognitive impairment, adjusted for educational level. Mrs Kwan's performance was significantly impaired in orientation to time (0/5) and place (0/5), delayed recall (0/3), calculation (0/5), and visuospatial relationship (0/1). She performed fairly in three-

	step commands (2/3) and normal in registration (3/3) and language (5/5). Abnormal clock face drawing with inaccurate denotation (reversal of numbers) and impaired executive function, conceptual deficits, visual-spatial deficits, and preservation errors were noted on the Clock Drawing Test (Figure 3.1).
ADL/IADL	Mrs Kwan was independent in the most basic ADL (Barthel Index 99/100), except for a need for supervision in bathing due to cognitive impairment. Instrumental activities of daily living (Lawton IADL Scale 10/56) were dependent.
Depressive symptoms	No indication of depression (GDS-15 score 1/15).
Staging and clinical rating	Results suggested a Global Deterioration Scale stage 6, indicating moderately severe dementia. She was largely unaware of all recent events and experiences in her daily life. No behavioural or psychological symptoms of dementia were noted.

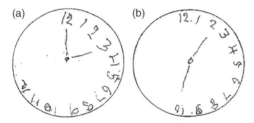

Figure 3.1 Findings from Mrs Kwan's Clock Drawing Test. (a) Clock Drawing (3 o'clock). (b) Clock Copying (10 past 10)

History Taken with Carer by Primary Care Physician

Mrs Kwan's daughter reported noticing memory problems in her mother that had concerned her for about two years, although no delusional ideations were reported. Using the GPCOG Informant Interview, the following areas were noted to show more trouble (✗) or were preserved (○) compared to about two years ago:

✗ Remembering recent events
✗ Recalling recent conversations
○ Word finding
✗ Managing money and finances
✗ Managing medication independently
✗ Using transport

Clinical features of overeating, especially sweet food (including chocolate and candy), suggestive of possible non-Alzheimer's dementia (bvFTD), were noted. Comorbidities of hypertension, diabetes mellitus, and hypercholesterolemia were reported. No family history of psychiatric disorders or dementia was reported. She had received secondary education.

Investigations

CBP, R/LFT, VDRL, vitamin B_{12}, folate, fasting sugar, fasting lipids, and TFT were ordered. Except for the negative VDRL value and elevated fasting sugar level, all other investigations were normal. A brain CT scan revealed vascular dementia.

Diagnosis

Vascular dementia. Differential diagnoses: frontotemporal dementia and a frontal variant of Alzheimer's disease.

Management

Donepezil 5 mg daily was prescribed. Mrs Kwan was recommended to join a centre-based programme with cognitively stimulating activities to maintain cognitive and self-care functioning and was encouraged to do regular exercise, have a healthy diet and mental stimulation, and maintain an active social life for general health and quality of life.

Suggestions for the Primary Care Team

Mrs Kwan showed unusually low MMSE and Lawton IADL scores, with a liking for sweet food. In view of the multiple domains of cognitive deficits, Mrs Kwan may have vascular dementia, frontotemporal dementia, or the frontal variant of Alzheimer's disease. Physicians can observe cognitive and personality changes as well as mood swings over time and response to medication; in cases of declining cognition, memantine can be added on top of donepezil.

In terms of her residual cognitive functions, attention and language appeared to be her areas of strength, and therefore communication and social activities should be maintained and encouraged for as long as possible. In cases of frontotemporal dementia, it is foreseeable that language comprehension and expression will deteriorate further, with mood and behavioural symptoms affecting ADLs, although in this case Mrs Kwan's ADLs were still independent at the present time. The primary care team should work with Mrs Kwan and her family to encourage her to maintain her existing lifestyle and routine as much as possible, while at the same time enriching her social activities. For her overeating problem, the family will need to be educated that strict restrictions or prohibitions may trigger mood problems, especially in the case of frontotemporal dementia. They should be provided with appropriate care tips for the situation, such as preparing for Mrs Kwan healthy finger food/snacks with low calories decreasing meal size but increasing the frequency of meals.

Case 083 Long History of Post-Stroke Cognitive Impairment

Mr Tang, a 91-year-old gentleman, presented with concerns raised by his wife about his cognitive problems, which started about six years ago after a cerebrovascular accident. His wife complained of his declining memory for recent events and misplaced items, which seemed to be worsening in the past two to three years.

Findings from Screening Assessments by Allied Healthcare and Social Care Team

Cognitive functioning	Scored 24/30 on MMSE, suggesting no cognitive impairment, after adjusting for education level. On MoCA, Mr Tang scored 21/30, indicating mild cognitive impairment. He showed impairments in executive function, verbal fluency, and delayed recall (free recall 0/5, categorical 2/5, and multiple choice 3/5). The Clock Drawing Test result was normal.
ADL/IADL	Mr Tang needed moderate help in toileting, bathing, stair climbing, and dressing and minimal help in bed/chair transfers, ambulation, and bowel

and bladder control. He was independent in other basic ADLs (Barthel Index 73/100). For IADL, he was dependent in meal preparation, laundry, and housekeeping; needed assistance in community access, handling finances, and grocery shopping; and needed supervision in taking medications (medications were prepared by a domestic helper; he would forget if not reminded), and external communication (able to pick up phone calls, but rarely calls) (Lawton IADL Scale 22/56).

| Staging and clinical rating | Results suggested a Global Deterioration Scale stage of 4, indicating mild dementia. He showed decreased knowledge of current and recent events and a concentration deficit on serial subtractions, and the carer reported a decreased ability to travel and handle finances. |

History Taken with Carer by Primary Care Physician

Mr Tang's wife reported noticing memory problems in her husband that had concerned her for about five to six years. No delusional ideations were reported. Using the GPCOG Informant Interview, the following areas were noted to show more trouble (×) or were preserved (○) compared to about two years ago:

× Remembering recent events
× Recalling recent conversations
○ Word finding
○ Managing money and finances
× Managing medication independently
× Using transport

There was no additional clinical feature to consider for non-Alzheimer's dementia. Comorbidities of hypertension, diabetes mellitus, hypercholesterolemia, and a cerebrovascular accident (six years ago) were reported. No family history of psychiatric disorders or dementia was reported. He has received tertiary education.

Investigations

Calcium, VDRL, vitamin B_{12}, and TSH were ordered. All investigations were normal, except for vitamin B_{12} deficiency.

Diagnosis

Vascular dementia with possible age-related cognitive impairment.

Management

Donepezil 5 mg daily and vitamin B_{12} were prescribed. He was also recommended to join a centre-based programme with cognitively stimulating activities for at least 18 months to maintain cognitive function.

Suggestions for the Primary Care Team

With rather intact visuospatial function as shown on the Clock Drawing Test and cognitive impairment after a stroke at an older age, the history is indicative of vascular (post-stroke) dementia with possible age-related cognitive impairment likely due to vitamin B_{12} deficiency. However, it should be noted that cardiovascular risk factors may also lead to Alzheimer's disease (1). Memantine may be considered an add-on therapy or when donepezil cannot be tolerated.

At the relatively old age of 91, Mr Tang's cognitive performance was satisfactory and appeared well maintained. His ADL and IADL performance, however, appeared inconsistent and worse than expected relative to his cognitive functional level: it is common for people with vascular dementia to have their physical functions affected at the same time as their cognitive performance. Maintenance of physical functions, including balance, mobility, and muscle strength, are equally important as cognitively stimulating activities at this moment to prevent future complications, such as falls and muscle wasting.

Case 084   Difficulties in Word Finding

Mr Fung, a 75-year-old gentleman, presented with concerns raised by his wife about his declining cognitive functions. His wife noticed difficulties in word finding, remembering recent events, misplacing items, being slow in his reactions, and problems finding his way after a minor stroke.

Findings from Screening Assessments by Allied Healthcare and Social Care Team

Cognitive functioning	Scored 21/30 on MMSE, indicating cognitive impairment after adjusting for educational level. Mr Fung showed impairment in calculation (1/5), three-step commands (1/3), visuospatial relationship (0/1), a slight problem in orientation to time (4/5), and delayed recall (2/3). He was, however, normal in orientation to place (5/5), registration (3/3), and language (5/5). The Clock Drawing Test (Figure 3.2) indicated dementia; he showed executive function deficits in planning and organisation, and conceptual deficits.
ADL/IADL	He was independent in basic ADLs (Barthel Index 100/100). For IADL, he was dependent in taking medications, modified dependent in external communication and handling finances, and needed supervision in meal preparation, doing laundry, housekeeping, and community access (Lawton IADL Scale: 40/56).
Depressive symptoms	Scored 1/15 on GDS-15, suggesting no indication of depression.
Staging and clinical rating	Results suggested a Global Deterioration Scale stage of 4, indicating mild dementia. He showed decreased knowledge of current and recent events, had got lost when travelling to unfamiliar locations, and had a concentration deficit evident on serial subtractions. His basic activities of daily living were, however, maintained, and he was able to select proper clothing to wear.

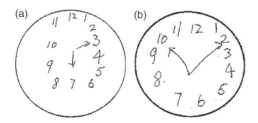

Figure 3.2 Findings from Mr Fung's Clock Drawing Test. (a) Clock Drawing (3 o'clock). (b) Clock Copying (10 past 10)

History Taken with Carer by Primary Care Physician

Mr Fung's wife reported noticing memory problems in her husband that had concerned her for about one and a half years after a minor stroke. However, the decline had become more significant in the last two months. Using the GPCOG Informant Interview, the following areas were noted to show more trouble (✘) or were preserved (○) compared to about two years ago:

- ✘ Remembering recent events
- ✘ Recalling recent conversations
- ○ Word finding
- ✘ Managing money and finances
- ✘ Managing medication independently
- ○ Using transport

There were no additional clinical features to consider for non-Alzheimer's dementia. Comorbidities of hypertension, diabetes mellitus, hypercholesterolemia, and a previous cerebrovascular accident were reported. No family history of psychiatric disorders or dementia was noted. He had received five years of primary education.

Investigations

CBP, R/LFT, calcium, fasting sugar, and fasting lipids were ordered. All investigations were normal except for the elevated fasting sugar. A CT brain scan two years ago revealed multiple bilateral cerebral hypodensities, which can be ischaemic changes or infarction.

Diagnosis

Dementia, likely vascular dementia (mixed dementia could not be ruled out), with no distressed behaviours and neuropsychiatric symptoms of dementia.

Management

At the time of the report, no medication was prescribed, as a blood work-up was awaited. He was encouraged to do regular exercise, have a healthy diet and mental stimulation, manage stress, maintain an active social life, and continue joining social activities classes (e.g., English class and Chinese class) at locations close to his residence. Mr Fung was also recommended to join a centre-based programme for cognitively stimulating activities to maintain his cognitive function and quality of life.

Suggestions for the Primary Care Team

The memory and language problems were mainly related to stroke, with a lot of vascular elements in the history. The CT brain scan can be repeated to characterise the speech impairment, which might be caused by conduction dysphasia in superior angular gyrus syndrome. A cholinesterase inhibitor in combination with memantine may be considered.

There are features suggestive of Alzheimer's disease; therefore, mixed dementia is the differential diagnosis: Mr Fung presented with a cognitive impairment pattern that is compatible with early Alzheimer's disease, with higher cognitive functions being impacted first (as shown in his Clock Drawing Test, with worse performance on the drawing part and improving on the copying part), as well as memory and orientation, while ADL performance was more preserved compared with IADL ability. Mr Fung had a relatively active social life, which is a strength. The primary care team, however, needs to remind his family about the need for adaptive strategies to help Mr Fung maintain his social life for as long as possible, for example by using a GPS tracking device or smartphone for safety measures when he goes out, cue cards or reminders in his wallet, and regular telephone contact by carers for caring and safety.

Case 085 Intact Visuospatial Performance

Mr Lo, a 79-year-old gentleman, presented with concerns raised by his wife about his memory decline. He was noted to have problems with finding his way in familiar places, forgetting recently learned materials such as things read and people met, and in verbal expression and word finding.

Findings from Screening Assessments by Allied Healthcare and Social Care Team

Cognitive functioning	Scored 23/30 on MMSE, suggesting no indication of cognitive impairment after adjusting for educational level. Results on MoCA (19/30) indicated mild cognitive impairment after adjusting for education. Mr Lo's performance was impaired in attention (3/6), abstraction (0/2), and orientation (3/6). Performance was fair in naming (2/3), language (2/3), and delayed recall (3/5). The Clock Drawing Test result was normal.
ADL/IADL	Mr Lo was largely independent in the basic ADLs (Barthel Index 93/100), except for minimal help required in ambulation, stair climbing, and dressing. For IADL, he needed assistance in meal preparation, external communication, doing laundry, housekeeping, and grocery shopping, and he needed supervision/a reminder in taking medications, community access (able to go out to nearby areas only), and handling finances (Lawton IADL Scale: 30/56).
Staging and clinical rating	Results suggested a Global Deterioration Scale stage of 4, indicating mild dementia. He showed decreased knowledge of current and recent events; a concentration deficit on serial subtractions; and a decreased ability to travel and handle finances; he was able to recall an address given to him for memorising, although he may not be able to select appropriate clothing for the weather.

History Taken with Carer by Primary Care Physician

Mr Lo's wife reported noticing memory problems in her husband that had concerned her for about two to three years, although no delusional ideations were reported. Using the GPCOG Informant Interview, the following areas were noted to show more trouble (✗) or were preserved (○) compared to about two years ago:

○ Remembering recent events
✗ Recalling recent conversations
✗ Word finding
✗ Managing money and finances
✗ Managing medication independently
✗ Using transport

No additional clinical feature of non-Alzheimer's dementia was noted. Comorbidities of hypertension, hypercholesterolemia, and old haematologic stroke were reported. No family history of psychiatric disorders or dementia was reported. He has received a secondary education.

Investigations

CBP, ESR, R/LFT, calcium, vitamin B_{12}, folate, fasting sugar, fasting lipid, MSU X R/M and culture test, HbA1C, PSA, and urine albumin/creatinine ratio were ordered. MRI revealed old haemorrhagic insult/cystic change, small vessel ischaemia, lacunar infarct, and mild to moderate cerebral atrophy.

Diagnosis

Mixed vascular and Alzheimer's disease.

Management

Rivastigmine transdermal system 5 mg was prescribed. Mr Lo was also recommended to join a centre-based programme with cognitively stimulating activities for the maintenance of cognitive function and quality of life.

Suggestions for the Primary Care Team

This is a typical case of vascular dementia with or without Alzheimer's disease with intact visuospatial function. The response to the cholinesterase inhibitor should be watched. On top of the cholinesterase inhibitor, memantine may also be considered. A CT brain scan can be considered to confirm the vascular burden.

Mr Lo had satisfactory performance in his cognitive functions in general, although his impairment in verbal expression early in the course of the disease – which was noted in both cognitive assessment and reports on daily living – was atypical of Alzheimer's disease and may reflect the location where the small vessel ischaemia has happened. Mr Lo's difficulties in ADL/IADL tasks were mainly caused by his short-term memory deterioration. At this stage, therefore, the primary care team could focus on working with Mr Lo and his family to identify the best ways to minimise the impact of short-term memory decline and maintain his ADL/IADL functioning. For example, Mr Lo may be allowed more time to perform his ADL/IADL tasks, with a carer providing only verbal cues. A carer should accompany Mr Lo in using public facilities, transportation, shopping, etc., to encourage him to stay in touch with the community in a safe manner. The primary care team should also advise the family to take safety precautions to enable Mr Lo to go out of nearby areas, for example, by using a location-tracking device.

3.2 Pseudodementia

Case 086 Significant Depression and Questionable Dementia

Mrs Yip, an 83-year-old lady, presented with concerns raised by her daughter about her memory decline. Mrs Yip also complained about her own memory decline.

Findings from Screening Assessments by Allied Healthcare and Social Care Team

Cognitive functioning	Scored 14/30 on MMSE, indicating cognitive impairment after adjusting for educational level. Mrs Yip's performance was significantly impaired in delayed recall (0/3) and calculation (0/5); poor in orientation to time (2/5) and place (1/5); and she had a slight problem in three-step commands (2/3). Her performance was, however, normal in registration (3/3), language (5/5), and visuospatial relationship (1/1). The Clock Drawing Test showed obvious impairment in executive function (Figure 3.3).

Activities of daily living:	Mrs Yip was independent in the most basic ADLs, except for ambulation and stair climbing (Barthel Index 95/100). For IADLs, she was dependent in taking medication; needed supervision or occasional assistance in external communication, housekeeping, and community access; and needed modified independence in meal preparation (Lawton IADL Scale: 43/56).
Depressive symptoms	Scored 11/15 on GDS-15; significant depressive mood was noted.
Staging and clinical rating	Scored 0.5/3 on Clinical Dementia Rating, indicating questionable dementia. She showed mild impairment in memory, judgement and problem-solving, and orientation; questionable impairment in home and hobbies; and was normal in personal care and community affairs aspects.

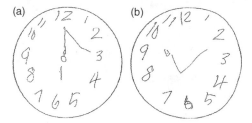

Figure 3.3 Findings from Mrs Yip's Clock Drawing Test. (a) Clock Drawing (3 o'clock). (b) Clock Copying (10 past 10)

History Taken with Carer by Primary Care Physician

Mrs Yip's daughter reported noticing memory problems in her mother that had concerned her for half a year, although no delusional ideations were reported. Using the GPCOG Informant Interview, the following areas were noted to show more trouble (✗) or were preserved (○) compared to about two years ago:

✗ Remembering recent events
✗ Recalling recent conversations
○ Word finding
○ Managing money and finances
✗ Managing medication independently
○ Using transport

There were no additional clinical features to consider for non-Alzheimer's dementia. She was known to a geriatric medicine outpatient clinic for hypertension. She was on a daily dosage of methyldopa 500 mg, atenolol 50 mg, hydrochlorothiazide 25 mg, and valsartan 160 mg. No family history of psychiatric disorders or dementia was reported. She had received one year of primary education.

Physical Examination Findings

General examination revealed a depressive-looking mood/affect problem, but no hygiene problem. No significant CVS or CNS findings.

Investigations

CBP, TSH, and Vitamin B$_{12}$ were ordered. Results were normal.

Diagnosis

Dementia with depression.

Management

Lexapro 5 mg daily was prescribed. She was also recommended to join a specialised day care service for two days per week to receive structured and tailored intervention programmes with cognitively stimulating activities to delay deterioration and maintain quality of life.

Suggestions for the Primary Care Team

Mrs Yip showed a typical pattern of Alzheimer's disease with severe depression. It is recommended to focus treatment on the depression first, arrange social support, and reassess to see if cognition improves with improvements in depressive symptoms ('pseudodementia'). Methyldopa should be stopped as it can lead to or exacerbate underlying depression. Physicians may review Mrs Yip's condition two to three months later after stopping methyldopa.

In this case, inconsistency among different assessments can be observed: Mrs Yip's ADL/IADL performance was higher than would be expected from her cognitive assessment findings on MMSE; at the same time, the Clinical Dementia Rating results suggested mild cognitive impairment only. It is likely that Mrs Yip's depressive mood has significantly masked her actual performance in the cognitive assessment, but not so much in affecting her daily life. The primary care team should explore further the reasons for the discrepancy: whether it was related to her level of motivation or denial of impairment and refusal to respond and answer properly; finding out would help develop a proper care plan. Mrs Yip should also be reassessed as her mood improves, to find out the actual level of her existing strengths and weaknesses. The primary care team should also note that 11/15 on GDS-15 suggests quite a significant level of depressive mood; the causes and factors contributing to her high level of depressive symptoms should be investigated.

Case 087 My Son Doesn't Care

Mrs Lam, a 90-year-old lady, presented with concerns raised by her social worker from the district elderly community centre about her memory problem. She was noted to have impaired short-term memory, with episodes when she has forgotten about appointments/event dates, misplaced items, and repeated questioning.

Findings from Screening Assessments by Allied Healthcare and Social Care Team

Cognitive functioning	Scored 25/30 on MMSE, suggesting no indication of cognitive impairment after adjusting for educational level. Results on MoCA (14/30) suggested mild cognitive impairment after adjusting for education. Mrs Lam's performance was impaired in visuospatial/executive performance (1/5), naming (1/3), attention (1/2), language fluency (0/1), abstraction (0/2), and delayed recall (0/5). The Clocking Drawing Test result was normal.
ADL/IADL	Mrs Lam was independent in all ADL and IADL tasks.
Depressive symptoms	Mild depression was noted (no GDS-15 rating available as Mrs Lam refused to complete it).
Staging and clinical rating	Results suggested a Global Deterioration Scale stage of 3, indicating questionable dementia. Impairment in sustained attention was evident during the assessment, accompanied by a mild to moderate anxiety symptom, although she seemed to have fair motivation in completing the assessment.

History Taken with Carer by Primary Care Physician

Mrs Lam's social worker reported noticing memory problems in her client that had concerned her for a few years, although no delusional ideations were reported. Using the GPCOG Informant Interview, the following areas were noted to show more trouble (✗) or were preserved (○) compared to about two years ago:

○ Remembering recent events
✗ Recalling recent conversations
○ Word finding
✗ Managing money and finances
✗ Managing medication independently
✗ Using transport

There were no additional clinical features of non-Alzheimer's dementia. Mrs Lam lived alone and had poor social support. She is known to a geriatric medicine outpatient clinic for hypertension. Comorbid trachoma was also reported. She did not receive any formal education.

Physical Examination Findings

No significant findings, except that Mrs Lam denied depressive thoughts during the general physical examination but became teary when talking about her son who was distant from her.

Investigations

No acute or subacute cerebral infarction was found on brain MRI. Cerebral atrophy (GCA score 2) was noted, with more prominent frontoparietal lobe atrophy, MTL R = 15.8 L + 13.6, Scheltens R = L = 1, and ARWMC 3. Possible subclinical hyperthyroidism, pending review at a general outpatient clinic.

Diagnosis

Mixed dementia, vascular dementia, and SVD subtype +/− limbic sparing-type Alzheimer's disease, with mild depression.

Management

Donepezil 5 mg daily was prescribed. Mrs Lam was also recommended to join a centre-based programme to receive cognitively stimulating activities to maintain her cognitive function and quality of life.

Suggestions for the Primary Care Team

This is a typical case of mood problems (anxiety and/or depression) mimicking dementia in an older person with poor social support. In view of the age of onset, with significant symptoms observed in her late 80s, negative Clock Drawing Test results, and acceptable visuospatial functioning, the mild cognitive impairment could also be age-related. A trial of donepezil 2.5 mg daily can be considered, while an antidepressant, such as escitalopram, can be considered on top of donepezil.

Given her general low score on cognitive assessments, it is out of expectation that Mrs Lam's ADL/IADL functioning was independent. There is a possibility that her poor cognitive performance was a result of her depressive mood and low motivation. In Mrs Lam's case, while a depressive mood can be observed, the GDS-15 result was not available. The primary care team should note that it is common for older people with depressive mood to be unwilling to share their problems/feelings with others. A social worker from the team would be in a good position to explore further and intervene as necessary, ensuring rapport building and a trusting relationship. Building on Mrs Lam's insight into her mood, the team can work with Mrs Lam to identify the best support/intervention, which could include counselling for Mrs Lam to accept the fact that her relationship with her son is beyond repair, as well as family intervention, conflict resolution, or other psychotherapies tailored to Mrs Lam's situation.

Case 088 Drinking Problem and Quetiapine

Mr Leung, an 82-year-old gentleman, presented with concerns raised by his wife about his memory change. He was noted to have repeated questioning and functional decline.

Findings from Screening Assessments by Allied Healthcare and Social Care Team

Cognitive functioning	Scored 14/30 on MMSE, indicating cognitive impairment after adjusting for educational level. Mr Leung's performance was impaired in orientation to time (1/5) and place (2/5), delayed recall (0/3), calculation, and three-step commands (1/3). His performance was, however, normal in registration (3/3), language (5/5), and visuospatial relationship (1/1).
ADL/IADL	Mr Leung was independent in the basic ADLs (Barthel Index 100/100). For IADLs, he was dependent in meal preparation; relied on carers for laundry and housekeeping; needed assistance in community access, handling finances, and shopping; and needed supervision in taking medication (Lawton IADL Scale: 24/56).
Depressive symptoms	He scored 2/15 on GDS-15, with no indication of depression.
Staging and clinical rating	Results suggested a Global Deterioration Scale stage of 5, suggesting moderate dementia. He needed assistance in choosing proper clothing to wear and was unable to recall relevant aspects of his current life such as the names of his grandchildren and his telephone number. No distressed behaviours and neuropsychiatric symptoms of dementia were noted.

History Taken with Carer by Primary Care Physician

Mr Leung's wife reported noticing memory problems in her husband that had concerned her for about one to two years, although no delusional ideations were reported. Using the GPCOG Informant Interview, the following areas were noted to show more trouble (×) or were preserved (○) compared to about two years ago:

× Remembering recent events
× Recalling recent conversations
○ Word finding
× Managing money and finances
× Managing medication independently
× Using transport

There were no additional clinical features of non-Alzheimer's dementia. Comorbidities of hypertension, diabetes mellitus, hyperlipidaemia, and alcohol dependence history were reported. He was on quetiapine 25 mg at night. No family history of psychiatric disorders or dementia was reported. He did not receive any formal education.

Investigations

CBP, R/LFT, VDRL, vitamin B_{12}, folate, and CT scan were ordered.

Diagnosis

Alzheimer's disease.

Management

Vitamin B complex daily was prescribed. A short-term cognitive rehabilitation programme was arranged to maintain cognition and self-care functioning. Mr. Leung was also encouraged to do regular exercise, have a healthy diet and mental stimulation, and engage in an active social life. He was also recommended to join a centre-based programme with cognitively stimulating activities to maintain cognitive function and quality of life.

Suggestions for the Primary Care Team

Mr Leung's presentation and history are compatible with Alzheimer's disease, with the cognitive impairment possibly related to his drinking problem and the use of quetiapine. Enquiries into the reasons for a previous quetiapine prescription are suggested to find out if there is any history of hallucinations, delusions, sleep problems such as REM sleep disorder, or any parkinsonism features suggesting cerebral Lewy body disease. Given that his cognitive symptoms were noted to first occur in the last one to two years according to his wife, it is worth investigating the history of alcohol dependency and management. If the timelines coincide and quetiapine is prescribed as part of the management, Mr Leung's cognitive impairment may be related to his drinking problem, thus the unexpectedly poor performance on cognitive assessment. Another possibility that quetiapine was prescribed is REM sleep disorder, where a person affected may lose their temper during the night, which is interpreted as agitated behaviour. Donepezil 2.5 mg and thiamine 50 mg daily can be prescribed if the client is still on alcohol. However, it is advisable to observe the side effects of quetiapine and reduce the dosage after ascertaining the reason for the medication. Physicians may consider memantine if irritability is noted: alcohol has anxiolytic and sedative effects, and some patients with alcohol-drinking problems may have anxiety-prone personalities.

A strength in Mr Leung's case is that his ADL is still independent. The primary care team nevertheless needs to prevent further dysfunctions because of his psychiatric condition. Negative symptoms, such as demotivation, tiredness, and psychosomatic discomfort, may be easily induced. The primary care team should also assess carer stress and skills. It is possible that Mr Leung's wife is experiencing a high level of stress, which is common when caring for a spouse with cognitive impairment and possible psychiatric symptoms, and the primary care team should make sure that effective support is available when needed.

Case 089 Suicidal Ideation and Temper Tantrum

Mrs Yuen, a 67-year-old lady, presented with depressive mood, suicidal ideation, difficulty managing activities of daily living, and temper tantrums. Her husband complained about her stubbornness, easy temper tantrums, and irritability over minor matters. She was noted to scold her daughter, with whom she never had any problem previously; there was also an episode of her not being able to recognise her son, who has returned from overseas, and forgetting to collect rent for over three months for the properties she owns.

Findings from Screening Assessments by Allied Healthcare and Social Care Team

Cognitive functioning	Scored 26/30 on MMSE, with no indication of cognitive impairment. Mrs Yuen's performance was normal in orientation to time (5/5), fair to place (4/5), normal in registration (3/3) and delayed recall (3/3), language (5/5), and visuospatial relationship (1/1), but impaired in calculation (2/5), and poor in three-step commands (1/3). Impairment was noted in the Clock Drawing Test (Figure 3.4).
ADL/IADL	For basic ADLs, Mrs Yuen needed her husband to help prepare her toothbrush and towel for grooming in the morning, although she was reported to refuse his help sometimes. For IADLs, she needed assistance with medication and was unable to cook or handle finances.
Staging and clinical rating	Staging and clinical rating were not completed.

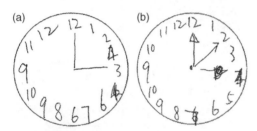

Figure 3.4 Findings from Mrs Yuen's Clock Drawing Test. (a) Clock Drawing (3 o'clock). (b) Clock Copying (10 past 10)

History Taken with Carer by Primary Care Physician

Mrs Yuen's husband reported noticing problems with money management for two years. She became passive and seldom talked to the family, developed a liking for sweets, and would sometimes ask for food non-stop. She gained weight recently and got lost once when she went out by herself. Using the GPCOG Informant Interview, the following areas were noted to show more trouble (✗) or were preserved (○) compared to about two years ago:

✗ Remembering recent events
○ Recalling recent conversations
✗ Word finding
✗ Managing money and finances
✗ Managing medication independently
✗ Using transport

Mrs Yuen used to work in a trading company. She had received secondary education.

Physical Examination Findings

Palmomental reflex positive.

Investigations

SPECT showed unilateral right frontotemporal hypoperfusion.

Diagnosis

Frontotemporal dementia.

Suggestions for the Primary Care Team

This is a case of frontotemporal dementia. The carer reported the mood and temper issues as the first symptoms. Mrs Yuen showed apraxia; it would be of moderate severity if it were an Alzheimer's disease; however, the MMSE score was not comparable with Alzheimer's disease. Her Clock Drawing Test result showed perseveration. Moreover, Mrs Yeung was apathetic. From the investigation, hypoperfusion in the right frontal lobe was noted, which matched the apathetic issue. Unilateral right frontotemporal hypoperfusion shown on SPECT is compatible with frontotemporal dementia, whereas symmetrical temporoparietal hypoperfusion would be expected in Alzheimer's disease. The MMSE score showed no impairment in language, yet the family carer reported the word-finding issue, showing that the MMSE is not sensitive in frontotemporal dementia. Therefore, the diagnosis is led by clinical symptoms and supported by psychometric testing and neuroimaging for atypical symptoms.

People with frontotemporal dementia may present at the onset with mood, behaviour, or personality changes, which can occur earlier than cognitive symptoms. Carers should be well prepared for the expected changes, including significant dysfunctions in verbal expression, mood swings, and rapid deterioration in cognitive functions (progressing much faster than typical Alzheimer's disease). The primary care team should work with the family to understand and become familiar with the person's habits, preferences, and character, so that when verbal expression becomes limited in the future, the family will still be able to understand her needs. Note that prohibiting eating can trigger an agitated mood; instead of stopping her from eating, providing finger food or snacks with low calories would help. Advance care planning with enduring powers of attorney (EPOA) appointed to handle the assets would be needed.

Case 090   Decline after Hospitalisation

Mr Ng, an 87-year old gentleman, presented with concerns raised by his brother about his memory problem. He was noted to have declining short-term memory (e.g., forgetting to take his medication) and difficulty navigating previously familiar places.

Findings from Screening Assessments by Allied Healthcare and Social Care Team

Cognitive functioning	Score 21/30 on MMSE, suggestive of cognitive impairment after adjusting for educational level. Mr Ng's performance was impaired in delayed recall (1/3) and calculation (2/5) and fair in orientation to time (3/5) and place (3/5); his performance was, however, normal in registration (3/3), language (5/5), three-step commands (3/3), and visuospatial relationship (1/1). He scored 13/30 on MoCA, suggesting cognitive impairment after adjusting for educational level. His performance was impaired in naming (1/3), abstraction (0/2), and delayed recall (0/5); fair in visuospatial/executive (3/5), attention (4/5), language (2/3), and orientation (3/6).
ADL/IADL	Mr Ng was independent in basic ADLs (Barthel Index 100/100). For IADLs, he needed supervision in taking medication (medications were prepared by the nurse weekly, and he needed to be reminded by calls) and community access; he was modified independent in handling finances and independent in other activities (Lawton IADL Scale: 51/56)

Staging and clinical rating	Results suggested a Global Deterioration Scale stage of 4, indicating mild dementia. He showed decreased knowledge of current and recent events; concentration deficit on serial subtractions; and a decreased ability to travel and handle finances. He seemed to be in denial of his deficits.

History Taken with Carer by Primary Care Physician

Mr Ng's brother reported noticing an insidious onset of memory problems in Mr Ng that had concerned him for about a year, with a more significant decline after his hospitalisation earlier this year. No delusional ideations were reported. Using the GPCOG Informant Interview, the following areas were noted to show more trouble (✗) or were preserved (○) compared to about two years ago:

○ Remembering recent events
✗ Recalling recent conversations
○ Word finding
✗ Managing money and finances
✗ Managing medication independently
✗ Using transport

There were no additional clinical features to consider for non-Alzheimer's dementia. Comorbidities of hypertension and spontaneous coronary artery dissection were reported. No family history of psychiatric disorders or dementia was reported. He had received secondary education.

Diagnosis

Delirium on cognitive frailty. Differential diagnosis: mild cognitive impairment.

Management

No medications were prescribed. He was recommended to join a centre-based programme with cognitively stimulating activities, for the maintenance of cognitive function and quality of life.

Suggestions for the Primary Care Team

As the deterioration happened after hospitalisation and the cognitive impairment appeared for only a year, with intact visuospatial function, Mr Ng's presentation is compatible with delirium on cognitive frailty: unresolved delirium could lead to post-operation cognitive decline. It would be useful to consider the time interval between his discharge and when the assessment was done: if the time interval is long, the likelihood that his performance was affected by delirium is lower. In any case, as delirium is usually reversible, it is recommended to observe for spontaneous improvement, with re-assessments, including cognitive tests, in three to six months' time. The team should also conduct a medication review.

At present, Mr Ng's cognitive performance on MMSE was satisfactory; although more obvious impairment was shown on MoCA, the Global deterioration scale rating showed only mild functional impairment, with largely independent ADL and IADL. Considering Mr Ng's relatively old age, the profile is more compatible with mild cognitive impairment or age-related cognitive frailty at this moment, although the condition could progress or worsen in the event of a change in his health condition. The primary care team is therefore advised to focus on maintaining a good health status, and physical health is a more important focus than other issues at this stage.

Case 091 Anticlockwise Clock

Ms Lo, an 89-year-old lady, presented with concerns raised by her daughter over her memory problems. Her daughter noted forgetfulness about recent events and frequent loss of personal belongings for about three years. Ms Lo has been aware of her own memory decline for about one year.

Findings from Screening Assessments by Allied Healthcare and Social Care Team

Cognitive functioning	Scored 20/30 on MMSE, suggesting cognitive impairment after adjusting for education level. Ms Lo's performance was impaired in delayed recall (0/3), visuospatial relationship (0/1), and orientation to time (2/5), fair in orientation to place (3/5), showed slight difficulties in calculation (4/5) but was normal in three-step commands (3/3), registration (3/3), and language (5/5). The Clock Drawing Test showed that she was unable to complete the drawing and placed the numbers anticlockwise (6/10). The clock copying task showed that she was able to read the clock (4/10) (Figure 3.5).
ADL/IADL	She was moderately dependent in basic ADLs (Barthel Index 87/100), walks with an umbrella, and was semi-independent in IADLs (Lawton IADL Scale 40/56): she needs assistance in taking medicine, meal preparation, and housekeeping; she needs company for community access, handling finances, and grocery shopping.
Depressive symptoms	Scored 9/15 on GDS-15, indicating significant depressive mood. She expressed worries about her health.
Staging and clinical rating	Scored 1/3 on Clinical Dementia Rating, suggesting mild dementia. She showed mild impairment in judgement and problem-solving, community affairs, home and hobbies, and personal care.

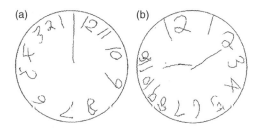

Figure 3.5 Findings from Ms Lo's Clock Drawing Test. (a) Clock Drawing (3 o'clock). (b) Clock Copying (10 past 10)

History Taken with Carer by Primary Care Physician

Ms Lo's daughter reported noticing memory problems in her mother that had concerned her for about one to two years. Delusional ideations were reported. Using the GPCOG

Informant Interview, the following areas were noted to show more trouble (×) or were preserved (○) compared to about two years ago:

× Remembering recent events
× Recalling recent conversations
○ Word finding
○ Managing money and finances
× Managing medication independently
× Using transport

There were no additional clinical features to consider for non-Alzheimer's dementia. Ms Lo had hypertension. She was on amlodipine 2.5 mg daily, enalapril 10 mg daily, aspirin 100 mg daily, piperidine 20 mg twice a day, and simvastatin 20 mg at night. No family history of psychiatric disorders or dementia was reported. Ms Lo currently lives with a domestic helper. She had received primary education.

Physical Examination Findings

General examination revealed no affect or hygiene problem. No significant CVS and CNS findings.

Diagnosis

Mild to moderate Alzheimer's disease.

Management

Rivastigmine transdermal system 4.6 mg daily was prescribed. Ms Lo was recommended to join a specialised day care service for two days per week to receive structured and tailored intervention programmes and cognitively stimulating activities to delay deterioration and maintain quality of life.

Suggestions for the Primary Care Team

Ms Lo presented at an old age (89 years) with a typical impairment pattern, although her MMSE performance was quite preserved. Her performance in all cognitive domains was generally satisfactory, except for short-term memory. Her impairments appeared more significant in basic ADLs than in IADLs, which is not typical in Alzheimer's disease, although the effects of age, depressive mood, and frailty should be taken into consideration. The obvious depression may be linked with cognitive frailty and thus should be treated. Further investigations into any relationship between her delusional ideations and depressive mood are also warranted. Pseudodementia is the differential diagnosis. An antidepressant, such as escitalopram 5 mg at night-time, can be prescribed. Social and leisure activities that are cognitively stimulating, such as card games, ball games, and board games (or Mahjong) tailored to her interests may be more appealing and thus effective and can be recommended instead of more formal cognitive training or exercise. Ms Lo's overall functions can be expected to improve along with improvements in mood.

3.3 Alzheimer's or Other Dementias? When to Refer

Case 092 Memory Decline in Three Months

Mrs Kong, a 72-year-old lady, presented with concerns raised by her daughter about her declining memory. She was reported to be misplacing items and forgetting about appointment dates soon after being told.

Findings from Screening Assessments by Allied Healthcare and Social Care Team

Cognitive functioning	Scored 26/30 on MMSE, suggesting no indication of cognitive impairment after adjusting for education level. Scored 20/30 on MoCA, suggesting mild cognitive impairment. Impairments were mainly noted in delayed recall. The Clock Drawing Test result was normal.
ADL/IADL	Mrs Kong is independent in all basic ADLs (Barthel Index 100/100) and most IADLs (Lawton IADL Scale 53/56), with modified independence in meal preparation, community access, and handling finances.
Staging and clinical rating	Results suggested a Global Deterioration Scale stage of 3, indicating mild cognitive impairment. Informants have become aware of the client's relatively poor performance in cognitive function. A concentration deficit was evident during assessment. She also showed a decreased ability to remember names when being introduced to new friends. There were mild to moderate anxiety symptoms.

History Taken with Carer by Primary Care Physician

Mrs Kong's daughter reported noticing memory problems in her mother that had concerned her for about two to three months, although no delusional ideations were reported. Using the GPCOG Informant Interview, the following areas were noted to show more trouble (×) or were preserved (○) compared to about two years ago:

× Remembering recent events
× Recalling recent conversations
○ Word finding
○ Managing money and finances
× Managing medication independently
× Using transport

There were no additional clinical features to consider for non-Alzheimer's dementia. Comorbidities of hypotension for over 30 years and osteoarthritis of the knees were reported. Mrs Kong lived alone. She had received a secondary education.

Diagnosis

Severe bradycardia on P/F with hypotension.

Management

Mrs Kong was already on memantine 5 mg prescribed by her private doctor. No further medication was prescribed pending the work-up. She was recommended to join a centre-based programme with cognitively stimulating activities, for the maintenance of cognitive function and quality of life.

Suggestions for the Primary Care Team

This case would require a case conference involving specialists. There are several points worth noting: the history of cognitive decline is short at only three months. Performance on MMSE was largely preserved, with intact visuospatial functioning and satisfactory performance in overall daily activities. Given the atypical presentations, a diagnosis of dementia cannot be given until other factors have been ruled out. Cognitive frailty may be involved, and poor attention and anxiety symptoms elicited during the clinical interview for staging suggest possible hidden mood problems. The primary care team should investigate further Mrs Kong's mental health, including her mood, by interviewing Mrs Kong and soliciting information from her family. Bradycardia and low blood pressure need further work-up, as a cholinesterase inhibitor is contraindicated. Review of medications, management of hypotension and bradycardia, neuroimaging, and close monitoring are recommended.

Case 093 No Concern for Personal Hygiene

Mr Cheng, an 82-year-old gentleman, presented with concerns raised by his daughter about his memory problem. He was noted to have a declining memory of recent events (e.g., whether he had eaten), difficulty finding his way, and showed little regard for his personal hygiene and attire.

Findings from Screening Assessments by Allied Healthcare and Social Care Team

Cognitive functioning	Scored 21/30 on MMSE, suggesting cognitive impairment after adjusting for education level. Mr Cheng's performance was impaired in orientation to place (1/5) and delayed recall (0/3), although he was able to recall items with cues (categorical); his performance was fair in orientation to time (3/5) and normal in registration (3/3), calculation (5/5), language (5/5), three-step commands (3/3), and visuospatial relationship (1/1). The Clock Drawing Test result was normal
ADL/IADL	Mr Cheng was independent in the most basic ADLs (Barthel Index 96/100) except for bladder control (leakage due to benign prostatic hyperplasia) and bowel control (occasional accident). He needed supervision in taking medication, meal preparation, and community access; was modified independent in housekeeping; and was independent in other IADLs (Lawton IADL Scale 49/56).
Staging and clinical rating	Results suggested a Global Deterioration Scale stage of 4, indicating mild dementia. He showed a concentration deficit on serial subtractions, and a decreased ability to travel and handle finances.
	Other behavioural symptoms were noted: for example, he was reported to often pick up dirty tissues and cigarette butts from the street and have poor hygiene and personal attire (urine and stool all over the flat, putting on dirty clothes, and dressing in rags). These occur frequently (once or more per day) at severe levels (the urge to hoard was very disturbing to him, and he had difficulty redirecting his attention), which also caused severe distress to others (his behaviours were described as very disruptive and a major source of distress for family members).

History Taken with Carer by Primary Care Physician

Mr Cheng's daughter reported noticing memory problems in her father that had concerned her for about a year. No delusional ideations were reported. Using the GPCOG Informant Interview, the following areas were noted to show more trouble (✗) or were preserved (○) compared to about two years ago:

○ Remembering recent events
✗ Recalling recent conversations

✗ Word finding
○ Managing money and finances
✗ Managing medication independently
○ Using transport

There were no additional clinical features to consider for non-Alzheimer's dementia. Comorbidities of benign prostatic hyperplasia and thalassemia trait were reported. He was on terazosin. No family history of psychiatric disorders or dementia was reported. He had received a secondary education.

Physical Examination Findings

Mr Cheng appeared to have fair hygiene on a general examination, which was unremarkable. The heart sounded normal, with no murmur or carotid bruit noted.

Investigations

CBC, MCV, platelet, FBS, LDL, UA, creatinine, and ALT were ordered. Resulted CBC Hb 12.2, MCV 69, platelet 114, FBS 5.2, LDL 2.5, UA 0.15, creatinine 81, and ALT 23. ECG and CSR revealed mild upper thoracic scoliosis.

Diagnosis

Mild dementia with hoarding behaviour.

Management

No medication was prescribed at this stage due to the pending work-up. Mr Cheng was recommended to join a centre-based programme with cognitively stimulating activities for the maintenance of cognitive function and quality of life.

Suggestions for the Primary Care Team

Mr Cheng showed intact visuospatial ability but rather prominent disinhibition symptoms and poor awareness of personal hygiene; the presentation is more compatible with frontotemporal dementia than Alzheimer's disease. Low MCV is also of note, which may be thalassemia minor or iron deficiency. It is advisable to check against his alcohol-drinking history and family history of psychiatric symptoms. The use of selective serotonin reuptake inhibitors and/or valproate for managing behavioural symptoms can be considered. This case would benefit from a case conference and psychiatric referral to rule out psychiatric disorders.

Distressed behaviours and neuropsychiatric symptoms that are related to habits, such as hoarding and poor hygiene, generally do not occur over a short period of time. They often start in the form of minor problems or issues, such as needing reminders to get changed, mistaking dirty clothes as clean, hiding their own belongings at home, and refusing to throw away trash. Hoarding behaviours may reflect an underlying sense of increasing insecurity, depression, or anxiety. In Mr Cheng's case, as the distressed behaviours and neuropsychiatric symptoms are severe and well established and considering his good cognitive functions, including judgement and problem-solving, with deteriorated/ deteriorating short-term memory, intervention strategies should be designed according to these strengths and weaknesses. Instead of aiming to correct and eliminate the well-established behaviours, the focus of intervention should be adaptive, with a goal to minimise the negative impact of these behaviours on Mr Cheng and his carers. Engaging Mr Cheng fully in well-structured, routine daily living activities, such as by offering full-day service in a day care centre for six days a week with scheduled activities, would help. Modifying the environment, such as by removing out of sight objects that are not needed (dirty clothes, unused utensils, etc.), can also be recommended. To minimise toileting behaviours in inappropriate places, the primary care team may advise the carers to ensure Mr Cheng can easily find his way to the toilet, with convenient accessible facilities, introduce a regular toileting schedule (e.g., toileting reminders at least once an hour), and scheduled showering or bathing at about the same time every day. For his habit of picking up dirty tissues and cigarette butts, carers may try to provide in-kind incentives and divert his attention by engaging him in activities that are meaningful to Mr Cheng.

Case 094 Hitting Wife in Sleep

Mr Chan, an 80-year-old gentleman, presented with memory impairment and aberrant behaviours over about two years. He was noted to have forgotten to switch off stoves, lost his way in the street, urinated in inappropriate places, and had visual hallucinations.

Findings from Screening Assessments by Allied Healthcare and Social Care Team

Cognitive functioning	Scored 21/30 on MMSE, suggestive of cognitive impairment after adjusting for education level. Mr Chan's performance was impaired in orientation to time (3/5) and place (3/5), calculation (3/5), three-step commands (1/3), and visuospatial relationship (0/1). His performance was, however, normal in registration (3/3) and delayed recall (3/3). The Clock Drawing Test showed significant impairment (Figure 3.6).
ADL/IADL	Mr Chan was independent in general ADLs; no incontinence was noted except that he would urinate suddenly in inappropriate places whenever in urge. He was modified independent in IADLs, had an incidence of getting lost when going out alone, and generally needed assistance in household tasks and meal preparation.
Staging and clinical rating:	Staging and clinical rating were not completed.

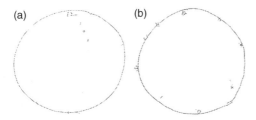

Figure 3.6 Findings from Mr Chan's Clock Drawing Test. (a) Clock Drawing (3 o'clock). (b) Clock Copying (10 past 10)

History Taken with Carer by Primary Care Physician

Mr Chan's daughter reported noticing memory impairment and aberrant behaviours for about two years and parkinsonism within one to two years. No delusional ideations were reported, although visual hallucinations were noted: Mr Chan would sometimes see children in his flat, which was not reported as a frightening experience. He was noted to have REM behaviour disorder for three years, and he would hit his wife (who has now passed away) in his sleep. Using the GPCOG Informant Interview, the following areas were noted to show more trouble (✗) or were preserved (○) compared to about two years ago:

✗ Remembering recent events
✗ Recalling recent conversations
○ Word finding
✗ Managing money and finances
✗ Managing medication independently
✗ Using transport

There were no additional clinical features to consider for non-Alzheimer's dementia. Comorbidities of hypertension and benign prostatic hyperplasia were reported. No family history of psychiatric disorders or dementia was reported. He had received two years of education.

Physical Examination Findings
On physical examination, Mr Chan showed parkinsonism features, a masked face, stooped posture, bradykinesia, and a shuffling gait.

Diagnosis
Cortical Lewy body disease.

Management
A cholinesterase inhibitor and low-dose carbidopa/levodopa were prescribed. Mr Chan is recommended to join a specialised dementia day care service, with structured activities and interventions for mood and quality of life, with carer support and education programmes.

Suggestions for the Primary Care Team
In cortical Lewy body disease, the primary symptoms can start with physical dysfunctions and psychiatric and psychological symptoms, which may occur earlier than cognitive symptoms. In the case of Mr Chan, his symptoms started in the form of aberrant behaviour, parkinsonism, and hallucinations, within the same time period (i.e., in the last one to two years) as memory problems were noted. At this stage, the primary care team should first attend to the impact of the disease on his physical functions, such as fall risk, sleeping quality, and safety. Mr Chan's deterioration in ADL functions may be caused by restricted mobility and slow reactions; giving him enough time to complete the ADL tasks may help. On the other hand, his condition would also be complicated by his physical impairments. For example, ongoing hallucinations and poor sleep quality can contribute to negative moods. The primary care team should pay attention to carer stress and intervene accordingly.

Case 095 Seeing Deceased Relatives
Mrs Yeung, a 92-year-old lady, presented with concerns raised by her husband about her memory problem, such as repeated questioning, misplacing items, forgetting whether she has eaten, and disorientation.

Findings from Screening Assessments by Allied Healthcare and Social Care Team

Cognitive functioning	Scored 12/30 on MMSE, indicating cognitive impairment after adjusting for education level. Mrs Yeung's performance was impaired in orientation to time (0/5), delayed recall (0/3), calculation (1/5), three-step commands (1/3), and visuospatial relationship (0/1) and fair in orientation to place (3/5) and registration (2/3). Her performance was, however, normal in language (5/5). The Clock Drawing Test showed obvious errors in time denotation (Figure 3.7).
ADL/IADL	Mrs Yeung was largely independent in basic ADLs (Barthel Index 98/100), except that she needed minimal help in stair climbing. For IADLs, she was dependent in meal preparation; needed assistance in taking medication, external communication (only able to pick up calls), laundry (able to handwash own clothes), housekeeping (able to finish simple cleaning only), handling finances, and grocery shopping; and needed supervision in community access (Lawton IADL Scale 24/56).
Staging and clinical rating	Results suggest a Global Deterioration Scale (GDS) stage of 5, indicating moderate dementia. She showed decreased knowledge of current and recent events; a deficit in memory of her personal history; and an inability to recall a major relevant aspect of her current life: she required prompting to provide her home address (named previous addresses) and was unable to recall names of close family members; she was reported to have frequent disorientation in time and occasional difficulty in choosing proper clothing to wear for the weather, and she forgets whether she has eaten.

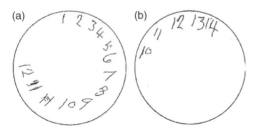

Figure 3.7 Findings from Mrs Yeung's Clock Drawing Test. (a) Clock Drawing (3 o'clock). (b) Clock Copying (10 past 10)

History Taken with Carer by Primary Care Physician

Mrs Yeung's husband reported noticing memory problems in his wife that had concerned him for more than a year. Delusional ideations were reported. Using the GPCOG Informant Interview, the following areas were noted to show more trouble (✗) or were preserved (○) compared to about two years ago:

- ○ Remembering recent events
- ✗ Recalling recent conversations
- ○ Word finding
- ✗ Managing money and finances
- ✗ Managing medication independently
- ✗ Using transport

A clinical feature of complex visual hallucinations (occasionally seeing deceased relatives) of non-Alzheimer's dementia (Lewy body dementia) was noted. Comorbid arrhythmia was reported. No family history of psychiatric disorders or dementia was reported. She had received three to four years of education.

Investigations

CBP, ESR, R/LFT, calcium, vitamin B_{12}, folate, fasting sugar, fasting lipid, MSU × R/M and culture test, CXR, and ECG were ordered. A Brain CT scan was also ordered.

Diagnosis

Mild Alzheimer's disease.

Management

No medications were prescribed at this stage. Mrs Yeung was recommended to join a centre-based programme with cognitively stimulating activities for the maintenance of cognitive function and quality of life.

Suggestions for the Primary Care Team

This is a case of Alzheimer's disease with significant cognitive frailty from age. Despite atypical presentation (presence of hallucinations and onset at a relatively older age), it is recommended to treat Mrs Yeung's case as in Alzheimer's disease. Donepezil 2.5 mg can be prescribed to observe any changes in hallucination and cognition. Antipsychotics are not indicated, as Mrs Yeung has no distress or other negative emotions associated with the visual hallucination.

The presence of hallucinations may be related to Alzheimer's disease pathology, cognitive frailty, or other reasons, which should be further explored. The description of seeing deceased relatives in this case appeared to be a complex hallucination, which is quite uncommon in Alzheimer's disease. Physicians could investigate further the nature of the hallucination; for example, more information is needed regarding the primary experience more compatible with a simple hallucination (e.g., shadow) that was interpreted as her deceased relatives; whether the hallucination happens within a certain context, and if so, whether any specific time, place, and triggering factors could be identified. The possibility of these hallucinations happening around sleep (hypnagogic and hypnopompic hallucinations), or confusion of memories from dreams with reality should also be explored, especially if they trigger any negative moods or behaviours.

The cognitive deterioration and other symptoms have likely been present for more than a year. Although Mrs Yeung's cognitive impairment level is compatible with mild dementia, her orientation to place is better than expected. Her attention and social communication are preserved, which are Mrs Yeung's strengths at the moment. Given her good ADL, satisfactory IADL, and remaining ability to handle simple household tasks, her family should be advised to continue to involve her in daily living activities. Social and leisure activities that are cognitively stimulating, as compared with cognitive training or exercises that focus only on cognitive improvement, are better choices to enhance both cognition and quality of life.

Case 096 Vascular or Vitamin?

Mrs Lau, an 89-year-old lady, presented with concerns raised by her daughter about her memory problems. She was noted to be emotional, unable to recognise her own family, and forgetting the content of a conversation, and there was an incident when she went to the kitchen instead of the toilet. Her daughter also reported difficulties in word finding and slurred speech.

Findings from Screening Assessments by Allied Healthcare and Social Care Team

Cognitive functioning	Scored 6/30 on MMSE, suggestive of cognitive impairment after adjusting for education level. Mrs Lau's performance was impaired in orientation to time (0/5) and place (0/5), registration (1/3), delayed recall (0/3), attention and calculation (0/5), and visuospatial relationship (0/1) and was fair in language (3/5) and three-step commands (2/3). Mrs. Lau was unwilling to complete the Clock Drawing Test and likely would have had difficulty completing it.
ADL/IADL	For basic ADLs, Mrs Lau was dependent in stair climbing; was unsafe in dressing; needed moderate help in bathing; and needed minimal help in bed/chair transfer, hygiene, toileting, ambulation, and bowel and bladder control (Barthel Index 67/100). For IADLs, she was dependent in meal preparation, laundry, housekeeping, handling finances, and grocery shopping and needed assistance in taking medications (medications were prepared by daughter), external communication (able to pick up calls occasionally), and community access (Lawton IADL Scale 14/56).
Staging and clinical rating	Results showed a Global Deterioration Scale stage of 5, indicating moderate dementia. She was unable to recall a major relevant aspect of her current life, such as the address of her long-term residence and the names of family members; she also showed frequent disorientation to time or place. She required no assistance with toileting or eating but had difficulty choosing proper clothing to wear and had difficulty counting from 1 to 10.

History Taken with Carer by Primary Care Physician

Mrs Lau's daughter reported noticing memory problems in her mother that had concerned her for about three to four years, with an acute decline for a few months although no delusional ideations were reported. Using the GPCOG Informant Interview, the following areas were noted to show more trouble (✗) or were preserved (○) compared to about two years ago:

✗ Remembering recent events
✗ Recalling recent conversations
✗ Word finding
✗ Managing money and finances
✗ Managing medication independently
✗ Using transport

There were no additional clinical features to consider for non-Alzheimer's dementia. Comorbidities of diabetes mellitus, hypertension, hypercholesterolemia, gout, cerebrovascular accidents, vitamin B_{12} deficiency, bilateral cataract, and hip replacement were reported. She was on a vitamin B_{12} supplement. No family history of psychiatric disorders or dementia was reported. She had received secondary education.

Investigations

CBP, R/LFT, calcium, vitamin B_{12}, folate, fasting sugar, and fasting lipids were ordered. CBP resulted in Hb 11.4, R/LFT Un 9.2 creatinine 151, calcium 2.27, vitamin B_{12} deficiency, fasting sugar 7.5, and fasting lipid TC 5.7 LDL 3.5, TG 2.8, and HDL 0.9. A CT scan revealed small vessel disease.

Diagnosis

Dementia, likely vascular dementia or due to low vitamin B_{12}; acute decline; probable delirium.

Management

No medications were prescribed due to pending further work-up. Mrs Lau was recommended to join a centre-based programme with cognitively stimulating activities, for the maintenance of cognitive function and quality of life.

Suggestions for the Primary Care Team

Mrs Lau's case is likely vascular (post-stroke) cognitive impairment or mixed dementia; the acute cognitive deterioration was potentially a small stroke, which showed improvement afterwards, while vitamin B_{12} deficiency may be a concomitant finding. Low-dose donepezil 2.5 mg can be started to observe any change in cognition and to replace vitamin B_{12} if the level is low. Memantine may also be considered on top of cholinesterase inhibitors for vascular dementia.

Slurred speech and other problems in verbal expression suggest that Mrs Lau is stepping into the late stage of dementia. At this stage, the focus should shift from improving functioning to enhancing the caring skills of carers and the quality of care for the person with dementia. Maintaining a stable mood, by engaging her in her interests through passive participation, such as playing her favourite songs at home, family gatherings, or outdoor activities such as a walk in the garden or a park, would help. Family carers should be equipped with caring skills for physical dysfunction as well, such as feeding and monitoring for any choking while eating, transferring skills (e.g., from bed to chair), and skin condition monitoring.

Case 097 Aggression as Key Complaint

Mr Yan, a 92-year-old gentleman, presented with concerns raised by his wife about his cognitive and temper problems. His wife complained of his use of offensive language and physical aggression, misplacing items and blaming others for stealing, forgetting to take medications, and being forgetful of events that happened the day before. He was also noted to have difficulty comprehending conversations.

Findings from Screening Assessments by Allied Healthcare and Social Care Team

Cognitive functioning	Scored 17/30 on MMSE, suggestive of cognitive impairment after adjusting for education level. Mr Yan's performance was impaired in orientation to time (1/5), delayed recall (1/3), and calculation (1/5) and was fair in orientation to place (3/5) and three-step commands (2/3). His performance was, however, normal in registration (3/3), language (5/5), and visuospatial relationship (1/1).
ADL/IADL	Mr Yan needed minimal help in feeding, ambulation, and stair climbing and was independent in other basic ADLs (Barthel Index 93/100). For IADLs, he was dependent in meal preparation (usually having lunch and dinner in a centre), laundry (unable to use the washing machine), housekeeping, handling finances (rarely using money), and grocery

	shopping and needed assistance in taking medications (medications were prepared by wife), external communication (due to difficulty hearing), and community access (Lawton IADL Scale 14/56).
Staging and clinical rating	Results suggested a Global Deterioration Scale stage of 4, indicating mild dementia. He showed decreased knowledge of current and recent events, a concentration deficit on serial subtractions, and decreased ability to travel and handle finances.

History Taken with Carer by Primary Care Physician

Mr Yan's wife reported noticing memory problems in her husband that had concerned her for about two to three years. Delusional ideations were reported (others stealing from him). Using the GPCOG Informant Interview, the following areas were noted to show more trouble (✗) or preserved (○) compared to about two years ago:

✗ Remembering recent events
✗ Recalling recent conversations
✗ Word finding
○ Managing money and finances
○ Managing medication independently
○ Using transport

There were no additional clinical features to consider for non-Alzheimer's dementia. Comorbidities of hypertension, hypercholesterolemia, benign prostatic hyperplasia, cerebral vascular accident (approximately 40 years ago; informant was uncertain about date), and osteoarthritis (informant was unsure) were reported. No family history of psychiatric disorders or dementia was reported. He had received two to three years of education.

Investigations

Calcium, VDRL, and vitamin B_{12}, folate, and a CT scan were ordered.

Diagnosis

Frontotemporal dementia.

Management

No medications were prescribed due to pending further work-up. Mr Yan was recommended to join a centre-based programme with cognitively stimulating activities, for the maintenance of cognitive function and quality of life.

Suggestions for the Primary Care Team

As behavioural problems were the key symptoms in this case, with delusional ideations, a frontal type of dementia rather than Alzheimer's disease should be considered. Management of this case would benefit from a case conference involving specialists.

In Mr Yan's case, the carer's stress is a concern. Considering that his wife is an older person herself, she may not be able or suitable to remain in the primary carer role, especially with the verbal and physical aggression that can cause great distress to her. The primary care team should discuss with the family regarding the need to refer to social services for long-term care arrangements. His delusional ideations can be helped with the use of antipsychotics together with a caring strategy. Antipsychotics or valproate are indicated for severe behavioural symptoms. His family should also be advised on strategies that can minimise the distressed behaviours and neuropsychiatric symptoms of dementia, such as by providing him with a locked cupboard or drawer where he can place his belongings. The primary care team should explore family support and relationships in tailoring the care plan.

Case 098 Soft Tissue Mass on MRI

Mrs Chan, a 77-year-old lady, presented with concerns raised by her son about her memory problem. She was reported to be forgetful about conversation content and appointment dates, misplacing personal items and being suspicious of others, and having slight difficulties in money management. Mrs Chan was also aware of her own memory decline.

Findings from Screening Assessments by Allied Healthcare and Social Care Team

Cognitive functioning	Scored 16/30 on MMSE, suggestive of cognitive impairment after adjusting for education level. Mrs Chan's performance was impaired in orientation to time (1/5) and place (2/5), calculation (1/5), and visuospatial relationship (0/1) and was fair in delayed recall (2/3) and three-step commands (2/3). Her performance was, however, normal in registration (3/3) and language (5/5). In the Clock Drawing Test, she refused to draw 3 o'clock arms and showed difficulty in executive function (6/10), but improved in clock copying (2/10) (Figure 3.8).
ADL/IADL	Mrs Chan was independent in all basic ADLs (Barthel Index 100/100) and IADLs (Lawton IADL Scale 56/56).
Depressive symptoms	Scored 4/15 on GDS-15; no suggestion of significant depressive mood.
Staging and clinical rating	Scored 0.5/3 on Clinical Dementia Rating, indicating questionable dementia. She had mild impairment in the memory, orientation, and community affairs domains.

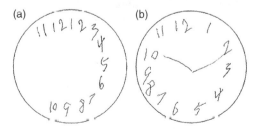

Figure 3.8 Findings from Mrs Chan's Clock Drawing Test. (a) Clock Drawing (3 o'clock). (b) Clock Copying (10 past 10)

History Taken with Carer by Primary Care Physician

Mrs Chan's son reported noticing memory problems in his mother that had concerned him for about a year. Delusional ideations were reported (others stealing things from her). Using the GPCOG Informant Interview, the following areas were noted to show more trouble (✗) or were preserved (○) compared to about two years ago:

✗ Remembering recent events
○ Recalling recent conversations
○ Word finding
○ Managing money and finances
○ Managing medication independently
○ Using transport

There were no additional clinical features to consider for non-Alzheimer's dementia. No comorbidity or family history of psychiatric disorders or dementia was reported. She did not receive any formal education.

Physical Examination Findings

General examination revealed no depressive-looking mood/affect problem, but showed general hygiene problems. CVS findings revealed BP 114/65 mm Hg.

Investigations

CBP, ESR, R/LFT, calcium, VDRL, vitamin B_{12}, fasting sugar, MSU × R/M and culture test, CXR, and ECG were ordered. All investigations were normal, except that CXR revealed cardiomegaly, and ECG revealed LVH and ST depression. An MRI plain scan revealed a 2.4 cm × 1.5 cm lobulated soft tissue mass over the cerebellopontine angle extension to the right medial temporal extra acid region and possible meningioma.

Diagnosis

Intracranial tumour.

Management

No medications were prescribed due to pending further work-up. Mrs Chan was recommended to join a specialised day care service for two days per week, with structured and tailored intervention programmes and cognitively stimulating activities to delay cognitive deterioration and maintain her quality of life.

Suggestions for the Primary Care Team

With the abnormal MRI results and considering the relatively young age of Mrs Chan, her clinical suspiciousness, unusual symptoms, and self-awareness, Alzheimer's disease is unlikely. Advanced imaging is recommended. This case would benefit from a case conference involving specialists, and a referral to a neurosurgeon is indicated. Mrs Chan's support appeared to be good, likely with good care and a high level of awareness from her son, which explained the satisfactory overall functions and very mild impairment, including cognition, physical, and ADL/IADL functioning. The primary care team is recommended to observe her cognition until a clear picture of the brain tumour is available and reassess after Mrs Chan's brain tumour is treated, to find out the actual impact of the tumour on her functioning.

Case 099 Shouting at TV

Mr Chan, a 65-year-old gentleman, presented with complaints from his wife about his personality change since around two years ago. He was noted to have mood swings and easy temper outbursts. He was also reported to be forgetful, asking questions repeatedly, and unable to recall recent events such as what he had for lunch.

Findings from Screening Assessments by Allied Healthcare and Social Care Team

Cognitive functioning	Scored 18/30 on MMSE, indicating cognitive impairment after adjusting for educational level. Mr Chan's performance was impaired in orientation to place (2/5), calculation (1/5), and was fair in delayed recall (2/3) in orientation to time (3/5), and three-step commands (2/3). His performance was, however, normal in registration (3/3), language (5/5), and visuospatial relationship (1/1). The Clock Drawing Test showed some impairment (Figure 3.9).
ADL/IADL	For basic ADL, Mr Chan was walking with a stick and needed assistance in bathing, changing clothes, and grooming (domestic helper prepares towel and toothbrush). For IADLs, it was noted that his wife handles all financial matters for him.
Staging and clinical rating	Staging and clinical rating were not completed.

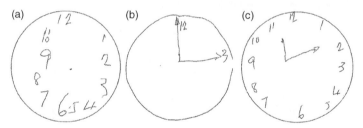

Figure 3.9 Findings from Mr Chan's Clock Drawing Test. (a) Clock Drawing (3 o'clock). (b) Clock Drawing (3 o'clock). (c) Clock Copying (10 past 10)

History Taken with Carer by Primary Care Physician

Mr Chan's wife reported noticing personality changes and temper outbursts that had concerned her for about two years, although no delusional ideations were reported. There were episodes when Mr Chan's behaviours appeared abnormal to his wife: he would shout at the TV when it was showing a violent scene, use an umbrella to hit his wife, and take a lot of toilet paper whenever he went to the toilet. He was also noted to be wandering and unable to sit still for more than 30 minutes. He had a minor stroke five years ago. He received a secondary school (F.3) level of education. Using the GPCOG Informant Interview, the following areas were noted to show more trouble (✗) or were preserved (○) compared to about two years ago:

- ✗ Remembering recent events
- ✗ Recalling recent conversations
- ○ Word finding
- ✗ Managing money and finances
- ✗ Managing medication independently
- ○ Using transport

No family history of psychiatric disorders or dementia was reported. Mr Chan was a merchant and owned an advertising company. He was retired, and the company was passed down to one of his two sons. He lived with his wife and a domestic helper. His wife expressed a high level of stress. Mr Chan had received approximately nine years of formal education.

Diagnosis

Frontotemporal dementia.

Suggestions for the Primary Care Team

In this case of younger-onset dementia (at the age of 65 years), the first symptom observed is personality related; impaired visuospatial ability was also evident in the Clock Drawing Test. The carer reported that the violence and emotional reactions were triggered after watching a violent scene. This is a case of frontotemporal dementia, and a referral to secondary care is recommended for a work-up with advanced neuroimaging, usually requiring a functional scan (e.g., SPECT). In frontotemporal dementia, primary symptoms are often related to mood and behaviours instead of cognitive impairment. Although the general functioning of Mr Chan remained satisfactory, the primary care team should work with his carers to ensure preparedness for future changes in his condition, including the onset of various dysfunctions such as language, mood swings, and rapid deterioration of cognitive and other functions, as compared with the gradual decline that would be expected in Alzheimer's disease.

References

1. Livingston G, Huntley J, Sommerlad A, Ames D, Ballard C, Banerjee S, et al. Dementia prevention, intervention, and care: 2020 report of the Lancet Commission. The Lancet. 2020;396 (10248): 413–46.

Useful Tools and Resources in Early Intervention Services

This chapter covers a selection of tools and resources for dementia diagnosis and management in primary care based on the experience of a community-based dementia early detection service (see Section 1.5) for use by trained allied health and social care professionals (1) and primary care physicians to promote communication across disciplines. Considering the large and growing number of validated tools available for outcome assessment and detection of dementia, our goal here is to share useful materials for quick reference rather than a comprehensive summary of available tools and resources (see Box 4.1 for some useful resources for further reading).

Box 4.1 Useful resources available for early intervention services

- **Dementia Revealed: What Primary Care Needs to Know. A Primer for General Practice**
  www.england.nhs.uk/wp-content/uploads/2014/09/dementia-revealed-toolkit.pdf
  An educational tool for general practitioners and practice nurses who have no experience in diagnosing and treating dementia prepared in partnership with NHS England and Hardwick CCG with the support of the Department of Health and the Royal College of General Practitioners in the UK. It covers topics such as identification and diagnosis of dementia, assessing cognition, ADL, brain scans, when to refer, drugs and other treatment, social services, and carers' assessment.
- **Dementia Toolkit for Primary Care, Sinai Health**
  www.mountsinai.on.ca/care/psych/patient-programs/geriatric-psychiatry/prc-dementia-resources-for-primary-care/dementia-toolkit-for-primary-care
  A toolkit and resources specifically designed for primary care with documents available for downloading from Mount Sinai Hospital in Canada. Covers assessment and screening tools, diagnosis of dementia, delirium, medication management, depression, responsive behaviours in dementia, driving safety, carer support, and palliative care.
- **Dementia Outcomes Measurement Suite (DOMS)**
  https://dementiaresearch.org.au/doms/
  A compendium of validated tools for the assessment of various aspects of dementia. A user-friendly website focused on clinical practice covering different types of dementia, severities of impairment, clinical settings (including primary care), and assessment modalities. Dementia outcome measures reviewed on this website may be used to screen for dementia signs and symptoms, monitor progression and treatment effects, and facilitate service planning. Updated web links and directories to many tools recommended in this chapter (e.g., Clinical Dementia Rating and Functional Assessment Staging Test) can be found in DOMS.

4.1 A Sample Form to Facilitate History-Taking

Box 4.2 shows a sample form to facilitate the recording of essential information during a help-seeking or first consultation with the primary care team.

The information included in this sample form is essential for the following reasons.

Age

Dementia is an age-related disease, with its age-specific prevalence ranging from 2 per cent to 41 per cent across countries in people aged 65 years or above (3). Finding out the age of the person with suspected dementia therefore provides some information about the likelihood of a person having dementia:

- 65–69 years old: 2 per cent
- 70–74 years old: 4 per cent
- 75–79 years old: 7 per cent
- 80–84 years old: 12 per cent
- 85–89 years old: 20 per cent
- 90+ years old: 41 per cent

For young-onset dementia (defined as onset before age 65), the estimated prevalence ranges between 42 and 98 per 100,000 people (4).

Education

Education forms an important part of the history because of its role as the main proxy for cognitive reserve (5, 6). A higher education level is associated with a lower risk of developing dementia (7). According to the cognitive reserve theory (8), for a person with a higher education level (thus reserve) to present with a functional impairment that exceeds the clinical threshold, s/he will have to sustain a bigger lesion compared with someone with a lower education. Likewise, a person with a higher reserve presenting with mild Alzheimer's disease symptoms would have more severe underlying pathology compared with someone presenting with a similar symptom level but a lower reserve. Education thus provides estimates about the severity of brain pathology given similar presentations. Education also significantly impacts cognitive assessment performance (see Section 4.3), and years of education is needed to interpret these test results.

Occupational Attainment

Like education, occupation is also a major proxy for cognitive reserve (5, 6). Thus, the above comments regarding symptoms/impairment presentation and underlying pathology also apply to the person's work history, specifically work complexity and occupational attainment.

Marital Status, Living Arrangements, and Relationship with the Informant

Marital status, living arrangements, and relationship with the informant are needed for a quick assessment of the person's support and safety in community living. Understanding the living arrangements and the person's relationships would provide information about a knowledgeable informant's and potential carers' stress and burden.

Box 4.2 Sample record form for help-seeking/first consultation of an early intervention service

Seen by _____ Date   dd / mmm / yyyy

Personal particulars

Name _____ Age _____

Gender _____ Education level _____ Education years _____

Marital status   single   married   widowed/separated/divorced   Occupational attainment _____

Living arrangement   living alone   with spouse only   with family / others, specify _____

Seen with (informant's name) _____ Relationship _____

Key complaints   (noticed for how long?)

Subjective _____ for _____

By informant _____ for _____

Interview with informant (modified from GPCOG) [note]	Yes	No	Don't know	N/A
1. Remembering recent events Does s/he have more trouble remembering things that have happened recently than s/he used to?				
2. Recalling recent conversations Does s/he have more trouble recalling conversations a few days later?				
3. Word finding When speaking, does s/he have more difficulty in finding the right word or tend to use the wrong words more often?				
4. Managing money and finance Is s/he less able to manage money and financial affairs (e.g., paying bills, budgeting)?				
5. Managing medication independently Is s/he less able to manage his or her medication independently?				
6. Using transport Does s/he need more assistance with transport (either private or public)? (if due only to physical problems, e.g., limb weakness, tick "no")				

Interview with informant (other history)

7. Delusions
   Does s/he show any delusional ideas (e.g., complaints of things being stolen by others when it is unlikely?). Specify:

8. Family history of dementia
   Does his/her immediate family member have any history of dementia? Specify:

9. Psychiatric history
   Does his/her have any history of psychiatric disorder? If yes, is s/he on any medication or other treatment? Specify:

10. Medical history
    Does his/her have any other medical conditions? If yes, is s/he on any medication or other treatment? Specify:

[note]Questions 1–6 are part of the General Practitioner Assessment of Cognition (GPCOG) (2)

Key Complaints (Open-Ended)

The open-ended method is an unstructured/unprompted way to capture spontaneous complaints. The type and pervasiveness of symptoms that informants report spontaneously predict the clinical severity (9). This may provide a quick reference for triage (see Section 4.4).

Interview with Informant (Modified from GPCOG)

The General Practitioner Assessment of Cognition (GPCOG) was designed as a brief and efficient screening tool for dementia for use in primary care (2). The rationale for developing the tool was due to the great need to detect and diagnose dementia by primary care physicians or general practitioners, which was not satisfactorily addressed by existing screening tests. The original GPCOG consists of items for cognitive tests and history-taking with the informant. Included in this sample form is only the informant's history-taking part; as we recommend in a multidisciplinary primary care team setting for early intervention in dementia, cognitive tests can be performed by trained allied health and social care professionals, with results shared within the team (see Section 4.3). The informant section of GPCOG was also found to be free of bias due to age, education, or depressive mood (10). Note that in the item about using transport, a remark is added to differentiate difficulties not due to cognitive but physical problems.

Delusions

Delusions are generally defined as fixed beliefs that are incorrigible despite conflicting evidence (11). They are key neuropsychiatric symptoms in dementia or neuropsychiatric symptoms (see Section 4.4 for examples). A common presentation of delusion in dementia is the person insisting that others are trying to steal from him/her (12). Exploring the presence of delusions can be helpful in screening, staging, and prioritising management, as they are often a trigger for help-seeking and a source of stress for the family, while their episodic nature provides anchors for estimating the time frame.

Family and Personal History

These would include current and past histories of psychiatric illness and physical health problems (such as stroke and head injury), recent hospitalisation, sensory problems, and alcohol and drug use.

Clinical Features Suggestive of Non-Alzheimer's Dementia

Apart from the above basic information on history-taking, the primary care team should pay attention to some of the following commonly reported clinical features that may suggest non-Alzheimer's dementia (see Box 4.3).[1]

---

[1] For more detailed discussions about clinical features of common non-Alzheimer's dementia, readers may refer to textbooks or review articles, such as the series 'Non-Alzheimer's dementia' from The Lancet (13), or an introduction to the common dementias in resources such as the Promoting Psychological Wellbeing for People with Dementia and Their Carers: An Enhanced Practice Resource (14), for health and social care staff.

Box 4.3 Additional clinical features to consider for non-Alzheimer's dementia

Feature	Consider possible
☐ Complex visual hallucinations	→ DLB, PDD
☐ Apraxia in self-care (e.g., inability to get dressed or use feeding utensils)	→ CBD
☐ Pain and rigidity on one side	→ CBD
☐ Inability to control mood and aggression	→ bvFTD
☐ Overeating, especially sweet food	→ bvFTD
☐ Early speech problems without evidence of stroke or SOL	→ PPA/tvFTD
☐ Early swallowing problem	→ PSP

SOL = space-occupying lesion; DLB = dementia with Lewy bodies; PDD = Parkinson's disease dementia; CBD = corticobasal degeneration; bvFTD = behavioural variant of frontotemporal dementia; PPA = primary progressive aphasia; tvFTD = temporal variant of frontotemporal dementia; PSP = progressive supranuclear palsy

Complex Visual Hallucinations

Visual hallucination is the clinical feature that most specifically distinguishes Lewy body from Alzheimer's disease in early-stage dementia (15). In dementia with Lewy body, as compared to Alzheimer's disease, the visual hallucinations are more likely to be multiple, speaking, and persistent (16). The core features of dementia with Lewy bodies (DLB) include fluctuating levels of attention and alertness, well-formed and detailed recurrent visual hallucinations, which are generally present in the early course of the disease, and spontaneous features of parkinsonism, such as bradykinesia and rigidity (17, 18). As Parkinson's disease dementia (PDD) and DLB have overlapping features and similar hallucination characteristics (19), PDD should also be considered. Another telltale symptom is the presence of rapid eye movement (REM) behaviour disorder (RBD), which could precede the dementia symptoms by some years (20). In clinical settings, people with DLB may have hallucinations preceded by hospitalisation, in the form of delirium, which may be understood as an overflow of dream content into the consciousness and experienced as hallucinations.

Apraxia in Self-care

Deficits in basic self-care (such as getting dressed) are a feature in the moderate rather than early stages of Alzheimer's disease (21). Apraxia in self-care is, however, a feature that can be seen in both progressive supranuclear palsy (PSP) and corticobasal degeneration (CBD) and is more severe in the latter (22). Thus, in a person presenting with apraxia in self-care with assessment findings suggestive of early dementia, non-Alzheimer's dementia such as CBD should be considered.

Pain and Rigidity on One Side

Apart from apraxia in self-care, asymmetric stiffness or rigidity and pain are other common features of CBD (23), with limb clumsiness and tremors commonly observed before unilateral limb rigidity.

Inability to Control Mood and Aggression

Mood and anxiety symptoms can be present in early Alzheimer's disease, which may increase as the disease progresses (24). However, excessive mood swings and aggressive behaviour are uncommon in the early stages of Alzheimer's disease, but may represent features of behavioural variants of frontotemporal dementia (bvFTD) (25), which is characterised by personality changes, behavioural disinhibition, and apathy.

Box 4.4 Variants of FTD

Frontotemporal dementia can be further classified into the following:

- behavioural variant frontotemporal dementia (bvFTD);
- non-fluent variant primary progressive aphasia (nfvPPA);
- semantic-variant primary progressive aphasia (svPPA).

Overeating, especially sweet foods

Binge eating and a preference for sweet foods are common features of bvFTD, which may be seen in 25 per cent to over 80 per cent of people with bvFTD (25). Disinhibition of impulse and basic needs control can be understood by frontal and executive dysfunction, which could also manifest as sexual disinhibition, poor hygiene, and early incontinence. In early dementia, especially in those presenting at a younger age (e.g., in their 50s or 60s), non-Alzheimer's dementia involving frontal lobe pathology should be considered.

Early speech problems without evidence of stroke or space-occupying lesion (SOL)

Speech problems are usually present in the advanced stage of Alzheimer's disease (21). If speech problems are present early – dementia with early speech involvement – primary progressive aphasia (PPA) or temporal variant FTD (tvFTD) should be considered (25).

Early swallowing problem

Swallowing problems occur very late in Alzheimer's disease (21). The presence of an early swallowing problem and parkinsonism suggests possible progressive supranuclear palsy (PSP). Other presentations of PSP include gaze palsy and postural instability (26).

Box 4.5 The non-Alzheimer's dementias

Belonging to one group of disorders with similar pathology, FTD, PPA, PSP, and CBD have varying symptoms. Put in a simplified way, they are characterised as follows:

- FTD: behaviour- and speech-related symptoms;
- PPA: speech-related symptoms;
- PSP: gaze- and swallow-related symptoms;
- CBD: apraxia symptoms.

As these dementias may evolve into a secondary diagnosis, a referral to secondary and tertiary care is needed.

Box 4.6 Midlife and later-life risk factors for dementia

Midlife
☐ Hearing loss
☐ Traumatic brain injury
☐ Hypertension
☐ Alcohol (>21 units per week)
☐ Obesity

Later life
☐ Smoking
☐ Depression
☐ Social isolation
☐ Physical inactivity
☐ Air pollution
☐ Diabetes

Other Information to Consider Collecting

Apart from 'passive' cognitive reserve (with education level and occupation attainment as proxy) covered above, understanding other known and modifiable risk factors would also provide information about the likelihood of neuropathological damage (e.g., vascular or inflammatory) and the potential of increasing 'active' cognitive reserve (e.g., increasing social contact) (7). Box 4.6 (based on (7)) lists the key risk factors in midlife and later life. In areas where driving is an important aspect of daily life, information about the person's current driving habits is also needed for an assessment of safety. For care planning, assessing family structure, relationships, and other support networks would be useful.

4.2 Physical Examination and Investigation Checklist for Suspected dementia

Box 4.7 shows a suggested order for relevant investigations for suspected dementia. For specific recommendations of tests and examinations, please refer to locally relevant clinical guidelines, such as the UK National Institute for Health and Care Excellence (NICE) guidance on Dementia: Assessment, management and support for people living with dementia and their carers (27). Briefly, in non-specialist settings, blood and other tests are undertaken to exclude reversible causes of cognitive impairments. Further tests such as fluorodeoxyglucose-positron emission tomography-computed tomography (FDG-PET-CT) should be considered only if they would facilitate dementia subtyping and the subtype would inform management. Primary care physicians should note that tests and brain imaging results are only for reference to guide clinical judgement. For example:

- Findings of vitamin B_{12} deficiency do not necessarily mean vitamin B_{12} deficiency is the cause of dementia symptoms.
- Alzheimer's disease should not be ruled out based solely on CT or MRI findings.
- Vascular dementia cannot be diagnosed based solely on vascular lesion burden.

4.3 Sample Cognitive and Functioning Report of an Early Intervention Service

Box 4.8 shows a sample brief report for quick communication of the cognitive and functioning assessment findings within the primary care team. Whenever possible,

Box 4.7 Checklist of investigations for the primary care physician to consider

☐ CBP   ☐ MSU x R/M and culture test
☐ ESR   ☐ CXR
☐ R/LFT   ☐ ECG
☐ Calcium   ☐ Others (specify: _____)
☐ VDRL   ***Brain imaging***
☐ Vitamin B$_{12}$, folate   ☐ CT
☐ Fasting sugar   ☐ MRI
☐ Fasting lipids   ☐ Further tests (specify: _____)

CBP = complete blood picture; ESR = erythrocyte sedimentation rate; R/LFT = renal and liver function tests; VDRL = venereal disease research laboratory test; MSU x R/M = midstream urine routine microscopy; CXR = chest X-ray; ECG = electrocardiography; CT = computed tomography; MRI = magnetic resonance imaging

Note: neuroimaging can be considered in case of abnormal clinical signs, e.g., (i) a space-occupying lesion (SOL) is suspected; (ii) onset is of short duration (3–4 months) especially if a history of head injury is obvious (to exclude subdural haematoma); (iii) MRI is indicated for non-Alzheimer's disease (to look for brainstem involvement, e.g., FTD frontal atrophy, and PSP hummingbird sign); and (iv) PiB PET in young-onset Alzheimer's disease.

the detailed assessment results should be included as appendices as part of the service record.

Cognitive Functioning

For early detection services, quick cognitive screening tests are needed with good psychometric properties, validated in normative samples locally (to understand 'normal' performance in a population), with good sensitivity and specificity in detecting cognitive impairment across the spectrum of mild cognitive impairment, early Alzheimer's disease, and other dementias (such as post-stroke cognitive impairment). They also need to be easy to administer by trained personnel across disciplines to allow for scaled-up services and communication.

Traditionally, the Mini-Mental State Examination (MMSE) (28) is one of the commonly used tools for these reasons. The Montreal Cognitive Assessment (MoCA; see www.mocatest.org/) is another popular tool (29). They are therefore included in this sample report form, although the selection of tests should also take into consideration the service context (e.g., level of specialisation and care pathway) and other local factors. In reporting, the following should be noted:

- Education level
  Scores for both MMSE and MoCA need to be adjusted for the education level (30). Especially with MoCA, very different cut-off scores have been reported for people with different education levels (31), and in some populations, a single cut-off was

Box 4.8 Sample report of the cognitive and functioning assessment

Name & ID [   ]   Date   dd / mmm / yyyy

Seen by [   ]   with informant [   ]
                                    (relationship)

	Assessment	Score	Remarks
Cognitive functioning	MMSE	__ /30	
	MoCA		
	CDT	__ / 10	
	Others		
ADL/IADL	BI	__ /100	
	Lawton	__ /56	
	Others		
Depressive symptoms	GDS-15	__ /15	
	PHQ-9	__ /27	
	Others		
Staging & clinical rating	GDS	Stage __	
	CDR	__ / 3	
	Others		

MMSE=Mini-Mental State Examination; MoCA=Montreal Cognitive Assessment; CDT=Clock Drawing Test; ADL=activities of daily living; IADL=instrumental activities of daily living; BI=Barthel Index; GDS-15=15-item Geriatric Depression Scale; PHQ-9=Patient Health Questionnaire-9; GDS=Global Deterioration Scale; CDR=Clinical Dementia Rating

found to risk misclassification (32). In the report, include a locally validated cut-off if available and always explain whether the score has been adjusted for the person's education level.

- Performance by cognitive domains
  As illustrated in Chapters 2 and 3, impairment pattern by cognitive domains provides important information about possible Alzheimer's disease, other dementias, and conditions (33) and for tailoring care and intervention strategies.

Reporting only the total score with a cut-off – a binary approach to cognitive impairment – means losing useful information that would be useful for triage and service planning. Reporting the domain scores is therefore recommended in the report. As age-related changes are not uniform across cognitive domains (34), ideally, neuropsychological assessments with population-specific normative cut-offs by domain (35) would give more accurate information, although time and test burden should be considered. Brief screening assessments that emphasise domain profiling, such as the Oxford Cognitive Screen-Plus (OCS-Plus) (36, 37), can be considered to address this need.

• Details that are remarkable

The assessor will often observe details in the process that can facilitate results interpretation. For example, the person's understanding of the assessment may be affected by language, mobility, mood, and physical discomfort. Was s/he motivated and cooperative in the assessment? Were there noticeable cognitive impairments during the test (e.g., difficulty remembering the instructions, or easily distracted)? Some of the screening tools (e.g., MoCA) include items that are not scored but contain useful information about the person's cognitive performance, such as delayed recall with cues or by recognition, which suggests whether information storage is intact by testing if performance is improved by reducing retrieval demands.

The Clock Drawing Test is another widely used test in clinical practice and research. In some of the screening tools, such as MoCA, a simplified version of clock drawing is incorporated as part of the test. It should be noted that many studies compared head-to-head copying and drawing under instructions (38, 39) and found that clock drawing under the instruction condition is more challenging than the copying condition and is thus more sensitive to early changes in cognitive functioning.

ADL/IADL

A commonly used tool for assessing activities of daily living (ADL) is the Barthel Index (40), which consists of 11 items on basic self-care tasks such as feeding, toileting, and bathing (score range, 0–100). For instrumental activities of daily living (IADL), the Lawton's IADL Scale (41) can be used, which consists of eight self-care items required for independent community living, such as meal preparation, handling finance, and housekeeping. These are tools often used in other aged care services/geriatric medicine fields, allowing for easy communication across services, and are therefore useful in dementia screening and early detection services. Tools that provide ADL/IADL information specific to dementia include the Alzheimer's Disease Cooperative Study – Activities of Daily Living Scale (ADCS-ADL) (42) and the Disability Assessment for Dementia (DAD) (43).

Communicating information about the person's ADL and IADL functioning within the primary care team will be useful for diagnostic, staging, and care/intervention planning purposes. For the latter, based on the biopsychosocial model of dementia (44), such information could be used to guide the identification of excess disability and tractable factors to intervene (see Section 1.5). When reporting, it would be helpful to remark whether the ADL/IADL impairment is likely due to physical frailty/medical conditions other than cognitive impairment.

Depressive Symptoms

Clinically significant depressive symptoms are prevalent among older people (approximately 10 per cent to 15 per cent, depending on settings) (45) and can complicate diagnosis, care, and intervention, as illustrated in previous chapters. Routine screening for depressive symptoms is therefore recommended among those seeking help for suspected dementia. The 15-item Geriatric Depression Scale (GDS) (46) is commonly used in geriatrics/aged care in view of its sensitivity and specificity in identifying depression in older people (a cut-off score of 8 out of 15 indicates clinically significant depressive symptoms). Other assessment tools not specific to older people that are also useful include the Patient Health Questionnaire (PHQ-9) (45), a nine-item tool that incorporates depression diagnostic criteria into the items, thereby also providing information about the presence and severity of individual depressive symptoms.

Staging and Clinical Rating

This part of the assessment would require interviewing with a knowledgeable informant. The Clinical Dementia Rating (CDR) (47) is a structured interview schedule involving both the person with suspected dementia and an informant to estimate performance in memory, orientation, judgement and problem-solving, community affairs, home and hobbies, and personal care (see https://knightadrc.wustl.edu/cdr/cdr.htm for details about training, scoring, and versions). It has a global rating ranging from 0 (normal) to 5 (severe dementia). The Global Deterioration Scale (GDS) (48) is a widely used scale to reflect the clinical characteristics of dementia, with stages 1–3 denoting pre-dementia stages and stages 4–7 denoting dementia stages. For a more specific staging assessment, the Functional Assessment Staging (FAST) in Alzheimer's Disease (21, 49) can be considered (see Section 1.3).

4.4 Common Symptoms Reported by Carers and People with Suspected Dementia

In Section 4.1, a sample form to facilitate history-taking in an unstructured, open-ended way to capture spontaneous complaints is suggested. This is considering the help-seeking population in an early intervention service setting, in which symptoms that have prompted help-seeking have clinical significance (as compared with symptoms elicited in structured interviews). The type of symptoms noted by an informant and the number of symptoms noted in these simple open-ended questions are linked with the clinical stage assessed using CDR (9), thus providing a quick indicator for triage and further investigations. These spontaneously reported symptoms can be grouped into categories as suggested in Box 4.9.

While memory problems are frequently reported, they are less discriminating as compared to language and orientation symptoms noted by an informant (9). The number of symptom categories spontaneously reported by the informant would also suggest more severe dementia when assessed in a more structured way (e.g., using CDR).

Box 4.9 Classification of common spontaneously reported symptoms from an early intervention service (9)

Symptom	Examples
☐ Memory	'he only remembers things that happened a long time ago'
☐ Executive function	'she cannot manage to cook any more'
☐ Language	'sometimes I cannot understand what she is trying to say'
☐ Orientation	'he was unable to find the way from home to a nearby restaurant'
☐ Neuropsychiatric	'he is always paranoid'
☐ Mood	'she always talks about sad things'
☐ Avolition	'she has decreased motivation in participating in leisure activities'

4.5 Infographic and Educational Material for Explaining Dementia Diagnosis and Management

Apart from the widely known resource centres such as Alzheimer's Disease International (ADI, www.alzint.org/), Dementia Alliance International (DAI, www.dementiaalliancei nternational.org/), and the Alzheimer's Association (www.alz.org/), various educational materials and helpful infographics have been developed and are available online. Box 4.10 lists a few useful examples that can be incorporated into a primary care practice for dementia early intervention.

Box 4.10 Some useful infographics and educational material for use in primary care

- **Visual summary of updated NICE guidance *Dementia: assessment, management and support***
  www.bmj.com/content/bmj/suppl/2018/06/27/bmj.k2438.DC1/Dementia_v19_web.pdf
  This plain language summary (50) available from *The BMJ* includes a one-page visual summary on pharmacological treatment – donepezil, galantamine, rivastigmine, and memantine – that can be offered as part of the management of Alzheimer's and other dementias according to disease stage, tolerance, and existing medications.
- **Dementia infographic by the US National Institute of Aging**
  www.nia.nih.gov/research/alzheimers-dementia-outreach-recruitment-engagement-resources/dementia-infographics-madrc
  Single-page infographics covering various topics in Alzheimer's disease and related dementias were developed by the Michigan Alzheimer's Disease Research Center (MADRC) for free download. Resources available include infographics explaining the difference between Alzheimer's disease and other dementia types, and whether Alzheimer's disease is genetic.
- **World Health Organization (WHO) Infographic on Dementia**
  www.who.int/health-topics/dementia#tab=tab_1
  A simple two-page infographic explaining the symptoms of dementia, its causes, and the number of people affected. It also provides information about the global action plan and highlights dementia as a public health priority.

References

1. Tang JY, Wong GH, Ng CK, Kwok DT, Lee MN, Dai DL, et al. Neuropsychological profile and dementia symptom recognition in help-seekers in a community early-detection orogram in Hong Kong. Journal of American Geriatric Society. 2016;64 (3):584–9.

2. Brodaty H, Pond D, Kemp NM, Luscombe G, Harding L, Berman K, et al. The GPCOG: A new screening test for dementia designed for general practice. Journal of American Geriatric Society. 2002;50(3):530–4.

3. OECD. Dementia Prevalence. Health at a Glance 2017: OECD Indicators. Paris: OECD Publishing. 2017.

4. Rossor MN, Fox NC, Mummery CJ, Schott JM, Warren JD. The diagnosis of young-onset dementia. Lancet Neurology. 2010;9(8):793–806.

5. Stern Y. Cognitive reserve. Neuropsychologia. 2009;47 (10):2015–28.

6. Meng X, D'Arcy C. Education and dementia in the context of the cognitive reserve hypothesis: A systematic review with meta-analyses and qualitative analyses. PLOS ONE. 2012;7(6):e38268.

7. Livingston G, Huntley J, Sommerlad A, Ames D, Ballard C, Banerjee S, et al. Dementia prevention, intervention, and care: 2020 report of the Lancet Commission. The Lancet. 2020;396 (10248):413–46.

8. Stern Y. What is cognitive reserve? Theory and research application of the reserve concept. Journal of the International Neuropsychological Society 2002;8(3):448–60.

9. Xu JQ, Choy JCP, Tang JYM, Liu TY, Luo H, Lou VWQ, et al. Spontaneously reported symptoms by informants are associated with clinical severity in dementia help-seekers. Journal of American Geriatric Society. 2017;65 (9):1946–52.

10. Brodaty H, Kemp NM, Low LF. Characteristics of the GPCOG, a screening tool for cognitive impairment. International Journal of Geriatric Psychiatry. 2004;19 (9):870–4.

11. American Psychiatric Association. Diagnostic and Statistical Manual of Mental Disorders 5th ed.) Arlington, VA: American Psychiatric Association. 2013.

12. Kaufer DI, Cummings JL, Ketchel P, Smith V, MacMillan A, Shelley T, et al. Validation of the NPI-Q, a brief clinical form of the neuropsychiatric inventory. Journal of Neuropsychiatry Clinical Neuroscience. 2000;12 (2):233–9.

13. The Lancet. Dementia – not all about Alzheimer's. The Lancet. 2015;386 (10004):1600.

14. NHS Education for Scotland. Promoting Psychological Wellbeing for People with Dementia and Their Carers: An Enhanced Practice Resource. Edinburgh: NHS Education for Scotland. 2012. Available from: www.nes.scot.nhs .uk/media/mvwlrvdt/enhanced_resource_ fullv2.pdf.

15. Tiraboschi P, Salmon DP, Hansen LA, Hofstetter RC, Thal LJ, Corey-Bloom J. What best differentiates Lewy body from Alzheimer's disease in early-stage dementia? Brain. 2006;129(Pt 3):729–35.

16. Ballard C, McKeith I, Harrison R, O'Brien J, Thompson P, Lowery K, et al. A detailed phenomenological comparison of complex visual hallucinations in dementia with Lewy bodies and Alzheimer's disease. International Psychogeriatric. 1997;9 (4):381–8.

17. McKeith IG, Boeve BF, Dickson DW, Halliday G, Taylor J-P, Weintraub D, et al. Diagnosis and management of

dementia with Lewy bodies: Fourth consensus report of the DLB Consortium. Neurology. 2017;89 (1):88–100.

18. Postuma RB, Berg D, Stern M, Poewe W, Olanow CW, Oertel W, et al. MDS clinical diagnostic criteria for Parkinson's disease. Movement Disorders: Official Journal of the Movement Disorder Society. 2015;30 (12):1591–601.

19. Mosimann UP, Rowan EN, Partington CE, Collerton D, Littlewood E, O'Brien JT, et al. Characteristics of visual hallucinations in Parkinson disease dementia and dementia with lewy bodies. American Journal of Geriatric Psychiatry. 2006;14 (2):153–60.

20. Genier Marchand D, Postuma RB, Escudier F, De Roy J, Pelletier A, Montplaisir J, et al. How does dementia with Lewy bodies start? Prodromal cognitive changes in REM sleep behavior disorder. Annals of Neurology. 2018;83 (5):1016–26.

21. Reisberg B. Functional assessment staging (FAST). Psychopharmacological Bulletin. 1988;24(4):653–9.

22. Pharr V, Uttl B, Stark M, Litvan I, Fantie B, Grafman J. Comparison of apraxia in corticobasal degeneration and progressive supranuclear palsy. Neurology. 2001;56 (7):957–63.

23. Mahapatra RK, Edwards MJ, Schott JM, Bhatia KP. Corticobasal degeneration. Lancet Neurology. 2004;3 (12):736–43.

24. Kazui H, Yoshiyama K, Kanemoto H, Suzuki Y, Sato S, Hashimoto M, et al. Differences of behavioral and psychological symptoms of dementia in disease severity in four major dementias. PLOS ONE. 2016;11(8): e0161092.

25. Bang J, Spina S, Miller BL. Frontotemporal dementia. The Lancet. 2015;386(10004):1672–82.

26. Williams DR, Lees AJ. Progressive supranuclear palsy: Clinicopathological concepts and diagnostic challenges. Lancet Neurology. 2009;8(3):270–9.

27. National Institute for Health and Care Excellence. Dementia: Assessment, management and support for people living with dementia and their carers 2018. Available from: www.nice.org.uk/ guidance/ng97/chapter/ Recommendations#diagnosis.

28. Folstein MF, Folstein SE, McHugh PR. "Mini-mental state". A practical method for grading the cognitive state of patients for the clinician. Journal of Psychiatric Research. 1975;12 (3):189–98.

29. Nasreddine ZS, Phillips NA, Bédirian V, Charbonneau S, Whitehead V, Collin I, et al. The Montreal Cognitive Assessment, MoCA: A brief screening tool for mild cognitive impairment. Journal of the American Geriatrics Society. 2005;53 (4):695–9.

30. Luo H, Andersson B, Tang JYM, Wong GHY. Applying item response theory analysis to the Montreal Cognitive Assessment in a low-education older population. Assessment. 2020;27 (7):1416–28.

31. Lu J, Li D, Li F, Zhou A, Wang F, Zuo X, et al. Montreal Cognitive Assessment in detecting cognitive impairment in Chinese elderly individuals: A population-based study. Journal of Geriatric Psychiatry and Neurology. 2011;24(4):184–90.

32. Wong A, Law LS, Liu W, Wang Z, Lo ES, Lau A, et al. Montreal Cognitive Assessment: One cutoff never fits all. Stroke. 2015;46(12):3547–50.

33. Salmon DP, Bondi MW. Neuropsychological assessment of dementia. Annual Review Psychology. 2009;60:257–82.

34. Glisky EL. Changes in cognitive function in human aging. In: Riddle DR, editor.

Brain Aging: Models, Methods, and Mechanisms. Frontiers in Neuroscience. Boca Raton, FL: CRC Press/Taylor & Francis. 2007.

35. Robotham RJ, Riis JO, Demeyere N. A Danish version of the Oxford cognitive screen: A stroke-specific screening test as an alternative to the MoCA. Neuropsychology Development Cognitive B Aging Neuropsychology Cognition. 2020;27 (1):52–65.

36. Humphreys GW, Duta MD, Montana L, Demeyere N, McCrory C, Rohr J, et al. Cognitive function in low-income and low-literacy settings: Validation of the tablet-based Oxford cognitive screen in the health and aging in Africa: A Longitudinal Study of an INDEPTH Community in South Africa (HAALSI). Journal of Gerontology B: Psychological Science and Social Science. 2017;72 (1):38–50.

37. Demeyere N, Haupt M, Webb SS, Strobel L, Milosevich E, Moore M, et al. The Oxford Cognitive Screen – Plus (OCS-Plus): A digital, tablet-based, brief cognitive assessment 2020. Available from: https://doi.org/10.31234/osf.io/b2vgc.

38. Rouleau I, Salmon DP, Butters N, Kennedy C, McGuire K. Quantitative and qualitative analyses of clock drawings in Alzheimer's and Huntington's disease. Brain Cognition. 1992;18(1):70–87.

39. Cacho J, Garcia-Garcia R, Arcaya J, Vicente JL, Lantada N. A proposal for application and scoring of the Clock Drawing Test in Alzheimer's disease. Review Neurology. 1999;28 (7):648–55.

40. Collin C, Wade D, Davies S, Horne V. The Barthel ADL Index: A reliability study. International Disability Studies. 1988;10(2):61–3.

41. Barberger-Gateau P, Commenges D, Gagnon M, Letenneur L, Sauvel C,

Dartigues JF. Instrumental activities of daily living as a screening tool for cognitive impairment and dementia in elderly community dwellers. Journal of American Geriatric Society. 1992;40 (11):1129–34.

42. Galasko D, Bennett D, Sano M, Ernesto C, Thomas R, Grundman M, et al. An inventory to assess activities of daily living for clinical trials in Alzheimer's disease: The Alzheimer's Disease Cooperative Study. Alzheimer Diseases Association Disorders. 1997;11 Suppl 2: S33–9.

43. Gelinas I, Gauthier L, McIntyre M, Gauthier S. Development of a functional measure for persons with Alzheimer's disease: The disability assessment for dementia. American Journal of Occupational Therapy. 1999;53 (5):471–81.

44. Spector A, Orrell M. Using a biopsychosocial model of dementia as a tool to guide clinical practice. International Psychogeriatrics. 2010;22 (6):957–65.

45. Kroenke K, Spitzer RL, Williams JB. The PHQ 9: Validity of a brief depression severity measure. Journal of General Internal Medicine. 2001;16 (9):606–13.

46. Yesavage JA, Brink TL, Rose TL, Lum O, Huang V, Adey M, et al. Development and validation of a geriatric depression screening scale: A preliminary report. Journal of Psychiatric Research. 1982;17 (1):37–49.

47. Morris JC. The Clinical Dementia Rating (CDR): Current version and scoring rules. Neurology. 1993;43 (11):2412–14.

48. Reisberg B, Ferris SH, de Leon MJ, Crook T. The Global Deterioration Scale for assessment of primary degenerative dementia. American Journal of Psychiatry. 1982;139 (9):1136–9.

49. Sclan SG, Reisberg B. Functional assessment staging (FAST) in Alzheimer's disease: reliability, validity, and ordinality. International Psychogeriatrics. 1992;4 Suppl 1:55–69.

50. Pink J, O'Brien J, Robinson L, Longson D, Guideline C. Dementia: Assessment, management and support: Summary of updated NICE guidance. BMJ. 2018;361: k2438.

Take-Home Messages and Further Readings

5

From the 99 cases presented in the previous chapters, we have touched on issues related to advance care planning, carer stress in different case scenarios and the support needed, practical tips about disclosing a dementia diagnosis, issues surrounding management, home safety, and dementia-friendly communities – with recommendations for the primary care team. In Section 1.3, we gave an overview of dementia work-up, diagnosis, and management. This chapter is a summary of the key lessons learned from the cases and a discussion of the recommended actions and further reading materials for consolidation and continued studies. These key lessons are grouped into five topics: advance care planning (Section 5.1); Carer Stress and Support (Section 5.2); Formulating and Disclosing the Dementia Diagnosis (Section 5.3); Issues Surrounding Management (Section 5.4); and Dementia-Friendly Communities and Prevention (Section 5.5).

5.1 Advance Care Planning

Advance care planning is a process of communication (1). When it is foreseeable that a person may lose the ability to make decisions, advance care planning is important for the person, their families, care providers, and others to communicate appropriate care. In Section 1.5, we allude to the need for advance care planning for people living with dementia. This is especially the case in Alzheimer's disease: its typical trajectory with relatively predictable functioning and needs allows planning, while the multidimensional needs at different disease stages require coordinated services.

Key Considerations in Primary Care

- The process of advance care planning in dementia is far from straightforward.
  As dementia progresses, the ability to consider future thoughts and actions becomes compromised, affecting decision-making abilities. Family carers may increasingly find themselves in a position where they need to inform, or directly make, decisions on behalf of the person with dementia (2).
- No high-quality guidelines are currently available for advance care planning in dementia (3). Evidence of planning's effectiveness for people with cognitive impairment/dementia is limited but growing. Although most evidence of how advance care planning can improve outcomes (such as end-of-life outcomes) for people living with dementia and their carers has come from Western cultures (4), increasing evidence is becoming available from Asian areas such as Taiwan (5) and Singapore (6).
- There are, however, key barriers to the uptake of advance care planning in dementia: uncertainties with planning and communication problems could reduce carers'

willingness to engage in active decision-making (7, 8); providers may have insufficient knowledge about dementia, lack confidence, and be uncertain about when to initiate advance care planning, how to assess decisional capacity, and how to accommodate changing preferences.

- In general, an early introduction of advance care planning when the person's cognitive impairment is still mild is facilitative. A community setting would be appropriate for advance care planning, as it would be too late in terms of the person's capacity when he/she is already institutionalised (9). There are different views as to whether the time of diagnosis is a good time to initiate advance care planning discussion, as it could depend on the person and their family's readiness, and the primary care team should consider receptiveness or reluctance carefully using a family- and person-centred approach.
- Inclusion of all stakeholders, discussions that focus on both medical *and* social issues with an aim to maintain a normal life, and supporting the integration of emotional and technical issues are required for good practice (10). The use of educational strategies that enable shared decision-making for future care can enhance advance care planning discussions (11).

Practice Point 1: Care Needs for the Next Stage

Family carers need to think ahead about how to prepare for the next stage of the disease. Advance care planning is a communication process (instead of static documentation of decisions made earlier). Primary care providers should maintain communication and support the family to prepare for new needs that are expected to arise in the next stage (see Box 5.1 for a case illustration). For people with Alzheimer's disease, this could be done considering the expected change in ADL and IADL functioning (see FAST staging in Section 1.3). For example, as the person develops dressing apraxia, suggesting a moderate stage, we could expect the need for assistance in bathing and toileting problems to follow. When the person starts to have speech problems, suggesting an advanced stage of dementia, the family may need to consider a care home arrangement. A care planner could guide the family through these typical disease progression stages and provide information to support better living for the person and their family carers.

Box 5.1 Case Illustration

In our Case 050 (How Did I Spend that Money?), Mr Hui is a typical case of early Alzheimer's disease. With his current difficulties in handling money and finances as his disease progresses and the expected further cognitive decline, financial management could become a key problem, and conflicts and abuse are potential risks to avoid. On the other hand, the family carer reported that Mr Hui has an unimpaired ability to use transportation, while based on a typical disease trajectory we can expect impairment in these more complex IADL tasks soon. This is a good time to discuss with Mr Hui and the family about future care planning, providing education on areas of functioning where the family already has concerns (i.e., financial management in this case), while explaining other areas with predicted deterioration and risks (e.g., using transport and getting lost in this case), to initiate the advance care planning communication process.

Practice Point 2: Is the Person Mentally Incapacitated?

Whether a person has the mental capacity to make certain decisions should be judged case by case: mental capacity (or mental incompetence) is always relative to the subject matter to be decided on. A person living with dementia, for example, could have the capacity to make a decision about what to have for a meal, but may lack the capacity to manage their property. Livingston et al. (12) provided a succinct summary of the key principles in assessing mental capacity, which include the following:

- Assuming capacity until proven otherwise;
- All feasible steps have been taken to support the person in making a decision;
- Making an unwise decision does not equal a lack of capacity; and
- Mental capacity assessment should be based on the person's ability to understand, retain in their mind, use or weigh the relevant information, and communicate their decision.

In general, people in the early stages of dementia are often still mentally competent to instruct a lawyer to draw up their will and power of attorney. This should therefore be considered in advance care planning, and the primary care team should find the opportunity to discuss with the family member and the person on these matters.

Practice Point 3: Powers of Attorney

Legal planning can be a complicated matter for the person living with dementia and the family, where counselling and advice from the primary care team may be necessary to identify the most suitable help. This advice may include the legal instruments available and what can be done to facilitate decisions and choices with the person's remaining legal capacity and autonomy (13). One of the legal instruments relevant to dementia care is a power of attorney. Depending on the local laws, an enduring power of attorney (EPA) or lasting power of attorney (LPOA) generally allows the person, while s/he still has the mental capacity to do so, to appoint someone to take care of his/her financial matters in the future when s/he becomes mentally incapacitated (see Box 5.2 for a case illustration). Sufficient counselling and early planning are important, due to the complexity of the decision (of handing over one's power to a trusted other) and risks (e.g., a new risk of financial abuse under an EPA or LPA (14)) that require sufficient mental capacity.

Box 5.2 Case Illustration

In our Case 089 (Suicidal Ideation and Temper Tantrum), Mrs Yuen's cognitive impairment has already affected her ability to take medication, cook, or handle finances independently. The reported incidents of her forgetting to collect rent for the properties she owns suggest that it could be beneficial for an attorney to be appointed to take care of her financial matters when necessary. In this case, should Mrs Yuen still have the mental capacity to make such a decision, an EPA or LPA could be an option to protect Mrs Yuen's rights and benefits. This case also illustrates the potential advantage of early advance care planning, to avoid unnecessary losses (and possible disputes) that have resulted from Mrs Yuen's current state of reduced ability to handle finances.

Practice Point 4: Advance Directive

Compared with those with other terminal diseases, people living with dementia are more likely to receive aggressive interventions during the end stage of their life, and this appears to be especially true in Eastern cultures compared with the West (15). At the same time, carers might regret their care decisions made on behalf of the person at their end-of-life stage, even when the decision was based on medical advice (16). It is now known that decisional conflicts and regrets could be minimised, carer satisfaction could be improved, and end-of-life care quality could be enhanced, if there is advance care planning discussion during early dementia (5, 6) involving the person, the family carers, and health and social care professionals.

As such, an advance directive should be considered a means towards an end, providing an opportunity to engage a person in communicating their preferences in advance care planning, from alpha to omega, including a discussion on end-of-life issues (17). The person and their family members benefit from the communication to get prepared cognitively, behaviourally, and most importantly, emotionally. Early and ongoing practical and emotional support is essential to prepare the family for potential changes and aid decision-making in the context of the realities of care towards the end of life (18). Given the uncertainty surrounding death in dementia, agreement on end-of-life care and interventions tends to be low even among families with good relationships. The emphasis here is therefore the communication opportunity and socioemotional aspect of the process of drawing up an advance directive while the person still has capacity, instead of having a mere legal document, to ensure family consensus and minimise regret.

Practice Point 5: Advance Proxy Care Planning

While an advance directive is applied if the person has decision-making capacity at the time when the directive is completed, advance proxy care planning would be needed for those who have already lost such capacity (19). A proxy decision-maker can be a next of kin, a close family member/friend, a designated power of attorney for care, or a guardian who is trusted to make decisions on the person's behalf. Some salient points for facilitating the development of a proxy plan include (19) careful consideration of the person's expressed goals, values, and preferences; regularly reviewing and updating the plan; and conflict resolution mechanisms.

See Box 5.3 for further reading and useful material on advance care planning in dementia.

Box 5.3 Further reading and useful material on advance care planning in dementia

- **Harrison Dening et al. (2019), Advance care planning in dementia: Recommendations for healthcare professionals (2)**
  discusses the context and importance of a palliative care approach and recommends rationales and strategies for healthcare professionals to support families affected by dementia to better plan for their future care.
- **Piers et al. (2018) Advance care planning in dementia: Recommendations for healthcare professionals (3)**
  contains 32 recommendations covering eight domains: (1) initiation of advance care planning, (2) mental capacity assessment, (3) holding advance care planning conversations, (4) the role and importance of those close to the person living with dementia, (5) advance care planning when it is difficult or no longer possible to communicate verbally, (6) documentation of wishes and preferences, including information transfer, (7) end-of-life decision-making, and (8) preconditions for optimal implementation.

5.2 Carer Stress and Support

Carer support is core to dementia management, with carer outcomes linked to many dementia outcomes, including disease progression and mortality (20, 21). Family carers are key partners in dementia care, while their own health (including mental health) and well-being can greatly influence the outcomes of the person living with dementia – to the extent that some carers could be the 'invisible second patients' (22). While caring for a person living with dementia can be associated with positive gains (23), dementia carers have an increased risk of having a high care burden (24) and other poor psychological and physical health outcomes (e.g., depression, infection, and death) (25–27). The primary care team should therefore pay attention to the burden and stress associated with dementia care, which are widely documented phenomena (28, 29). Evidence-based interventions are available to minimise the negative consequences of caregiving and delay institutionalisation, and the primary care team have a role to provide education, psychological support, and mobilise support networks (30).

Key Considerations in Primary Care

- The caring experience is diverse. Carer stress is influenced by a range of factors/stressors, including service accessibility, distressed behaviours and neuropsychiatric symptoms, functioning of the person living with dementia, their existing relationship, and the carer's coping and social support (28). Many of these factors are modifiable and targets of interventions.
- Among these factors, distressed behaviours and neuropsychiatric symptoms have a significant and complex relationship with carer stress and burden. They tend to interact with each other: neuropsychiatric symptoms and personality change can be hard for carers to make sense of or come to terms with; they can increase carer stress and negative emotions (31). These could in turn trigger or worsen distressed behaviours, especially when the carers cope with non-adapting strategies and have a low sense of competence in managing distressed behaviours (32).
- Current guidelines recommend not just one single protocol of carer intervention, but psychoeducation and skills training that are tailored and easily accessible for carers (33).
- There can be more than one carer. Family care is sometimes shared among multiple family members (34). Whenever possible, the primary care team should engage the primary carer as well as other family members to facilitate communication and family support.
- Caring can happen in the pre-diagnostic and help-seeking periods (35). In primary care settings, carers who seek help could have been struggling for a long period of time. Carer burden can be evident during this period (36). In some cases, because of the denial and resistance of the person with suspected dementia and a lack of support from other family members, the carer who first noticed symptoms of dementia may be faced with moral dilemmas and conflicts. Support from the primary care team can help address the burden and stress of help-seekers.

Practice Point 1: Supporting Positive Communication and Understanding

The nature of some common distressed behaviours and neuropsychiatric symptoms, such as delusion of theft and agitation, has a close relationship with psychosocial needs

Box 5.4 Case Illustration

In our Case 009 (Where is My Wife?), Mr Tam's son has noted that he keeps asking about his wife's whereabouts, forgetting that she is in hospital. While it is a normal reaction for family members to correct or sometimes confront the person with facts, a more helpful way of communication here would be to promote carers' understanding of the emotional or psychosocial needs or motives behind the behaviour. By allowing Mr Tam to express and by listening to his feelings, opinions, and needs – things that are 'beyond the realm of fact and correction' (38) – better communication, relationships, and well-being could result.

In many cases when a family member is targeted, it could be distressing and communication could be challenging. For example, in our Case 006 (Forgotten Home Address), Mrs Cheung suspects that her daughter steals money from her; we can expect her daughter to have negative emotions (e.g., anger and depression) even when the behaviour is recognised as a symptom with treatment indicated. The primary care team could support the carer to understand the behaviour from the person's perspective through psychoeducation that could help address carer stress: in this case, the behaviour (suspicion of the daughter for stealing) could be understood as a reasonable response, when Mrs Cheung has no recollection of where her money is, and in that situation, it is perhaps logical to suspect someone close (a spouse, child, or in some areas a domestic helper) to be involved. With this understanding, family carers may have greater acceptance of using adaptive coping and communication strategies (e.g., reminders and a safety box) to support the person, rebuilding trust and relationships, which could in turn reduce the behaviour.

(e.g., social interaction, positive regard, occupation, and identity). Psychoeducation with carers could focus on ways to address these needs, by improving communication skills and creating a positive social environment at home, which should also include fostering self-care in family carers (see Box 5.4 for case illustrations).

Based on the experience from evidence-based multicomponent carer interventions, some common factors in these intervention programmes can be identified (37), including promoting affective expression, enhancing empathy, and increasing tolerance of the person's neuropsychiatric symptoms. Encouraging carers to validate the person's feelings behind certain behaviours, instead of focusing on correcting his/her mistakes and confusion, can be helpful (38).

Practice Point 2: Meaningful Activities for Behaviours

Family members can also be encouraged to facilitate meaningful activity for the person living with dementia, which, when tailored to their abilities and interests could create a positivity and fulfilment. Participation in meaningful activities could be useful for maintaining social roles and self-identity, encouraging positive expression, and promoting feelings of connectedness. Evidence from individualised, family-centric programmes has shown that family carers can be coached to introduce meaningful activities, communicate effectively, break down tasks, and create a suitable and simplified environment to promote engagement with the person living with dementia, which can reduce distressed behaviours while promoting well-being in both the person living with dementia and family carers (39).

> **Box 5.5** Further reading and useful material on carer stress and support
>
> - **NHS Education for Scotland (2020). Promoting Psychological Wellbeing for People with Dementia and their Carers: An Enhanced Practice Resource (38)**
>   an easy-to-read resource designed to enhance the understanding of dementia from a psychological perspective, with practical tips and exercises to enable practitioners to apply the learning to supporting people living with dementia and their families.
> - **American Psychological Association (2011). Principles: Common Factors in Caregiving Interventions (37)**
>   a succinct summary of the key learnings from carer interventions, including characteristics of successful programmes, with reference to the US Resources for Enhancing Alzheimer's Caregiver Health Studies.
> - **World Health Organization (2019). iSupport for Dementia: Training and Support Manual for Carers of People with Dementia (44)**
>   a skills and training programme for carers of people living with dementia, with five modules and accompanying exercises.

Practice Point 3: Younger-Onset Dementia and Younger Carers

What we know about younger-onset dementia is still relatively little, including its impact on carers. It is likely that carers of both younger-onset dementia and older-onset dementia experience high stress and burden, which would necessarily interact with their life stage (40). For spouses, dependency could be a key concern (41). For children, the perception of severe threats in the future is similarly a common theme (42). This is understandable given that many people with younger-onset dementia are still working and could be the family's major breadwinner, when the children may still be under schooling.

In this group of carers, there may be increased barriers in accessing services, as very often dementia care services are designed to target older people; unmet needs could be common. Family members may also find it challenging to understand and accept the change in behaviours and personality in younger-onset dementia (43). The primary care team can be an important support to provide these families with information and address other unmet care needs. While aids to facilitate family role restructuring are important in dementia carer support in general (37), a reconfiguration of family relationships would probably take even higher priority in younger-onset dementia.

See Box 5.5 for Further reading and useful material on carer stress and support.

5.3 Formulating and Disclosing Dementia Diagnosis

As this book is about help-seeking cases and the initial encounter(s) with an early detection service and a primary care team, readers will now be accustomed to many of the considerations involved in formulating and disclosing a dementia diagnosis. What cannot be emphasised enough is that delay in help-seeking is common. Late help-seekers, however, have worse functioning and symptoms (45). The benefits and needs of a dementia diagnosis are clear, but timely diagnosis remains a major challenge globally (46, 47). Some primary care professionals may, understandably, have concerns over diagnosing and disclosing dementia to the person and their family carers, as some people may have a strong negative emotional response to the disclosure. Some argue against disclosing for fear of upsetting the person and potential consequences such as suicide. However, existing evidence and reports from primary care physicians suggest that many families are able to handle well the disclosed information (48), and the vast majority of people with or without cognitive impairment do want to have the information, for autonomy reasons (49), as the knowledge is essential for their future planning and decisions on treatment and care options. How to deliver the message with care is key.

Key Considerations in Primary Care

- Primary care professionals are in a good position to facilitate help-seeking and timely diagnosis because:
  - ○ there is an existing rapport with the family, before the presentation of dementia signs and symptoms. Trust in the professional could help the family go through the disclosure process;
  - ○ they have good knowledge of the person's other conditions, needs, and strengths/ resources, which are often important considerations in the diagnosis and subsequent care planning, including advice on legal matters;
  - ○ involvement of primary care may reduce fear and stigma surrounding the diagnosis;
  - ○ family physicians and care services have the advantage of working with the family as a unit, which is particularly important in dementia care;
  - ○ primary care physicians can function in the healthcare system to act as gatekeepers and seek specialist support when indicated.

Practice Point 1: Break Bad News with Care

The formulation and disclosure of a dementia diagnosis is a process rather than an encounter. The primary care team has an important role in ensuring this process is carried out in a way that minimises psychological harm and maximises the health benefits an early diagnosis can bring. Given that individuals have different preferences for accessing health information (their own or that of a person they are caring for), whenever possible, the primary care team should consult the person and the family at the outset to understand their preferences for disclosure, which could range from information-sharing to counselling and instrumental support. In any case, it is important to ensure clarity in the disclosure. Approaches that downplay the significance of the condition and potentially poor prognosis, sometimes motivated by an intention to preserve hope, may nevertheless compromise understanding and informed future planning (50). Some key behaviours in an appropriate disclosure of a dementia diagnosis include (51) preparing for the disclosure, involving the family, responding to the person's reactions, and communicating effectively.

Disclosing the diagnosis may be particularly challenging if the person lacks insight or when it is something exceedingly difficult for the person and/or some family members to accept (see Box 5.6). As the disease progresses, the person may lose insight into their cognitive impairment and may have fewer complaints than the carer. In some cases, the assessment and diagnostic consultation could be a source of conflict within the family when not all members share the same understanding of the condition. It is thus even more important to not leave the task of breaking bad news to a family carer alone. Having a trusted professional within the

> **Box 5.6 Case Illustration**
>
> Diagnosis disclosure may be particularly tricky when the person does not acknowledge any issues, as in our Case 017 (Time and Place Orientation, Mrs Yip) and Case 059 (Denial of Functional Decline and Dementia, Ms Tse). In both cases they denied having dementia: one was defensive and irritable during the assessment, while the other was aware of memory decline but denied other impairments. In these cases, finding out the level of insight may help in deciding the best way to communicate. For example, Mrs Yip's irritability and defensiveness could indicate either a complete lack of insight (and the assessment viewed as something ungrounded) or good awareness (and denial out of fear about what might happen when she has a confirmed diagnosis). For the latter, reassurance, signposting of post-diagnostic support, and patient education could help. In the former case, if insight is affected by cognitive impairment, confrontation with facts may not be the best strategy, whereas care and intervention that preserve dignity and focus on strengths would be helpful. Carers may also need support in developing communication skills that neither confront the person nor reinforce denial of his/her care needs.

primary care team explaining with patience what a diagnosis of dementia means, what the care and treatment options are, and what support will be available (see Section 4.5) can have a significant impact on the person's and the carers' outcomes.

Practice Point 2: Next Steps Are Part of the Process

Some practitioners may hold negative attitudes towards diagnosing dementia due to a perceived suboptimal post-diagnostic management (52). The same can be expected of family carers and the person. It is thus an essential component of the assessment and disclosure process that management options are provided. A focus on quality of life and well-being, as well as planning for the future, are therefore also considered part of the best practice in disclosing the diagnosis (51).

An individualised approach is important in tailoring the next steps based on assessment findings (e.g., whether the person's cognitive impairment level may benefit from cognitive stimulation/rehabilitation, whether other more acute conditions and safety should be prioritised, or if no diagnosis can be given at the moment and information/monitoring is advised). At the same time, some general information would be useful for the person and the family to consider the next steps:

- communicating the fact that dementia is a chronic condition and the possible prognosis;
- emphasising that both drugs and non-drug interventions can help in stabilising symptoms, delaying deterioration, and minimising complications;
- highlighting the role of continuing mental and social activities and daily routines.

Remember that a dementia diagnosis is a major life event, and the person and the family will need time to process the information and adjust. While information on treatment options and advance planning is important at this stage to induce hope, it can sometimes be overwhelming with too many other major decisions that need to be made within a short period of time. The primary care team can support by working with the family at the preferred pace and level of support needed in planning for the future, while reassuring them that help is available.

Practice Point 3: Typical Presentation and Assessment Findings

From the cases of Alzheimer's disease and other cases presented in Chapters 2 and 3, we hope that readers are now familiar enough with the characteristics of the assessment profile to be able to form a clinical impression of Alzheimer's disease or otherwise, when a person presents with suspected dementia (see Figure 5.1 for an illustration of a typical case presentation in this casebook). In particular:

- Age: although Alzheimer's disease can occur at different ages, the early 80s is the typical age of presentation.
- Cognitive assessment findings: while the overall performance (e.g., total score) would depend on age and education, the pattern of impairments should remain similar in people with Alzheimer's disease. These include better performance in immediate recall than delayed recall; in place orientation compared with time orientation;[1] and in clock copying versus clock drawing. Since MMSE is sensitive for Alzheimer's disease, if near-normal MMSE results are obtained alongside other dementia symptoms, frontotemporal dementia or other conditions should be suspected.
- Clinical examination findings: in typical Alzheimer's disease cases, the clinical examination usually shows normal findings, with typical symptomatology and presentation. In moderate Alzheimer's disease, apraxia in self-care is common. Note that while ADL performance tends to decline with age, in Alzheimer's disease IADLs should be more impaired than ADLs (unless there are non-cognitive reasons for specific ADL impairments, such as physical frailty). In people who present at a younger age (e.g., in their 50s and 60s), the primary presenting symptom may not be memory impairment, but could be behavioural, speech problems and apraxia; these should lead to the consideration of non-Alzheimer's dementia and suggest referral for secondary care assessment, including more advanced neuroimaging.

Practice Point 4: Complaints to Watch Out For

The importance of complaints spontaneously made by the person and/or a knowledgeable informant deserves more recognition: they are observations that are significant enough to prompt help-seeking. Evidence from community-based early detection services suggests that the type and pervasiveness of these complaints are associated with illness severity and can provide useful information for triage (53).

Common complaints from the carer seen in our cases of uncomplicated early Alzheimer's disease include repeated searching for belongings, losing items/money frequently, delusions of stealing, difficulty in finding their way, repeated questions, forgetfulness about appointments and recent events, and decreased motivation. Carers of a person with Alzheimer's disease would typically answer 'yes' to most of the questions covered in the GPCOG (on remembering recent events, recalling recent conversations, managing money and finances, managing medication independently, and using transport), except for word finding (see Box 4.2).

---

[1] This assumes the assessment is conducted in a venue familiar to the person, thus involving long-term memory that should be better preserved in the earlier stages of Alzheimer's disease; this pattern may not be observed if the venue is unfamiliar and requires short-term memory to orient. Similarly, within the time orientation test, performance should typically be better for years than months and days, with the latter reflecting short-term memory.

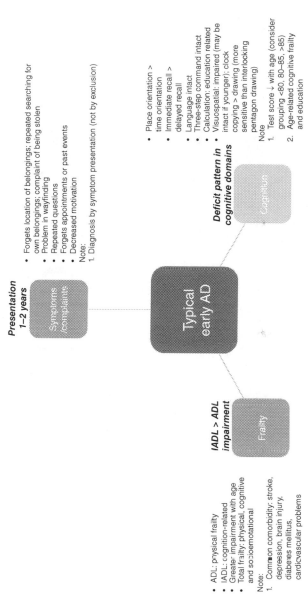

Presentation
1–2 years

Symptoms /complaints
- Forgets location of belongings; repeated searching for own belongings; complaint of being stolen
- Problem in wayfinding
- Repeated questions
- Forgets appointments or past events
- Decreased motivation

Note:
1. Diagnosis by symptom presentation (not by exclusion)

Deficit pattern in cognitive domains

Cognition
- Place orientation > time orientation
- Immediate recall > delayed recall
- Language intact
- Three-step command intact
- Calculation: education related
- Visuospatial: impaired (may be intact if younger); clock copying > drawing (more sensitive than interlocking pentagon drawing)

Note
1. Test score ↓ with age (consider grouping <80, 80–85, >85)
2. Age-related cognitive frailty and education

Typical early AD

IADL > ADL impairment

Frailty

- ADL: physical frailty
- IADL: cognition-related
- Greater impairment with age
- Total frailty: physical, cognitive and socioemotional

Note:
1. Common comorbidity: stroke, depression, brain injury, diabetes mellitus, cardiovascular problems

Figure 5.1 Typical presentation of early Alzheimer's disease: A summary of Cases 1–80

> **Box 5.7** Further reading and useful material on formulating and disclosing dementia diagnosis
>
> - **Dementia Australia. Informing the Person with Dementia (54)**
>   www.dementia.org.au/about-dementia-and-memory-loss/how-can-i-find-out-more/informing-the-person-with-dementia
>   a plain-language guide explaining how to prepare for disclosing a dementia diagnosis.
> - **Dementia: Timely diagnosis and early intervention (55)**
>   a *BMJ* clinical review with discussion on the role of primary care in dementia diagnosis, investigation, and assessment tools in primary care, assessment of mental capacity, and other tips for non-specialists.
> - **Dementia Diagnosis and Management: A Brief Pragmatic Resource for General Practitioners (56)**
>   www.england.nhs.uk/wp-content/uploads/2015/01/dementia-diag-mng-ab-pt.pdf
>   a resource pack by the UK NHS aiming to support general practitioners in identifying and appropriately managing people living with dementia in the primary care environment, with case scenarios illustrating when referral is justified and when cases can be safely diagnosed by a general practitioner.

Considering that there can be discrepancies between the complaints from the person and the carer, a point to note is to arrange time for separate interviewing. With decreasing levels of insight, the carer's report is often more important, although the primary care team should always bear in mind how 'knowledgeable' the carer is (e.g., whether living together and awareness of the person's functioning level) in evaluating the validity of the complaint (or the lack of it). In some cases (e.g., Case 003), there may also be insufficient information from a carer, and reports from other informants (e.g., a formal carer or home helper) should also be sought as far as possible.

Practice Point 5: Remember It's a Clinical Diagnosis

One of the key advantages of the primary care team in the diagnostic process of uncomplicated Alzheimer's disease is that it is a clinical diagnosis in an older person, who would typically be known to the team for other chronic illnesses and care needs, with clinical symptoms of early Alzheimer's disease usually presenting for one to two years before help is sought. In considering a dementia diagnosis, comprehensive information about frailty, co-occurring conditions, and family relationships is an important context, which should be taken into account in understanding findings from assessments and examinations, such as the person's ADL and IADL performance. These other conditions and age-related physical, cognitive, and socioemotional changes could mean that presenting symptoms and assessment results may be modified.

See Box 5.7 for futher reading and useful material on formulating and disclosing dementia diagnosis.

5.4 Issues Surrounding Management

Post-diagnostic management is multidisciplinary and multicomponent, as 'good dementia care spans medical, social, and supportive care; it should be tailored to unique individual and cultural needs, preferences, and priorities and should incorporate support for family carers' (12).

Important themes surrounding management go beyond treatment (including drug and non-pharmacological interventions); a unique combination of care and support services, which may cover emotional and psychological well-being and practical and integrated support, is needed for the person and/or their family members (57). We have discussed family carer support in Section 5.2; here we will focus on disease management that directly involves the person with dementia.

Key Considerations in Primary Care

- The multidisciplinary and multicomponent nature of dementia management means that a team approach is necessary. Depending on the country and local service system context, the primary care team would

  ○ need to partner with other service providers to facilitate access and adherence to the recommended interventions, care, and support

  ○ need support from relevant specialist/specialised care services as the disease progresses or when complications arise. Understanding when to refer in line with local collaborative care practice is important

Practice Point 1: Both Pharmacological and Non-Pharmacological Interventions Are Needed

It is increasingly recognised that pharmacological and non-pharmacological interventions, when given early, have equal roles in maintaining cognition, functioning, and quality of life in people with dementia. Cognitive, physical, and social activities have potential benefits (58): there is dissociation between brain pathology and cognitive symptom presentation (59, 60), and cognitive functioning is malleable throughout life even in the context of brain diseases and lesions, which can be altered by everyday experience, including cognitive, physical, and social activities (61).

For drug treatment, in the case of deteriorating cognition in mild to moderate Alzheimer's disease, physicians may escalate the dose of a cholinesterase inhibitor or add memantine (e.g., Case 025). Memantine may also be prescribed when there is irritability (e.g., Case 017) or in cases of mixed dementia (e.g., Case 020). Response to drug treatment can also be helpful in diagnosis, such as in cases presenting with features of Alzheimer's disease but when vascular or mixed dementia cannot be ruled out entirely (e.g., Case 010). The presence of neuropsychiatric symptoms does not necessarily indicate antipsychotics and specialist care; for example, the delusional ideas in Case 005 can be handled by non-pharmacological means such as the provision of cues. However, in cases where significant delusion is present, a specialist referral and neuroleptics may be needed. Other situations where referral is indicated include the presence of rigidity (e.g., Case 042) and urgent psychiatric referral in the case of imminent suicide risk (e.g., Case 041).

For non-pharmacological interventions that target cognition and quality of life, group cognitive stimulation that involves social interaction and cognitive processing can be used (62, 63). Cognitive stimulation has been recommended in England's National Institute for Health and Care Excellence (NICE) guidelines and by Alzheimer's Disease International (64, 65). A manualised version of cognitive stimulation therapy (CST) with evidence of effectiveness and cost-effectiveness when used alone or in combination with medication as maintenance therapy (66, 67) is available in 35 countries (see www.ucl.ac.uk/international-cognitive-stimulation-therapy/international-cognitive-stimulation-therapy-cst-centre). Mental stimulation is therefore one of the most commonly recommended management strategies in the typical Alzheimer's disease cases presented in this book. Apart from mental stimulation, other common recommendations are regular exercise, a healthy diet, and an active social life. In fact, social interaction is an integral part of CST and may account for some of its benefits. Physical exercise improves activities of daily living and cognitive functioning (especially executive function) (68, 69). Locally developed interventions based on these principles and evidence may be available; for example, in China, an approach integrating cognitive stimulation, physical exercise, and social relationships into traditional Chinese culture has been developed (70) for use as an intervention or as a lifestyle approach available from community service providers (see www.eng.hkada.org.hk/about6arts).

Practice Point 2: Managing Distressed Behaviours and Neuropsychiatric Symptoms

Sometimes referred to as 'challenging behaviours' and 'behavioural and psychological symptoms of dementia (BPSDs)' previously – terms that are now regarded as less helpful (71) – distressed behaviours and neuropsychiatric symptoms can be managed and sometimes prevented. Distressed behaviours that more commonly prompt family carers to seek help include resistance to care, paranoia/suspiciousness, aggression, and restlessness/wandering (71). In the cases presented in this book, for example, suspiciousness of others stealing things from oneself is a common presenting problem (e.g., Cases 025, 035, 047, and 068). Other neuropsychiatric symptoms such as sexual disinhibition, hallucinations, and nocturnal disturbances, on the other hand, may not be easily understood by family carers as related to dementia. These could lead to distress and other undesirable consequences such as premature institutionalisation. The primary care team can help manage and reduce the occurrence of some of these behaviours and symptoms.

Many educational materials and resources are available on managing distressed behaviours and neuropsychiatric symptoms; some non-pharmacological approaches currently being used involve the family carer (see Section 5.2) and include

- the Activating event, Behaviour, Consequence (ABC) framework, which focuses on identifying the specific circumstances associated with the behaviour and developing targeted strategies. For example, underlying medical illness, pain, and other potentially modifiable triggers would be explored (72);
- A related Describe, Investigate, Create, Evaluate (DICE) approach that highlights a person–carer–environment triangle, to conceptualise factors related to the person (e.g., unmet needs), carer (e.g., communication issues), and environment (e.g., over-/under-stimulation) (73);
- preventive measures including person-centred care and meaningful activities (see Box 5.8), which may reduce agitation and other behavioural problems, thereby decreasing the use of chemical or physical restraints.

In some situations, when the agitation, aggression, and psychotic symptoms are causing severe distress or posing a threat to the person or others, clinicians may consider offering antipsychotics (65).

> **Box 5.8 Case Illustration**
>
> In our Case 093 (No Concern for Personal Hygiene), Mr Cheng has the habit of picking up dirty tissues and cigarette butts, which can be disturbing to the family. There can be many ways to understand this behaviour, and one possibility is that the hoarding provides some meaning to Mr Cheng: it could be filling a void, or perhaps he enjoys the feeling of being 'productive' and normal in some sense by collecting. Providing an alternative, more adaptive activity in such a case could be a win–win: Mr Cheng can lead a meaningful everyday life while the behaviour is less disruptive to the carer. A point to note is that what is meaningful varies from person to person, depending on factors such as capability, previous interests, identity, and roles. Family carers can be in a good position to identify appropriate activities that are meaningful to the person, with support from the primary care team.

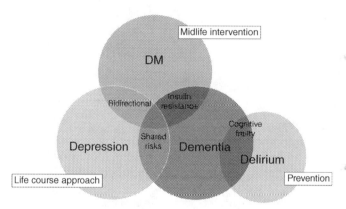

Figure 5.2 The four Ds – dementia, depression, diabetes mellitus, and delirium – as management targets

Practice Point 3: Optimising Safety, Physical Health, and Mental Health

In Section 1.4, we introduced the biopsychosocial model, which explains the need to intervene on tractable physical, psychological, and social health factors to reduce excess disability in dementia (74). We have seen cases in which the recommended management included prevention of health hazards (e.g., fall prevention in Case 002 with a history of hip replacement; home assessment for fire hazards in Case 055) and optimising the person's physical health (e.g., cardiovascular risks in Cases 001 and 048) and mental health (e.g., depression in Cases 028 and 035).

Figure 5.2 illustrates some important connections among the four 'Ds': dementia, depression, delirium, and diabetes mellitus. As their relationships are complex, management strategies should be individualised considering the person's comorbidity profile. In Case 013, for example, monitoring for mood problems and adjustment disorder is recommended, considering the person's insight into his cognitive problem. Whereas in Case 035 with comorbid depression at presentation, the temporal sequence between dementia and depression needs to be elucidated to inform the best management. In Case 036, the recommendation is to optimise treatment for the comorbid depression and

> **Box 5.9** Further reading and useful material on issues surrounding dementia management
>
> - **UCL Dementia Training Academy**
>   www.ucldementiatrainingacademy.org/
>   a web resource signposting to training for professionals on evidence-based psychological and social interventions for people with dementia, their carers, and care staff.
> - **Dementia Centre for Research Collaboration. Behaviour Management: A Guide to Good Practice (BPSD Guide)**
>   https://dementiaresearch.org.au/resources/bpsdguide/
>   a comprehensive overview of evidence- and practice-based management principles for distressed behaviours and neuropsychiatric symptoms of dementia for clinicians caring for people with dementia.
> - **Alzheimer's Association. Safety Assessment Checklist**
>   www.alz.org/media/Documents/safety-assess-checklist.pdf
>   an easy-to-use safety assessment guide covering safety issues such as driving, taking medication, and getting lost.
> - **National Collaborating Centre for Mental Health. The Dementia Care Pathway: Full Implementation Guidance**
>   www.rcpsych.ac.uk/docs/default-source/improving-care/nccmh/dementia/nccmh-dementia-care-pathway-full-implementation-guidance.pdf?sfvrsn=cdef189d_8
>   a resource pack by the UK NHS aiming to support general practitioners in identifying and appropriately managing people living with dementia in the primary care environment, with case scenarios illustrating when referral is justified and when cases can be safely diagnosed by a general practitioner.

diabetes on top of the cholinesterase inhibitor prescription, considering the contribution of both depression and diabetes to dementia.

See Box 5.9 for further reading and useful material on issues surrounding dementia management.

5.5 Dementia-Friendly Communities and Prevention

The functions and performance of the primary care team shape and are shaped by the community they are embedded in. A dementia-friendly community usually encompasses activities promoting wider community involvement of people with dementia, care and support services for them and family carers, awareness and education, and environmental design (75–77). Dementia-friendly communities are developed not only for people with dementia but for everyone ('what is good for dementia is good for everyone') (78, 79). Such an environment promotes early help-seeking, risk reduction, and primary prevention, with primary care having major roles.

Key Considerations in Primary Care

- Emphases of dementia-friendly communities centre around personhood, social inclusion, empowerment, stigma reduction, localised strategies, and community engagement and collaboration (75) – concepts and values that are in line with primary care (as compared with secondary or specialised care).

- In a dementia-friendly community, a wider collaborative network beyond health and social care providers works with the primary care team to support dementia care.
- As much as 40 per cent of dementia risk is potentially modifiable, mostly occurring in midlife and later life (12, 80), and can be addressed through primary care.

Practice Point 1: Dementia Awareness

Stigma and a lack of awareness are barriers to early help-seeking. Late presentation could mean more complications and an increased need for specialised care. Public education on early intervention and prevention is therefore essential for people with dementia to benefit most from primary care. The cases in this book presented to an early detection service in collaboration with primary care practitioners; as the public is generally unaware of the role of primary care in dementia diagnosis and care, there was a need to prepare society in identifying probable dementia as well as recognising primary care as a possible care pathway.

On the other hand, the level of dementia literacy and awareness in the community would affect the perception, experience, and report of the person with dementia and their carer, which should be considered when conducting clinical interviews and assessments. Some examples can be found in the case of Mr Hung (Case 030), where his wife might have missed (and thus under-reported) early signs and symptoms, which can be compared and contrasted with the case of Mrs Cheng (Case 068), where public awareness efforts might have prompted her to present at a preclinical or very early stage. The primary care team have to exercise discretion in weighing the informant's account.

Dementia awareness in the community is also relevant to social support (or the lack of it). In areas with a high level of awareness and easily accessible diagnostic services, late help-seeking could signal insufficient social support (which was identified as an area for further exploration in Case 019). Where public education targeted gatekeepers other than family carers (e.g., Case 030), people who would otherwise present late (e.g., living alone or with an older spouse only) may be able to access primary care in a timely manner.

Practice Point 2: Collaborative Network

Dementia-friendly communities promote partnerships across public/private sectors and between formal and informal carers for shared care (81, 82). These may include co-working to increase provision of evidence-based interventions and respite services, and training, coordination, and support for volunteers (83) – 'Dementia Friends Champions' – who would provide care navigation and lifestyle support (84).

Components of dementia-friendly communities concern people, organisations, communities, and partnerships (85).

- People: involving people with dementia; enhancing public understanding; enhancing caring skills.
- Organisations: promoting and providing timely diagnosis and post-diagnostic support by primary care
- Communities: for social environment, increasing awareness, reducing stigma, and improving engagement; for physical environment, it includes providing home services and public space.

> **Box 5.10** Further reading and useful material on dementia-friendly communities and prevention
>
> - **Livingston G et al. (2020). Dementia prevention, intervention, and care: 2020 report of the Lancet Commission (80)**
>   an update to the 2017 report, with estimates of early-life, midlife, and later-life risk factors.
> - **Risk reduction of cognitive decline and dementia: WHO guidelines**
>   www.who.int/publications/i/item/9789241550543
>   an evidence-based recommendation on lifestyle behaviours and interventions to delay or prevent cognitive decline and dementia.
> - **Towards a dementia inclusive society. WHO toolkit for dementia-friendly initiatives (DFIs)**
>   www.who.int/publications/i/item/9789240031531
>   a toolkit providing practical guidance and tools to support efforts in creating dementia-inclusive societies.

- Partnerships: including cross-sectional support with a collaborative approach and collective commitment.

The point about partnership can be illustrated with Case 002 (repeated buying of groceries), where education and community engagement (e.g., targeting shopkeepers) could potentially improve the disease management, reduce carer stress, and improve the quality of life (better autonomy) of the person with dementia. Case 025 highlighted the role of communities: Ms Wong's suspicions about her neighbours stealing her safety box key could lead to conflicts; improving understanding and acceptance of dementia in the neighbourhood may help avoid conflicts.

Practice Point 3: The Life Course Approach to Prevention

As mentioned in Section 1.3, Alzheimer's disease is characterised by a slow, gradual progression of neuropathology over many years. Like most chronic diseases, lifestyle factors contribute significantly to its prevention at different levels. For primary or secondary prevention, modifiable midlife risk factors identified include hearing loss, hypertension, alcohol (>21 units/week), obesity, and traumatic brain injury; in later life, these include smoking, depression, physical inactivity, diabetes, and social isolation (80). The primary care team is in a good position to advise middle-aged and older people on reducing these risks.

For people with dementia, good management of these factors could potentially reduce complications and slow progression as tertiary prevention measures. In some of the cases presented in this book, for example, management of hearing problems is recommended (e.g., Cases 060 and 067). As hearing impairment could reduce sensory and mental stimulation directly, or indirectly through its association with social isolation, it was recommended to consider otoscopic examination, the use of hearing aids, and/or referral to an otolaryngologist in these cases. The same can be said for other known risk factors, which could sometimes be just as important as drug treatment for dementia.

See Box 5.10 for further reading and useful material on dementia-friendly communities and prevention.

References

1. Mullick A, Martin J, Sallnow L. An introduction to advance care planning in practice. BMJ. 2013;347:f6064.

2. Harrison Dening K, Sampson EL, De Vries K. Advance care planning in dementia: Recommendations for healthcare professionals. Palliative Care. 2019;12:1178224219826579.

3. Piers R, Albers G, Gilissen J, De Lepeleire J, Steyaert J, Van Mechelen W, et al. Advance care planning in dementia: recommendations for healthcare professionals. BMC Palliative Care. 2018;17(1):88.

4. Dixon J, Karagiannidou M, Knapp M. The effectiveness of advance care planning in improving end-of-life outcomes for people with dementia and their carers: A systematic review and critical discussion. Journal of Pain and Symptom Management. 2018;55(1):132–50.e1.

5. Huang H-L, Lu W-R, Liu C-L, Chang H-J. Advance care planning information intervention for persons with mild dementia and their family caregivers: Impact on end-of-life care decision conflicts. PLOS ONE. 2020;15(10): e0240684.

6. Tay RY, Hum AYM, Ali NB, Leong IYO, Wu HY, Chin JJ, et al. Comfort and satisfaction with care of home-dwelling dementia patients at the end of life. Journal of Pain and Symptom Management. 2020;59(5):1019–32.e1.

7. Cresp SJ, Lee SF, Moss C. Substitute decision makers' experiences of making decisions at end of life for older persons with dementia: A systematic review and qualitative meta-synthesis. Dementia. 2018;19(5):1532–59.

8. Sellars M, Chung O, Nolte L, Tong A, Pond D, Fetherstonhaugh D, et al. Perspectives of people with dementia and carers on advance care planning and end-of-life care: A systematic review and thematic synthesis of qualitative studies. Palliative Medicine. 2019;33(3):274–90.

9. Robinson L, Dickinson C, Rousseau N, Beyer F, Clark A, Hughes J, et al. A systematic review of the effectiveness of advance care planning interventions for people with cognitive impairment and dementia. Age and Ageing. 2012;41(2):263–9.

10. Lee RP, Bamford C, Poole M, McLellan E, Exley C, Robinson L. End of life care for people with dementia: The views of health professionals, social care service managers and frontline staff on key requirements for good practice. PLOS ONE. 2017;12(6):e0179355.

11. Brazil K, Carter G, Galway K, Watson M, van der Steen JT. General practitioners perceptions on advance care planning for patients living with dementia. BMC Palliative Care. 2015;14:14.

12. Livingston G, Sommerlad A, Orgeta V, Costafreda SG, Huntley J, Ames D, et al. Dementia prevention, intervention, and care. Lancet. 2017;390(10113):2673–734.

13. Nikumaa H, Mäki-Petäjä-Leinonen A. Counselling of people with dementia in legal matters: Social and health care professionals' role. European Journal of Social Work. 2020;23(4):685–98.

14. Purser K, Cockburn T, Cross C, Jacmon H. Alleged financial abuse of those under an enduring power of attorney: An exploratory study. The British Journal of Social Work. 2018;48(4):887–905.

15. Chen YH, Ho CH, Huang CA-O, Hsu YW, Chen YC, Chen PA-O, et al. Comparison of healthcare utilization and life-sustaining interventions between elderly patients with dementia and those with cancer near the end of life: A nationwide, population-based study in Taiwan. Geriatrics & Gerontology International. 2017;17(12):2545–51

16. Supiano KP, Luptak M, Andersen T, Beynon C, Iacob E, Wong B. If we knew then what we know now: The preparedness experience of pre-loss and post-loss dementia caregivers. Death Studies. 2022;46(2):369–80.

17. Tilburgs B, Vernooij-Dassen M, Koopmans R, van Gennip H, Engels Y,

Perry M. Barriers and facilitators for GPs in dementia advance care planning: A systematic integrative review. PLOS ONE. 2018;13(6):e0198535.

18. Harrison Dening K, King M, Jones L, Vickerstaff V, Sampson EL. Advance care planning in dementia: Do family carers know the treatment preferences of people with early dementia? PLOS ONE. 2016;11 (7):e0159056.

19. Volicer L, Cantor MD, Derse AR, Edwards DM, Prudhomme AM, Gregory DC, et al. Advance care planning by proxy for residents of long-term care facilities who lack decision-making capacity. Journal of American Geriatric Society. 2002;50(4):761–7.

20. Lwi SJ, Ford BQ, Casey JJ, Miller BL, Levenson RW. Poor caregiver mental health predicts mortality of patients with neurodegenerative disease. Proceedings of the National Academy Science USA. 2017;114(28):7319–24.

21. Tschanz JT, Piercy K, Corcoran CD, Fauth E, Norton MC, Rabins PV, et al. Caregiver coping strategies predict cognitive and functional decline in dementia: The Cache County Dementia Progression Study. American Journal of Geriatric Psychiatry. 2013;21(1):57–66.

22. Brodaty H, Donkin M. Family caregivers of people with dementia. Dialogues Clinical Neuroscience. 2009;11 (2):217–28.

23. Carbonneau H, Caron C, Desrosiers J. Development of a conceptual framework of positive aspects of caregiving in dementia. Dementia. 2010;9(3):327–53.

24. Etters L, Goodall D, Harrison BE. Caregiver burden among dementia patient caregivers: A review of the literature. Journal of the American Association of Nurse Practitioners. 2008;20(8):423–8.

25. Schulz R, Boerner K, Shear K, Zhang S, Gitlin LN. Predictors of complicated grief among dementia caregivers: A prospective study of bereavement. The American Journal of Geriatric Psychiatry. 2006;14(8):650–8.

26. Sorensen S, Conwell Y. Issues in dementia caregiving: Effects on mental and physical health, intervention strategies, and research needs. American Journal of Geriatric Psychiatry. 2011;19(6):491–6.

27. Ory MG, Hoffman RR, 3rd, Yee JL, Tennstedt S, Schulz R. Prevalence and impact of caregiving: A detailed comparison between dementia and nondementia caregivers. Gerontologist. 1999;39(2):177–85.

28. Pearlin LI, Mullan JT, Semple SJ, Skaff MM. Caregiving and the stress process: An overview of concepts and their measures. Gerontologist. 1990;30(5):583–94.

29. Schulz R, O'Brien AT, Bookwala J, Fleissner K. Psychiatric and physical morbidity effects of dementia caregiving: Prevalence, correlates, and causes. Gerontologist. 1995;35(6):771–91.

30. Cohen CA, Pringle D, LeDuc L. Dementia caregiving: The role of the primary care physician. Canadian Journal of Neurological Science. 2001;28(Suppl 1): S72–S6.

31. Conde-Sala JL, Turró-Garriga O, Calvó-Perxas L, Vilalta-Franch J, Lopez- Pousa S, Garre-Olmo J. Three-year trajectories of caregiver burden in Alzheimer's disease. Journal of Alzheimers Diseases. 2014;42:623–33.

32. de Vugt ME, Stevens F, Aalten P, Lousberg R, Jaspers N, Winkens I, et al. Do caregiver management strategies influence patient behaviour in dementia? International Journal of Geriatric Psychiatry. 2004;19(1):85–92.

33. National Institute for Health and Care Excellence (NICE). Dementia: Assessment, Management and Support for People Living with Dementia and Their Carers. London: NICE; 2018.

34. Harvath TA, Mongoven JM, Bidwell JT, Cothran FA, Sexson KE, Mason DJ, et al. Research priorities in family caregiving: Process and outcomes of a conference on family-centered care across the trajectory of serious illness. The Gerontologist. 2020;60(Suppl 1):S5–S13.

35. van Vliet D, de Vugt ME, Bakker C, Koopmans RT, Pijnenburg YA, Vernooij-Dassen MJ, et al. Caregivers' perspectives on the pre-diagnostic period in early onset dementia: A long and winding road. International Psychogeriatry. 2011;23 (9):1393–404.

36. Ng CKM, Leung DKY, Cai X, Wong GHY. Perceived help-seeking difficulty, barriers, delay, and burden in carers of people with suspected dementia. International Journal of Environmental Research Public Health. 2021;18(6):2956.

37. American Psychological Association. Principles: Common Factors in Caregiving Interventions: American Psychological Association. Available from: www.apa.org/pi/about/ publications/caregivers/practice-settings/ intervention/principles.aspx.

38. NHS Education for Scotland. Promoting Psychological Wellbeing for People with Dementia and Their Carers: An Enhanced Practice Resource. Scotland: NHS Education for Scotland. 2020.

39. Gitlin LN, Winter L, Vause Earland T, Adel Herge E, Chernett NL, Piersol CV, et al. The Tailored Activity Program to reduce behavioral symptoms in individuals with dementia: Feasibility, acceptability, and replication potential. Gerontologist. 2009;49(3):428–39.

40. van Vliet D, de Vugt ME, Bakker C, Koopmans RT, Verhey FR. Impact of early onset dementia on caregivers: A review. International Journal of Geriatric Psychiatry. 2010;25 (11):1091–100.

41. Kaiser S, Panegyres PK. The psychosocial impact of young onset dementia on spouses. American Journal of Alzheimers Disease and Other Dementias. 2006;21 (6):398–402.

42. Allen J, Oyebode JR, Allen J. Having a father with young onset dementia: The impact on well-being of young people. Dementia. 2009;8(4):455–80.

43. Millenaar JK, Bakker C, Koopmans RT, Verhey FR, Kurz A, de Vugt ME. The care needs and experiences with the use of services of people with young-onset dementia and their caregivers: A systematic review. International Journal of Geriatric Psychiatry. 2016;31 (12):1261-76.

44. World Health Organization. iSupport for Dementia: Training and Support Manual for Carers of People with Dementia. Geneva: World Health Organization. 2019.

45. Tang JY, Wong GH, Ng CK, Kwok DT, Lee MN, Dai DL, et al. Neuropsychological profile and dementia symptom recognition in help-seekers in a community early-detection program in Hong Kong. Journal of American Geriatric Society. 2016;64(3):584–9.

46. Alzheimer's Disease International. Journey through the Diagnosis of Dementia: World Alzheimer's Report 2021. London: Alzheimer's Disease Interantional. 2021.

47. Alzheimer's Disease International. Early Diagnosis and Intervention: World Alzheimer's Report 2011. London: Alzheimer's Disease Interantional. 2011.

48. Connell CM, Boise L Fau, Stuckey JC, Stuckey Jc Fau, Holmes SB, Holmes Sb Fau, et al. Attitudes toward the diagnosis and disclosure of dementia among family caregivers and primary care physicians. The Gerontologist. 2004;44(4):500–7.

49. van den Dungen P, van Kuijk L, van Marwijk H, van der Wouden J, Moll van Charante E, van der Horst H, et al. Preferences regarding disclosure of a diagnosis of dementia: A systematic review. International Psychogeriatry. 2014;26(10):1603–18.

50. Dooley J, Bass N, McCabe R. How do doctors deliver a diagnosis of dementia in memory clinics? British Journal of Psychiatry. 2018;212(4):239–45.

51. Lecouturier J, Bamford C, Hughes JC, Francis JJ, Foy R, Johnston M, et al. Appropriate disclosure of a diagnosis of dementia: identifying the key behaviours of 'best practice'. BMC Health Service Research. 2008;8:95.

52. Giezendanner S, Monsch AU, Kressig RW, Mueller Y, Streit S, Essig S, et al. General practitioners' attitudes towards early diagnosis of dementia: A cross-sectional survey. BMC Family Practise. 2019;20(1):65.

53. Xu JQ, Choy JCP, Tang JYM, Liu TY, Luo H, Lou VWQ, et al. Spontaneously reported symptoms by informants are associated with clinical severity in dementia help-seekers. Journal of American Geriatric Society. 2017;65 (9):1946–52.

54. Dementia Australia. Informing the person with dementia. Available from: www .dementia.org.au/about-dementia-and-memory-loss/how-can-i-find-out-more/ informing-the-person-with-dementia.

55. Robinson L, Tang E, Taylor JP. Dementia: Timely diagnosis and early intervention. BMJ. 2015;350:h3029.

56 Dementia Diagnosis and Management: A Brief Pragmatic Resource for General Practitioners. Available from: www .england.nhs.uk/wp-content/uploads/ 2015/01/dementia-diag-mng-ab-pt.pdf.

57. Bamford C, Wheatley A, Brunskill G, Booi L, Allan L, Banerjee S, et al. Key components of post-diagnostic support for people with dementia and their carers: A qualitative study. PLOS ONE. 2021;16 (12):e0260506.

58. Burke D, Hickie I, Breakspear M, Gotz J. Possibilities for the prevention and treatment of cognitive impairment and dementia. British Journal of Psychiatry. 2007;190:371–2.

59. Stern Y. Cognitive reserve in ageing and Alzheimer's disease. Lancet Neurology. 2012;11(11):1006–12.

60. Stern Y, Gurland B, Tatemichi TK, Tang MX, Wilder D, Mayeux R. Influence of education and occupation on the incidence of Alzheimer's disease. JAMA. 1994;271(13):1004–10.

61. Fratiglioni L, Paillard-Borg S, Winblad B. An active and socially integrated lifestyle in late life might protect against dementia. Lancet Neurology. 2004;3(6):343–53.

62. Woods B, Aguirre E, Spector AE, Orrell M. Cognitive stimulation to improve cognitive functioning in people with dementia. The Cochrane Database of Systematic Reviews. 2012;2:CD005562.

63. Huntley JD, Gould RL, Liu K, Smith M, Howard RJ. Do cognitive interventions improve general cognition in dementia? A meta-analysis and meta-regression. BMJ Open. 2015;5(4): e005247.

64. Prince M, Bryce R, Ferri C, Alzheimer's Disease International. World Alzheimer Report 2011: The Benefits of Early Diagnosis and Intervention. London, UK: Alzheimer's Disease International; 2011.

65. National Institute for Health and Care Excellence. Dementia: Assessment, management and support for people living with dementia and their carers 2018 Available from: www.nice.org.uk/ guidance/ng97/chapter/ Recommendations#diagnosis.

66. Knapp M, Thorgrimsen L, Patel A, Spector A, Hallam A, Woods B, et al. Cognitive stimulation therapy for people with dementia: Cost-effectiveness analysis. British Journal of Psychiatry. 2006;188:574–80.

67. D'Amico F, Rehill A, Knapp M, Aguirre E, Donovan H, Hoare Z, et al. Maintenance cognitive stimulation therapy: An economic evaluation within a randomized controlled trial. Journal of American Medical Director Associates. 2015;16(1):63–70.

68. Forbes D, Thiessen EJ, Blake CM, Forbes SC, Forbes S. Exercise programs for people with dementia. The Cochrane Database of Systematic Reviews. 2013;12: CD006489.

69. Colcombe S, Kramer AF. Fitness effects on the cognitive function of older adults: A meta-analytic study. Psychological Science. 2003;14(2):125–30.

70. Adjepong M, Amoah-Agyei F, Du C, Wang W, Fenton JI, Tucker RM. Limited negative effects of the COVID-19 pandemic on mental health measures of Ghanaian university students. Journal of

Affected Disorders Report. 2022;7:100306.

71. NHS Education for Scotland. Promoting psychological wellbeing for people with dementia and their carers: An enhanced practice resource. Available from: www .nes.scot.nhs.uk/media/zw0o3utc/ promoting-psychological-wellbeing-for-people-with-dementia.pdf.

72. Gitlin LN, Kales HC, Lyketsos CG. Nonpharmacologic management of behavioral symptoms in dementia. JAMA. 2012;308(19):2020–9.

73. Kales HC, Gitlin LN, Lyketsos CG. Assessment and management of behavioral and psychological symptoms of dementia. BMJ. 2015;350:h369.

74. Spector A, Orrell M. Using a biopsychosocial model of dementia as a tool to guide clinical practice. International Psychogeriatry. 2010;22 (6):957–65.

75. Hebert CA, Scales K. Dementia friendly initiatives: A state of the science review. Dementia. 2019;18(5):1858–95.

76. Shannon K, Bail K, Neville S. Dementia-friendly community initiatives: An integrative review. Journal of Clinical Nursing. 2019;28(11–12):2035–45.

77. Buckner S, Darlington N, Woodward M, Buswell M, Mathie E, Arthur A, et al. Dementia friendly communities in England: A scoping study. International Journal of Geriatric Psychiatry. 2019;34 (8):1235–43.

78. Rahman S, Swaffer K. Assets-based approaches and dementia-friendly communities. Dementia (London). 2018;17(2):131–7.

79. Crampton J, Eley R. Dementia-friendly communities: What the project 'Creating a dementia-friendly York' can tell us. Working with Older People. 2013;17 (2):49–57.

80. Livingston G, Huntley J, Sommerlad A, Ames D, Ballard C, Banerjee S, et al. Dementia prevention, intervention, and care: 2020 report of the Lancet Commission. Lancet. 2020;396 (10248):413–46.

81. Twigg J. Models of carers: How do social care agencies conceptualise their relationship with informal carers? Journal of Social Policy. 1989;18(1):53–66.

82. Kemp CL, Ball MM, Perkins MM. Convoys of care: Theorizing intersections of formal and informal care. Journal of Aging Studies. 2013;27(1):15–29.

83. Cameron A, Johnson EK, Willis PB, Lloyd L, Smith R. Exploring the role of volunteers in social care for older adults. Quality in Ageing and Older Adults. 2020;21(2):129–39.

84. Malby R, Boyle D, Wildman J, Omar BS, Smith S. The Asset Based Health Inquiry: How Best to Develop Social Prescribing. London: London South Bank University; 2019.

85. Prince M, Comas-Herrera A, Knapp M, Guerchet M, Karagiannidou M. World Alzheimer report 2016: Improving healthcare for people living with dementia: Coverage, quality and costs now and in the future. London: Alzheimer's Disease International. 2016.

Glossary

ADI:	Alzheimer's Disease International
ADL:	Activities of daily living
ARWMC:	age-related white matter changes. ARWMC is a commonly used rating scale in MRI and CT
bvFTD:	Frontotemporal dementia, behavioural variant
CBD:	Corticobasal degeneration
CBP:	Complete blood picture
ChEIs:	Cholinesterase inhibitors
CNS:	Central nervous system
CT:	Computed tomography
CVS:	Cardiovascular system
CXR:	Chest X-ray
DLB:	Dementia with Lewy body
ECG:	Electrocardiography
ESR:	Erythrocyte sedimentation rate
FAST:	Functional Assessment Staging Test
FDG-PET-CT:	Fluorodeoxyglucose-positron emission tomography-computed tomography
GCA:	Global cortical atrophy scale
GDS:	Global Deterioration Scale
GDS-15:	15-item Geriatric Depression Scale
GPCOG:	General Practitioner Assessment of Cognition
HDL-C:	High-density lipoproteins-cholesterol
IADL:	Instrumental activities of daily living
LDL-C:	Low-density lipoproteins-cholesterol
MCV:	Mean corpuscular volume
MMSE:	Mini-Mental State Examination
MoCA:	Montreal Cognitive Assessment
MRI:	Magnetic resonance imaging
MSU x R/M:	Midstream urine routine microscopy
MTA/MTLA:	Medial temporal lobe atrophy
MTL:	Medial temporal lobe
nfvPPA:	Non-fluent variant primary progressive aphasia
PET:	Positron emission tomography
PiB:	Pittsburgh compound B
PPA:	Primary progressive aphasia
PSP:	Progressive supranuclear palsy
RBD:	Rapid eye movement (REM) sleep behaviour disorder
R/LFT:	Renal and liver function tests
Scheltens:	Medial temporal lobe atrophy (MTA) score, also known as Scheltens' scale
SDH:	Subdural haematoma
SL:	Sublingual
SOL:	Space-occupying lesion
SPECT:	Single-photon emission CT
SSRIs:	Selective serotonin reuptake inhibitors
TSH:	Thyroid-Stimulating Hormone-Sensitive
SVD:	Subcortical vascular dementia
svPPA:	Semantic variant primary progressive aphasia
TCHL:	Total cholesterol

TFT:	Thyroid function tests
TG:	Triglycerides
tSAH:	Traumatic subarachnoid haemorrhage
TSH:	Thyroid-stimulating hormone
VDRL:	Venereal disease research laboratory test

Index

Printed in the United States
by Baker & Taylor Publisher Services